# Multiple Sclerosis

*Editor*

CARRIE M. HERSH

# NEUROLOGIC CLINICS

www.neurologic.theclinics.com

*Consulting Editor*
RANDOLPH W. EVANS

February 2024 • Volume 42 • Number 1

**ELSEVIER**

1600 John F. Kennedy Boulevard • Suite 1800 • Philadelphia, Pennsylvania, 19103-2899

http://www.theclinics.com

**NEUROLOGIC CLINICS Volume 42, Number 1**
**February 2024 ISSN 0733-8619, ISBN-13: 978-0-323-93917-1**

Editor: Stacy Eastman
Developmental Editor: Varun Gopal



*Neurologic Clinics* (ISSN 0733-8619) is published quarterly by Elsevier Inc., 360 Park Avenue South, New York, NY 10010–1710. Months of issue are February, May, August, and November. Periodicals postage paid at New York, NY, and additional mailing offices. Subscription prices are $360.00 per year for US individuals, $100.00 per year for US students, $445.00 per year for Canadian individuals, $504.00 per year for international individuals, $210.00 for foreign students/residents, and $100.00 for Canadian students/residents. For institutional access pricing please contact Customer Service via the contact information below. To receive student/resident rate, orders must be accompanied by name of affiliated institution, date of term, and the *signature* of program/residency coordinator on institution letterhead. Orders will be billed at individual rate until proof of status is received. Foreign air speed delivery is included in all *Clinics* subscription prices. All prices are subject to change without notice. **POSTMASTER:** Send address changes to *Neurologic Clinics*, Elsevier Health Sciences Division, Subscription Customer Service, 3251 Riverport Lane, Maryland Heights, MO 63043. **Customer Service: Telephone: 1-800-654-2452 (U.S. and Canada); 314-447-8871 (outside U.S. and Canada). Fax: 314-447-8029. E-mail: journalscustomerservice-usa@elsevier.com (for print support); journalsonlinesupport-usa@elsevier.com (for online support).**

*Reprints.* For copies of 100 or more of articles in this publication, please contact the Commercial Reprints Department, Elsevier Inc., 360 Park Avenue South, New York, New York, 10010-1710; Tel.: +1-212-633-3874; Fax: +1-212-633-3820, and E-mail: reprints@elsevier.com.

*Neurologic Clinics* is also published in Spanish by Nueva Editorial Interamericana S.A., Mexico City, Mexico.

*Neurologic Clinics* is covered in *Current Contents/Clinical Medicine, MEDLINE/PubMed (Index Medicus), EMBASE/Excerpta Medica, and PsycINFO, and ISI/BIOMED.*

# Contributors


## CONSULTING EDITOR

**RANDOLPH W. EVANS, MD**
Clinical Professor, Department of Neurology, Baylor College of Medicine, Houston, Texas, USA

## EDITOR

**CARRIE M. HERSH, DO, MSc, FAAN**
Director, Multiple Sclerosis Health and Wellness Program, Director, Professional Engagement, Associate Program Director, Neuroimmunology and Multiple Sclerosis Fellowship, Cleveland Clinic Lou Ruvo Center for Brain Health, Las Vegas, Nevada, USA; Associate Professor of Neurology, Cleveland Clinic Lerner College of Medicine of Case Western Reserve University, Cleveland, Ohio, USA

## AUTHORS

**AHMAD ABDELRAHMAN, MD, MPH**
Department of Neurology, Rocky Mountain MS Center, University of Colorado Anschutz Medical Center, Aurora, Colorado, USA

**ALBERT ABOSEIF, DO**
Department of Neurology, Neurological Institute, Cleveland Clinic, Cleveland, Ohio, USA

**JEMIMA AKISANYA, DO, MD**
Assistant Professor, Department of Neurology, Georgetown University Medical Center, Washington, DC, USA

**ENRIQUE ALVAREZ, MD, PhD**
Department of Neurology, Rocky Mountain MS Center, University of Colorado Anschutz Medical Center, University of Colorado, Associate Professor of Neuroimmunology, Vice Chair of Clinical Research, Aurora, Colorado, USA

**LILYANA AMEZCUA, MD, MS, FAAN**
Associate Professor, Department of Neurology, University of Southern California, Keck School of Medicine of USC, Los Angeles, California, USA

**CHRISTINA J. AZEVEDO, MD, MPH**
Department of Neurology, Keck School of Medicine of USC, University of Southern California, Los Angeles, California, USA

**PAVAN BHARGAVA, MD**
Associate Professor of Neurology, Division of Neuroimmunology and Neurological Infections, Department of Neurology, Johns Hopkins School of Medicine, Baltimore, Maryland, USA

**NICOLE BOU RJEILY, MD**
Department of Neurology, Johns Hopkins School of Medicine, Baltimore, Maryland, USA

**RILEY BOVE, MD, MSc**
Associate Professor, UCSF Weill Institute for Neurosciences, San Francisco, California, USA

**LAURA CACCIAGUERRA, MD, PhD**
Department of Neurology, Mayo Clinic Center for Multiple Sclerosis and Autoimmune Neurology, Mayo Clinic, Rochester, Minnesota, USA

**ALISE K. CARLSON, MD**
Cleveland Clinic Mellen Center, Cleveland, Ohio, USA

**ANIBAL CHERTCOFF, MD**
Division of Neurology, Department of Medicine, St. Michael's Hospital, University of Toronto, Toronto, Ontario, Canada

**JEFFREY A. COHEN, MD**
Staff Neurologist, Mellen Center, Neurological Institute, Cleveland Clinic, Cleveland, Ohio, USA

**DEVON S. CONWAY, MD**
Mellen Center for Multiple Sclerosis, Neurological Institute, Cleveland Clinic, Cleveland, Ohio, USA

**ANNE H. CROSS, MD**
Professor, Department of Neurology, Washington University School of Medicine in St. Louis, St Louis, Missouri, USA

**EOIN P. FLANAGAN, MB, BCh**
Department of Neurology, Mayo Clinic Center for Multiple Sclerosis and Autoimmune Neurology, Laboratory Medicine and Pathology, Mayo Clinic, Professor of Neurology, Mayo Clinic College of Medicine, Rochester, Minnesota, USA

**ROBERT J. FOX, MD**
Cleveland Clinic Mellen Center, Cleveland, Ohio, USA

**JENNIFER S. GRAVES, MD, PhD, MAS**
Department of Neurosciences, University of California San Diego, Rady Children's Hospital, San Diego, California, USA

**BENJAMIN M. GREENBERG, MD, MHS**
Distinguished Teaching Professor, Vice Chair, Clinical and Translational Research, Department of Neurology, The University of Texas Southwestern Medical Center, Dallas, Texas, USA

**CARRIE M. HERSH, DO, MSc, FAAN**
Director, Multiple Sclerosis Health and Wellness Program, Director, Professional Engagement, Associate Program Director, Neuroimmunology and Multiple Sclerosis Fellowship, Cleveland Clinic Lou Ruvo Center for Brain Health, Las Vegas, Nevada USA; Associate Professor of Neurology, Cleveland Clinic Lerner College of Medicine of Case Western Reserve University, Cleveland, Ohio, USA

**LE H. HUA, MD**
Cleveland Clinic Lou Ruvo Center for Brain Health, Las Vegas, Nevada, USA

**LARISSA JANK, MD**
Postdoctoral Fellow, Division of Neuroimmunology and Neurological Infections, Department of Neurology, Johns Hopkins School of Medicine, Baltimore, Maryland, USA

**MARWA KAISEY, MD**
Assistant Professor, Department of Neurology, Cedars-Sinai Medical Center, Los Angeles, California, USA

**TOMAS KALINCIK, MD, PhD, PGCertBiostat, FRACP**
Professor, Department of Medicine, CORe, University of Melbourne, Department of Neurology, Neuroimmunology Centre, Royal Melbourne Hospital, Melbourne, Australia

**JONATHAN D. KRETT, MD**
Division of Neuroimmunology and Neurological Infections, Department of Neurology, Johns Hopkins School of Medicine, Baltimore, Maryland, USA

**STEPHEN KRIEGER, MD, FAAN**
Professor, Corinne Goldsmith Dickinson Center for Multiple Sclerosis, Icahn School of Medicine at Mount Sinai, New York, New York, USA

**ELLEN M. MOWRY, MD, MCR**
Departments of Neurology and Epidemiology, Johns Hopkins School of Medicine, Baltimore, Maryland, USA

**SCOTT D. NEWSOME, DO**
Division of Neuroimmunology and Neurological Infections, Department of Neurology, Johns Hopkins School of Medicine, Baltimore, Maryland, USA

**JACQUELINE NICHOLAS, MD, MPH**
System Chief Neuroimmunology and Multiple Sclerosis, OhioHealth Multiple Sclerosis Center, Columbus, Ohio, USA

**JIWON OH, MD, PhD**
Division of Neurology, Department of Medicine, St. Michael's Hospital, University of Toronto, Toronto, Ontario, Canada; Department of Neurology, Johns Hopkins University, Baltimore, Maryland, USA

**DANIEL ONTANEDA, MD, PhD**
Cleveland Clinic Mellen Center, Cleveland, Ohio, USA

**CHRISTOPHER ORLANDO, MD, MPH**
Clinical Instructor, Department of Neurology, University of Southern California, Keck School of Medicine of USC, Los Angeles, California, USA

**MARY RENSEL, MD**
Mellen Center for Multiple Sclerosis, Neurological Institute, Cleveland Clinic, Cleveland, Ohio, USA

**IZANNE ROOS, MBChB, MMed (Neurology), FRACP, PhD**
Department of Neurology, Neuroimmunology Centre, Royal Melbourne Hospital, Department of Medicine, CORe, University of Melbourne, Melbourne, Australia

**LINDSAY A. ROSS, MD, MSc**
Staff Neurologist, Mellen Center, Neurological Institute, Cleveland Clinic, Cleveland, Ohio, USA

**AMBER SALTER, PhD**
Section on Statistical Planning and Analysis, Department of Neurology, The University of Texas Southwestern Medical Center, Dallas, Texas, USA

**RAPHAEL SCHNEIDER, MD, PhD**
Division of Neurology, Department of Medicine, St. Michael's Hospital, University of Toronto, Toronto, Ontario, Canada

**AFSANEH SHIRANI, MD, MSCI**
Division of Multiple Sclerosis, Department of Neurological Sciences, University of Nebraska Medical Center, Omaha, Nebraska, USA

**NANCY SICOTTE, MD**
Department of Neurology, Cedars-Sinai Medical Center, Los Angeles, California, USA

**AREEBA SIDDIQUI, MD**
Cleveland Clinic Lou Ruvo Center for Brain Health, Las Vegas, Nevada, USA

**ANDREW J. SOLOMON, MD**
Professor and Division Chief, Department of Neurological Sciences, University of Vermont, Larner College of Medicine, University Health Center, Burlington, Vermont, USA

**LISA M. STROPP, MD**
Fellow, Mellen Center, Neurological Institute, Cleveland Clinic, Cleveland, Ohio, USA

**OLAF STUVE, MD, PhD**
Professor, Department of Neurology, The University of Texas Southwestern Medical Center, Dallas, Texas, USA

**AMY B. SULLIVAN, PSYD**
Mellen Center for Multiple Sclerosis, Neurological Institute, Cleveland Clinic, Cleveland, Ohio, USA

**PAIGE SUTTON, MD**
Neuroimmunologist, OhioHealth Multiple Sclerosis Center, Columbus, Ohio, USA

**MITZI J. WILLIAMS, MD, FAAN**
Medical Director, Joi Life Wellness Multiple Sclerosis Center, Adjunct Assistant Professor of Neurology, Morehouse School of Medicine, Atlanta, Georgia, USA

**JENNIFER H. YANG, MD**
Department of Neurosciences, University of California San Diego, Division of Pediatric Neurology, Rady Children's Hospital, San Diego, California, USA

# Contents

**Preface: Contemporary Topics in Multiple Sclerosis** xiii

Carrie M. Hersh

**Multiple Sclerosis Diagnostic Delay and Misdiagnosis** 1

Marwa Kaisey and Andrew J. Solomon

Multiple sclerosis (MS) misdiagnosis in the form of an incorrect diagnosis of MS, as well as delayed diagnosis in patients who do have MS, both influence patient clinical outcomes. Contemporary studies have reported data on factors associated with these diagnostic challenges and their frequency. Expediting diagnosis in patients with MS and reducing MS misdiagnosis in patients who do not have MS may be aided by educational efforts surrounding early MS symptoms and proper application of MS diagnostic criteria. Emerging novel MS diagnostic biomarkers may aid early and accurate diagnosis of MS in the future.

**Recent Advances in Diagnostic, Prognostic, and Disease-Monitoring Biomarkers in Multiple Sclerosis** 15

Anibal Chertcoff, Raphael Schneider, Christina J. Azevedo, Nancy Sicotte, and Jiwon Oh

Multiple sclerosis (MS) is a highly heterogeneous disease. Currently, a combination of clinical features, MRI, and cerebrospinal fluid markers are used in clinical practice for diagnosis and treatment decisions. In recent years, there has been considerable effort to develop novel biomarkers that better reflect the pathologic substrates of the disease to aid in diagnosis and early prognosis, evaluation of ongoing inflammatory activity, detection and monitoring of disease progression, prediction of treatment response, and monitoring of disease-modifying treatment safety. In this review, the authors provide an overview of promising recent developments in diagnostic, prognostic, and disease-monitoring/treatment-response biomarkers in MS.

**Pathophysiology, Diagnosis, Treatment and Emerging Neurotherapeutic Targets for Progressive Multiple Sclerosis: The Age of PIRA** 39

Alise K. Carlson and Robert J. Fox

More than one million individuals are impacted by progressive forms of multiple sclerosis. The literature examining the management of MS has focused primarily on relapsing forms of the disease, and effective therapies targeting progressive mechanisms in MS remains a significant unmet need. Despite this, there are several encouraging potential therapeutics on the horizon. Improved understanding of mechanisms underlying MS progression, identification and validation of biomarkers, identification of novel therapeutic targets, and improved trial design are needed to further propel progress in the management of individuals with progressive forms of MS.

sclerosis (RMS); it reduces progression to a lesser extent in nonrelapsing progressive MS. Mechanisms whereby anti-CD20 mAbs reduce MRI and clinical relapse activity in people with RMS are still being elucidated. Anti-CD20 agents do not fully protect from nonrelapsing disease progression, possibly due to their inability to cross the blood–brain barrier and inability to ameliorate the full extent of biology of MS progression. Anti-CD20 mAbs have a relatively favorable safety profile, at least in the short-term. Long-term safety studies are still needed.

**Bruton's Tyrosine Kinase Inhibitors for Multiple Sclerosis Treatment: A New Frontier** **155**

Benjamin M. Greenberg

Multiple sclerosis (MS) can cause significant disability to patients via relapse-associated worsening and progression independent of relapses. The causes of neuronal and myelin damage can include lymphocyte-mediated inflammation and microglial activation. Bruton's tyrosine kinase (BTK) is an enzyme that mediates B cell activation and the proinflammatory phenotype of microglia. Inhibiting BTK provides a novel therapeutic target for MS but also has a complicated pharmacology based on binding specificity, CNS penetration, half-life, and enzyme inhibition characteristics. Multiple agents are being studied in phase 3 trials, and each agent will have unique efficacy and safety profiles that must be considered individually.

**Autologous Hematopoietic Stem Cell Transplantation to Treat Multiple Sclerosis** **165**

Lindsay A. Ross, Lisa M. Stropp, and Jeffrey A. Cohen

In aggregate, the available data suggest autologous hematopoietic stem cell transplantation (AHSCT) has potent, durable efficacy to treat relapsing multiple sclerosis (MS). Safety issues and financial costs are significant but largely associated with the procedure itself. AHSCT is a reasonable option for patients with highly active relapsing MS and an inadequate response to the available disease therapies. The key question is where to place AHSCT in the overall relapsing MS algorithm relative to other high-efficacy therapies. Ongoing randomized trials will better characterize the benefit and risk of AHSCT compared with currently available high-efficacy disease therapies.

**Highly Effective Therapy Versus Escalation Approaches in Early Multiple Sclerosis: What Is the Future of Multiple Sclerosis Treatment?** **185**

Nicole Bou Rjeily, Ellen M. Mowry, Daniel Ontaneda, and Alise K. Carlson

Treatment options for patients newly diagnosed with multiple sclerosis (MS) are expanding with the continuous development and approval of new disease-modifying therapies (DMTs). The optimal initial treatment strategy, however, remains unclear. The 2 main treatment paradigms currently employed are the escalation (ESC) approach and the early highly effective treatment (EHT) approach. The ESC approach consists of starting a lower- or moderate-efficacy DMT, which offers a potentially safer approach, while the EHT approach favors higher-efficacy treatment early in the disease course, despite a potential increase in risk. Randomized

clinical trials aiming to directly compare these approaches in newly diagnosed MS patients are currently underway.

**Leveraging Real-World Evidence and Observational Studies in Treating Multiple Sclerosis** 203

Albert Aboseif, Izanne Roos, Stephen Krieger, Tomas Kalincik, and Carrie M. Hersh

Randomized controlled trials (RCTs) are essential for regulatory approval of disease-modifying therapies (DMTs), yet their strict selection criteria often lead to limited generalizability. Observational studies using real-world data (RWD) allow for more inclusive heterogeneous cohorts resulting in higher external validity to inform treatment practices. As reviewed in this article, well-designed comparative effectiveness studies are an important application of RWD. Although, like RCTs, observational studies have their own set of limitations, including various biases that may confound results, advanced statistical methods can mitigate many of these limitations. A focus on personalized treatment will continue to add value to individualize MS care.

**Health, Wellness, and the Effect of Comorbidities on the Multiple Sclerosis Disease Course: Tackling the Modifiable** 229

Devon S. Conway, Amy B. Sullivan, and Mary Rensel

Multiple sclerosis (MS) is a disease of the central nervous system characterized by inflammatory demyelination and neurodegeneration. Numerous disease-modifying therapies for MS exist but are only partially effective, making it essential to optimize all factors that may influence the course of the disease. This includes conscientious management of both mental and physical comorbidities, as well as a comprehensive strategy for promoting wellness in patients with MS. Thoughtful engagement of those living with MS through shared decision making and involvement of a multidisciplinary team that includes primary care, relevant specialists, psychology, and rehabilitation is likely to lead to better outcomes.

**Clinical and Treatment Considerations for the Pediatric and Aging Patients with Multiple Sclerosis** 255

Areeba Siddiqui, Jennifer H. Yang, Le H. Hua, and Jennifer S. Graves

Chronologic aging is associated with multiple pathologic and immunologic changes that impact the clinical course of multiple sclerosis (MS). Clinical phenotypes evolve across the lifespan, from a highly inflammatory course in the very young to a predominantly neurodegenerative phenotype in older patients. Thus, unique clinical considerations arise for the diagnosis and management of the two age extremes of pediatric and geriatric MS populations. This review covers epidemiology, diagnosis, and treatment strategies for these populations with nuanced discussions on therapeutic approaches to effectively care for patients living with MS at critical transition points during their lifespan.

**Women's Health and Pregnancy in Multiple Sclerosis** **275**

Riley Bove, Paige Sutton, and Jacqueline Nicholas

Multiple sclerosis has a 3:1 female-to-male predominance and commonly presents in young adult women. The hormonal changes in women throughout their lifetime do affect the underlying pathology of multiple sclerosis, and the needs of women therefore change with age. Although multiple sclerosis does not adversely affect fertility or pregnancy, there are many factors to consider when caring for women throughout family planning, pregnancy, and the postpartum period. The care of these women and complex decisions regarding disease-modifying therapy use in family planning should be individualized and comprehensive.

**Multiple Sclerosis in Black and Hispanic Populations: Serving the Underserved** **295**

Mitzi J. Williams, Christopher Orlando, Jemima Akisanya, and Lilyana Amezcua

Multiple sclerosis has historically been characterized as a disease that affects young women of European ancestry, but recent studies indicate that the incidence and prevalence of the disease is much higher in Black and Hispanic populations than previously recognized. There is evidence that there is a more severe disease course in these populations, but the intersection of genetic underpinnings and social determinants of health (SDOH) is poorly understood due to the lack of diversity in clinical research. Improving health disparities will involve multiple stakeholders in efforts to improve SDOH and raise awareness about research involvement and the importance of developing personalized health care plans to combat this disease.

**Era of COVID-19 in Multiple Sclerosis Care** **319**

Jonathan D. Krett, Amber Salter, and Scott D. Newsome

The unprecedented scope of the coronavirus disease 2019 (COVID-19) pandemic resulted in numerous disruptions to daily life, including for people with multiple sclerosis (PwMS). This article reviews how disruptions in multiple sclerosis (MS) care prompted innovations in delivery of care (eg, via telemedicine) and mobilized the global MS community to rapidly adopt safe and effective practices. We discuss how our understanding of the risks of COVID-19 in PwMS has evolved along with recommendations pertaining to disease-modifying therapies and vaccines. With lessons learned during the COVID-19 pandemic, we examine potential questions for future research in this new era of MS care.

# NEUROLOGIC CLINICS

## FORTHCOMING ISSUES

***May 2024***
**Current Advances and Future Trends in Vascular Neurology**
Michael J. Schneck, *Editor*

***August 2024***
**Secondary Headaches**
Randolph W. Evans, *Editor*

***November 2024***
**Neuropsychology for Neurologists**
Jane S. Paulsen and Carissa Gehl, *Editors*

## RECENT ISSUES

***November 2023***
**Functional Neurological Disorder**
David L. Perez and Sara A. Finkelstein, *Editors*

***August 2023***
**Medicolegal Issues in Neurology**
Joseph S. Kass and Michael A. Rubin, *Editors*

***May 2023***
**Neurological Disorders in Women: from Epidemiology to Outcome**
Rima M. Dafer, *Editor*

**ISSUES OF RELATED INTEREST**

*Neurosurgery Clinics*
https://www.neurosurgery.theclinics.com/
*Neuroimaging Clinics*
https://www.neuroimaging.theclinics.com/
*Psychiatric Clinics*
https://www.psych.theclinics.com/
*Child and Adolescent Psychiatric Clinics*
https://www.childpsych.theclinics.com/

# Preface

# Contemporary Topics in Multiple Sclerosis

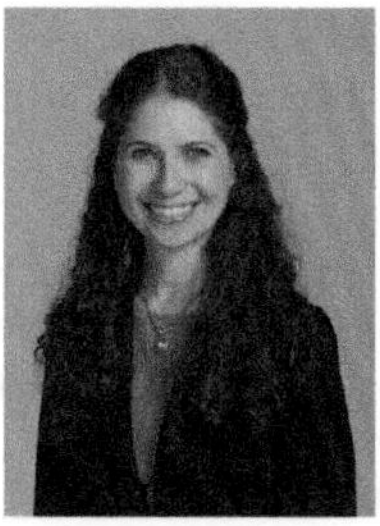

Carrie M. Hersh, DO, MSc, FAAN
*Editor*

Multiple sclerosis (MS) is a complex neurologic disorder that affects millions of people worldwide. As our understanding of this condition evolves, so too does the landscape of contemporary topics surrounding MS. In this issue of *Neurologic Clinics*, we explore advancements in the field, including emerging themes around diagnostics, special patient populations, and treatments.

One key area of exploration is the discovery of markers allowing for early diagnosis and accurate prognosis in persons with multiple sclerosis (PwMS), thereby facilitating treatment decisions. Similarly, prompt recognition of other autoimmune-mediated demyelinating disorders, such as neuromyelitis optica spectrum disorder and myelin oligodendrocyte glycoprotein antibody-associated disease, is paramount for early targeted treatment to improve long-term outcomes.

While the exact cause of MS remains unknown, growing evidence suggests a combination of genetic, epigenetic, environmental, infectious, nutritional, and immunologic factors contributes to its development. Unraveling the intricate mechanisms underlying MS pathogenesis and new targets for disease therapy are vital for improving therapeutic and preventive strategies. The lack of effective treatments for progressive MS is one of the most significant unmet needs in the field. In this context, concerted efforts are focused on understanding neurodegenerative pathology and tailoring approaches in drug development for progressive forms of the disease. Moreover, optimizing treatment of special populations across the lifespan—including the pediatric, reproductive, pregnant, postpartum, perimenopausal, and aging patient—is essential and is reviewed in this issue. Further, recognizing the complexities of managing MS in the era of COVID-19 is crucial for balancing safety with the need for effective disease control.

Neurol Clin 42 (2024) xiii–xv
https://doi.org/10.1016/j.ncl.2023.08.001
0733-8619/24/© 2023 Published by Elsevier Inc.
neurologic.theclinics.com

Another pivotal aspect of MS research is innovative therapeutic approaches. Disease-modifying therapies (DMTs) are instrumental in controlling the macroscopic neuroinflammatory features of MS (eg, reducing relapses and new MRI lesions and slowing disability accumulation mostly from incomplete relapse recovery), but new avenues are actively being investigated, especially for the neurodegenerative components of this disease. From emerging immunotherapies in various late-phase clinical trials, such as Bruton's Tyrosine Kinase inhibitors, to neuroprotective, regenerative, and remyelinating techniques, researchers are pushing the boundaries of treatment options. The pursuit of personalized medicine, in which treatments are tailored to individual patients based on their unique characteristics and disease course, has gained considerable attention in recent years and is discussed collectively in this MS-dedicated issue.

Beyond disease-focused interventions, the impact of MS on quality of life cannot be overlooked. Topics such as health and wellness, gut dysbiosis, nutrition, psychological evaluation, management, and support, and identification and treatment of comorbidities are crucial for enhancing the well-being of those living with MS.

Equity, access to care, and health disparities are also pivotal themes in the MS field. These topics highlight the need for equal opportunities and resources for individuals of diverse backgrounds affected by MS. In recent years, there has been a growing awareness of the importance of cultural competence in health care settings, ensuring that individuals receive care that is sensitive to their unique needs, beliefs, and values. In addition, the role of advocacy organizations, support networks, and patient-driven initiatives in fostering inclusive and equitable care has gained prominence. Furthermore, the rapid accessibility of telemedicine during the COVID-19 pandemic allowed for continued connections between the health care team, patient, and care partners and is expected to result in lasting changes in health care delivery for PwMS.

The convergence of MS research with emerging technologies from large registries and improved statistical approaches for optimizing the robustness of studies using real-world data present exciting prospects. These contemporary tools hold the potential to unlock new insights from harmonized real-world data, aiding evidence-based decisions around when to start, switch, and discontinue DMTs, tailoring therapy to individuals, and predicting disease outcomes in heterogeneous populations. Integration of cutting-edge precision medicine into MS research and clinical practice is an ever-evolving frontier.

With deep gratitude to the contributing authors, all of whom are renowned experts in the field, I am excited to present this collection of articles. These works delve into the contemporary topics in MS and related disorders with the aim of shedding light on the latest research, innovations, and challenges faced by the MS community. Experts from various disciplines share their insights, offering a comprehensive exploration of the multifaceted nature of MS and related disorders and their impact on individuals and the community at large.

As we embark on this journey, we invite readers to engage with these topics, challenge existing paradigms, and contemplate the future of MS research, care, and support. Through the collective exploration of these contemporary issues, we strive to foster a better understanding of MS and related disorders, inspire collaborative efforts, and ultimately improve the lives of those affected by these complex neurologic conditions.

Together, we can advance the frontiers of knowledge, unravel the mysteries of MS, and make meaningful strides toward a future where PwMS can live life to the fullest. The future of person-centered MS care is as bright as ever.

Let the exploration begin.

Carrie M. Hersh, DO, MSc, FAAN
Cleveland Clinic Lou Ruvo Center
for Brain Health
888 West Bonneville Avenue
Las Vegas, NV 89106, USA

*E-mail address:*
hershc@ccf.org

# Multiple Sclerosis Diagnostic Delay and Misdiagnosis

Marwa Kaisey, MD[a,*], Andrew J. Solomon, MD[b]

**KEYWORDS**

• Multiple sclerosis • Diagnosis • Diagnostic errors • McDonald criteria

**KEY POINTS**

- Misdiagnosis and delayed diagnosis of MS are both relatively common.
- Delayed diagnosis impacts prognosis by delaying treatment.
- Misapplication and misunderstanding of the McDonald criteria appear to contribute to MS misdiagnosis.
- Comprehensive educational efforts surrounding MS clinical presentations and the correct use of MS diagnostic criteria may prevent misdiagnoses.

## INTRODUCTION

Accurate interpretation of a patient's clinical presentation and radiologic studies, accompanied by knowledgeable and thoughtful application of the 2017 revised McDonald criteria (**Table 1**),[1] is necessary for the diagnosis of multiple sclerosis (MS). This diagnostic process can be fraught with error. As a consequence, a patient's diagnosis may be delayed; patients with MS often present months or even years before receiving a correct MS diagnosis. On the other hand, patients who do not have MS may be misdiagnosed incorrectly with MS. Both outcomes cause a host of problems, including increased morbidity. This article reports contemporary data concerning the frequency, causes, and consequences of delayed diagnosis and misdiagnosis of MS. Based on these data, the authors discuss strategies to curb diagnostic error.

## DELAYED DIAGNOSIS OF MULTIPLE SCLEROSIS

Disease-modifying therapies (DMTs) can prevent disability in patients with MS, particularly when initiated early in the disease course.[2] Thus, diagnostic delay and subsequent treatment delay in some patients with MS have prognostic consequences. For example,

[a] Department of Neurology, Cedars-Sinai Medical Center, 127 South San Vicente Boulevard, A6600, Los Angeles, CA 90048, USA; [b] Department of Neurological Sciences, University of Vermont, Larner College of Medicine, University Health Center, Arnold 2, 1 South Prospect Street, Burlington, VT 05401, USA
* Corresponding author.
*E-mail address:* Marwa.Kaisey@csmc.edu


https://doi.org/10.1016/j.ncl.2023.07.001

**Table 1**
**2017 McDonald criteria for the diagnosis of multiple sclerosis**

| Clinical Presentation | Additional Data Needed for a Diagnosis of MS |
|---|---|
| Typical clinical attack at onset and: | |
| ≥2 attacks with objective clinical evidence of ≥2 lesions | None |
| ≥2 attacks with objective clinical evidence of 1 lesion and historical evidence of prior attack with lesion in different anatomic location | None |
| ≥2 attacks and objective clinical evidence of 1 lesion | DIS demonstrated by any of the following:<br>• additional clinical attack implicating different CNS site<br>• MS-typical T2 lesion(s) in ≥2 areas of CNS: periventricular, cortical, juxtacortical, infratentorial, or spinal cord |
| 1 attack and objective clinical evidence of ≥2 lesions | DIT demonstrated by any of the following:<br>• Additional clinical attack or<br>• Simultaneous presence of both enhancing and nonenhancing MS-typical MRI lesions or<br>• New T2 or enhancing MRI lesion compared with baseline scan (without regard to timing of baseline scan)<br>• CSF-specific oligoclonal bands |
| 1 attack and objective clinical evidence of 1 lesion | DIS demonstrated by:<br>• additional clinical attack implicating different CNS site or<br>• MS-typical T2 lesion(s) in ≥2 areas of CNS: periventricular, cortical, juxtacortical, infratentorial, or spinal cord<br>And<br>DIT demonstrated by:<br>• Additional clinical attack or<br>• Simultaneous presence of both enhancing and nonenhancing MS-typical MRI lesions or<br>• New T2 or enhancing MRI lesion compared with baseline scan (without regard to timing of baseline scan)<br>• CSF oligoclonal bands |
| Steady progression of disease since onset and: | |
| 1 year of disease progression (retro- or prospective) | DIS demonstrated by at least 2 of the following:<br>• ≥1 MS-typical T2 lesions in periventricular, cortical, juxtacortical, infratentorial<br>• ≥2 T2 spinal cord lesions<br>• CSF oligoclonal bands |

*Abbreviations:* CNS, central nervous system; CSF, cerebrospinal fluid; DIS, dissemination in space; DIT, dissemination in time; T2 lesion, hyperintense lesion on T2-weighted MR.

1 study demonstrated that for every year MS DMT was delayed, risk of reaching moderate disability level (Expanded Disability Status Scale[3] of 4) after 8 years was increased by 7.4%.[4] Even survival may be affected by early treatment. At follow-up 21 years after a pivotal DMT trial,[5] mortality rates were significantly higher in patients who presented with a first attack of MS and were initially randomized to 3 years of placebo compared with patients randomized to receive treatment.

Researchers investigating causes of delayed MS diagnosis face several challenges. Most importantly, any such study is necessarily retrospective, after a diagnosis of MS is confirmed. Patients' recollection of their diagnostic journey may be limited or influenced by recall bias and may not adequately capture health care system barriers that could have contributed to delayed diagnosis. Medical records documenting care before MS diagnosis may be incomplete or unobtainable, particularly in fragmented health care systems, and are often inadequate to capture clinical thought processes or decision making. Implicit and explicit biases within the health care system concerning race, gender, and other identifiers may contribute to delayed diagnosis[6,7] and are particularly difficult to assess. Administrative claims data utilizing diagnostic codes can estimate the scope of a diagnostic delay in MS care. Still, for optimal accuracy, this approach requires costly and time-consuming manual validation in the medical record, and claims data are typically inadequate alone for assessment of causation. Furthermore, revisions to MS diagnostic criteria over the last 3 decades – which have resulted in improved sensitivity for MS and earlier diagnosis – complicate any study focused on diagnostic delay. For example, in a cohort of patients with clinically isolated syndrome (CIS) in Spain from 1997 to 2020, time to MS diagnosis decreased with each new iteration of the diagnostic criteria.[8]

Few contemporary studies have interrogated the diagnostic journey for causes of delay[9] in MS care. A 2019 study of 285 patients from 5 MS tertiary referral centers in Portugal evaluated duration of delay and its contributing factors.[10] This study relied on patients' recollection of their symptoms and diagnostic process. The most significant delay, averaging 11 months, occurred between first symptom and first evaluation by a neurologist, echoing the main delay in a 2010 study conducted in Spain.[11] Motor symptoms at onset were often first evaluated by a non-neurologist, delaying evaluation by a neurologist and MS diagnosis. Older age and progressive MS subtype were significantly associated with diagnostic delay, as was presence of medical comorbidities. This is concordant with a population-based study in Denmark that also found that comorbidities, including cardiovascular disease and malignancy, delayed MS diagnosis.[12] A 2022 study of 70 patients in Italy with average diagnostic delay of almost 2 years similarly found motor symptoms at onset, age greater than 40 years, and lower education level were significant variables correlated with longer diagnostic delay.[13] A 2018 interrogation of the Swiss MS Registry found that progressive MS subtype was associated with significant increase in time to diagnosis.[14] Along with the previously mentioned study in Portugal and a 2010 Canadian study,[15] this highlights the particular challenge of diagnosing progressive-onset MS.

Although helpful to spur further research, these findings may not be generalizable to other regions or health care systems and do not capture patient-related or health care system-related barriers to care. Further studies are needed to rigorously interrogate factors resulting in MS diagnostic delay, including gender and racial biases in particular.[16] Although it was not designed to identify causes of delay, a 2011 retrospective evaluation of Hispanic patients with MS noted that their time to diagnosis was almost a full year longer than White patients treated at the same clinic.[17] A recent survey of African American women with MS reported delayed diagnosis occurred, because treating physicians considered MS, in the words of one woman, a "White people's disease" and as a result prioritized workup for "Black diseases" such as sickle cell disease and systemic lupus erythematous, thereby delaying evaluation for MS.[18] Several of the patients in this study also reported carrying this misconception themselves and did not seek care for early symptoms of MS. Of note, although a recent study of MS prevalence in a private healthcare maintenance organization in Southern California found similar rates of MS in White and Black patients,[19] another study including claims data from private, government, and military insurances across the United States found that the prevalence of MS was higher in the population of White Americans than Black Americans.[20] This study group reports that per 100,000 adults, 298 Black individuals and 375 White individuals have MS. Gender bias in MS diagnosis is another likely contributor that has not recently received extensive exploration. A study published in 2003 surveyed 50 patients with MS with an average diagnostic delay of 3.5 years; half were initially given another, incorrect diagnosis, with psychiatric diagnoses commonly suspected in women compared with orthopedic diagnoses in men.[21]

Multiple research approaches accounting for these limitations are necessary to fully understand the scope and causes of diagnostic delay in the care of MS. One method leverages administrative claims data. A key early study using this approach suggested that the delay from MS symptom onset to diagnosis was decreasing.[22] Yet contemporary studies seem to indicate that delay remains a substantial problem. Utilizing a dataset comprising 85% of the German population, Gasperi and colleagues compared ambulatory diagnosis billing codes between 2010 and 2017 for over 10,000 German individuals in the 5 years preceding MS diagnosis, with cohorts of almost 200,000 individuals with psoriasis, Crohn disease, or no autoimmune disease.[23] Codes more frequently identified in patients with MS appeared to reflect symptoms suggestive of unrecognized demyelinating events, indicating missed opportunities for earlier diagnosis in this population.[24] Similarly, a contemporary retrospective evaluation of a comprehensive registry in a Norwegian county showed that although the incidence of MS has steadily increased from 1990 to 2017, particularly among women, the median diagnostic delay remained stable at 1.5 years despite revisions to the MS diagnostic criteria during this period.[25] These data do not necessarily contrast with the previously mentioned CIS cohort-based study[7] evaluating revisions to the MS diagnostic criteria; while the time to diagnosis of MS in patients presenting with a clinical attack typical of MS has decreased over time, delays in the time to this initial clinical presentation for evaluation appear to have persisted.

Some types of initial clinical presentations of MS may be inherently associated with delayed diagnosis given that MS diagnostic criteria were not designed for application in such patients. For instance, patients with MS first presenting with an isolated tumefactive lesion[26] or single spinal cord lesion[27] pose diagnostic challenges that inevitably result in delay. Recent data also suggest that early MS may be associated with non-neurological prodromal symptoms[28] and asymptomatic radiological findings[29] that also would not fulfill MS diagnostic criteria. Future data may facilitate diagnosis of MS in patients presenting with atypical or non-neurological syndromes before a classic MS attack or the progression of neurologic disability at onset.

## MISDIAGNOSIS OF MULTIPLE SCLEROSIS

In contrast to patients who receive a delayed but accurate diagnosis of MS, patients with other disorders can be misdiagnosed as having MS. Particularly given the lack of a highly specific biomarker for MS, misdiagnosis has been a persistent problem in the field.[30] Several early studies of MS misdiagnosis[30–32] were completed before the current MS diagnostic criteria incorporating MRI, limiting application to current practice. However, several recent studies published between 2016 and 2022 reported data concerning patients misdiagnosed with MS (**Table 2**).[33–37] Notably, between 7% to 18% of patients in these cohorts were found to have been misdiagnosed with MS, indicating misdiagnosis remains a frequent problem. Indeed, in a 2012 survey of 122 neuorlogists,[38] 95% indicated they had evaluated misdiagnosed patients within the last year.

Although these data are influenced by several biases, including referral bias and hindsight bias, common findings concerning the clinical characteristics of misdiagnosed

**Table 2**
**Contemporary studies investigating patients identified as misdiagnosed with multiple sclerosis**

| Authors, Publication Year | Country (Number of Sites) | Study Design | Misdiagnosis % | Average Misdiagnosis Duration, Years | Five Most Frequent Alternate Diagnoses | DMT % |
|---|---|---|---|---|---|---|
| Solomon et al,[36] 2016 | Vermont, Oregon, Missouri and Minnesota, United States | Multicenter case series - prospective identification of *only* misdiagnosed patients at MS referral centers | 110/110 (100%) | 3–5 (median) | • Migraine<br>• Fibromyalgia<br>• Nonspecific neurologic symptoms with abnormal MRI<br>• Conversion or psychogenic disorder<br>• NMOSD | 70% |
| Kaisey et al,[33] 2019 | California, United States | Retrospective review of all new referrals to MS centers 2016–2017 | 43/241 (18%) | 4 (mean) | • Migraine<br>• RIS<br>• Cervical spondylosis<br>• Peripheral neuropathy<br>• Optic neuropathy (without neuritis) | 60% |
| Midaglia et al,[34] 2021 | Catalonia, Spain | Prospective review of all new referrals to MS center 2017–2018 | 8/112 (7%) | 7.2 (mean) | • Migraine<br>• Cerebrovascular disease<br>• Functional neurologic disorder<br>• Inflammatory disease<br>• Nonspecific sx | 75% |
| Abdula et al,[37] 2021 | Kurdistan, Iraq | Expert committee review of randomly selected current MS center patients 2019–2020 | 9/106 (8.4%) | Not reported. DMT exposure was 4 y (mean) | • CIS[a]<br>• Possible CADASIL<br>• Solitary Sclerosis<br>• Stroke with polycythemia vera<br>• Undiagnosed | 100% |
| Gaitan et al,[35] 2022 | Buenos Aires, Argentina | Retrospective review of new referrals to MS center presenting for second opinion 2013–2021 | 89/572 (16%) | 0.33 (median) | • Cerebrovascular disease<br>• RIS<br>• Headache<br>• Peripheral vestibular syndrome<br>• [illegible] | 61% |

*Abbreviations:* CADASIL, cerebral autosomal dominant arteriopathy with subcortical infarcts and leukoencephalopathy; CIS, clinically isola[illegible]e; DMT, disease modifying therapy, % of study misdiagnosed patients who at some point received MS DMT; NMOSD, neuromyelitis optica spe[illegible]er; RIS, radiologically isolated syndrome.

[a] CIS was excluded as a misdiagnosis category in other studies.

...cross these studies may guide practice and prevention efforts. MS has ...s mimics,[39] many of which are rare and challenging to recognize; these studies ...ning MS misdiagnosis[33–37] report that certain common disorders are frequently ...ken for MS. Cerebrovascular disease, or white matter ischemic disease, and ...raine were the most frequent correct alternative diagnoses identified (see ...able 2). The acuity, symptoms, and clinical findings associated with these diagnoses ...iffer from the typical clinical syndromes associated with MS, suggesting clinicians may ...e neglecting or misunderstanding this key element of the McDonald criteria (**Table 3**). ...ig. 1 provides examples of imaging findings that fulfill dissemination in space criteria for periventricular, juxtacortical, infratentorial, and spinal cord MS lesions, as well as examples of lesions that do not fulfill these criteria or raise red flags that there may be an alternate diagnosis.

Care provided by a clinician with MS subspecialty expertise does not appear to eliminate MS misdiagnosis. Specialists had previously cared for a quarter of the misdiagnosed patients in the 2019 study by Kaisey and colleagues, the same proportion as in the 2016 study by Solomon and colleagues.[36] Misinterpretation of MRI (see **Fig. 1**) is an issue among specialists and nonspecialists.[40,41]

The consequences of misdiagnosis are varied and can be serious. Most of the identified misdiagnosed patients received MS disease-modifying therapy (DMT). In a study of misdiagnosed patients presenting to 2 MS centers, the 43 misdiagnosed patients received a mean of 2.6 years of unnecessary DMT.[33] These medications are associated with risks and adverse effects such as injection site or infusion reactions, potentially fatal infections, and malignancy.[42] In a multicenter case series of patients misdiagnosed with MS, 70% had received MS DMT, and 25% of that group experienced treatment-related adverse outcomes.[36] Furthermore, the unnecessary monetary cost of DMT and the imaging and laboratory studies associated with their routine surveillance add to the financial burden of patients and the health care system.[43,44] In 1 study, misdiagnosed patients received 110 total patient-years of costly DMT.[33]

Misdiagnosis of MS also delays diagnosis and creates a missed opportunity for appropriate treatment of a patient's true underlying disease, often increasing risk for disease progression and disability. For example, in patients with neuromyelitis optica spectrum disorder (NMOSD) or stroke misdiagnosed as MS, a recurrent neurologic

**Table 3**
**Red flags that should prompt consideration of diagnoses other than multiple sclerosis**

| | |
|---|---|
| Demographic and Clinical presentation | • Onset after age 50 years<br>• Hyperacute onset (within minutes)<br>• Simultaneous bilateral optic neuritis or unilateral optic neuritis with minimal recovery<br>• Complete transverse myelitis<br>• Encephalopathy<br>• Headache or meningismus<br>• Intractable hiccups, nausea or vomiting<br>• Duration of neurologic symptom(s) <24 hours |
| Paraclinical findings | • Absence of CSF IgG oligoclonal bands<br>• Greater than 50 CSF leukocytes/μL<br>• Spinal cord lesions extending >2 vertebral levels<br>• Contrast enhancement persisting longer than 3 months<br>• Absence of brain lesions<br>• Predominantly subcortical or deep white matter brain MRI lesions, without juxtacortical, infratentorial, or spinal cord lesions |

*Abbreviations:* CSF, cerebrospinal fluid; IgG, immunoglobulin G.

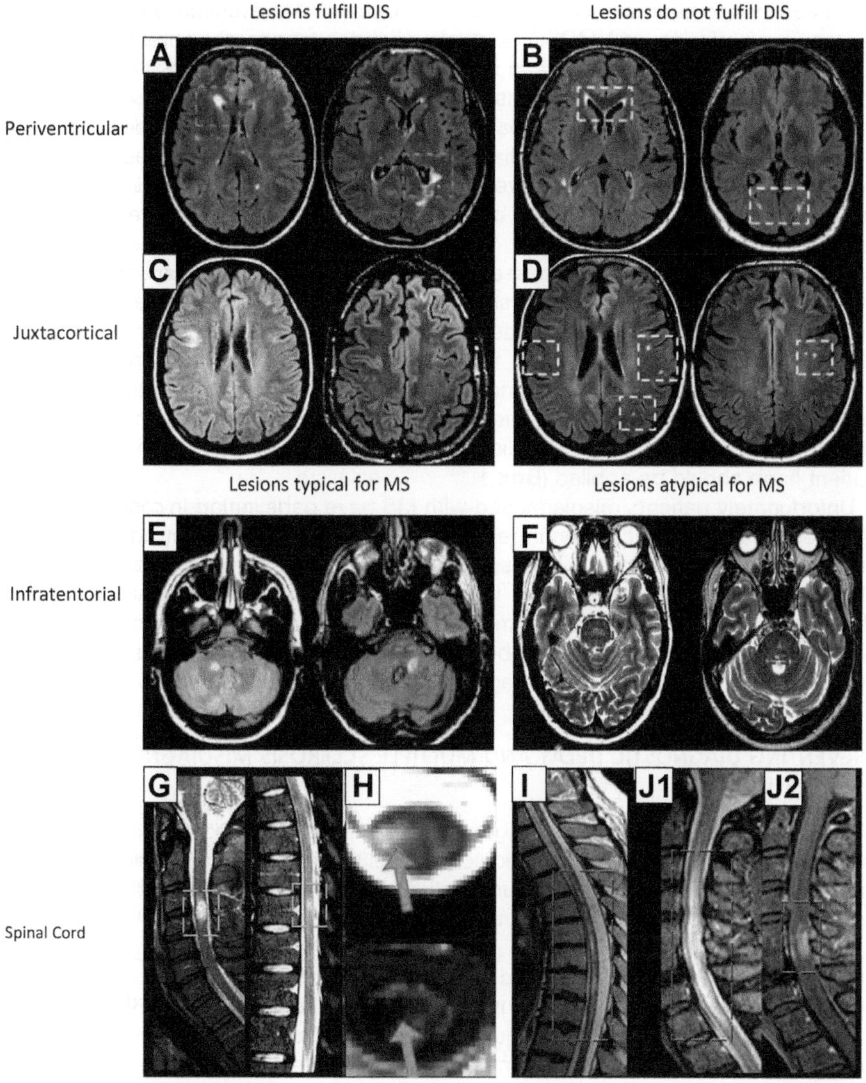


**Fig. 1.** Evaluation of MRI lesions for MS diagnosis. (*A*) periventricular lesions suggestive of MS; (*B*) anterior and posterior symmetric periventricular capping, a nonspecific, common finding associated with aging; (*C*) juxtacortical lesions suggestive of MS; (*D*) subcortical lesions (do not touch cortex), can be found in several conditions including small-vessel disease; (*E*) infratentorial lesions suggestive of MS; (*F*) symmetric lesions involving central pons in small-vessel disease; (*G*) cervical and thoracic spinal cord lesions in MS; (*H*) cervical cord lesion involving lateral column and central gray matter in MS; (*I*) longitudinally extensive transverse myelitis (LETM, extending over $\geq$3 vertebral segments) in neuromyelitis optica spectrum disorder; (*J1*) LETM with (*J2*) leptomeningeal and spinal cord contrast-enhancement in neuro-sarcoidosis. Images A–F: fluid attenuated inversion recovery (FLAIR) brain MRI. Images G, I, J1: short-tau inversion recovery sequence (STIR) on cervical and thoracic spinal cord MRI, H: T2-weighted and phase sensitive inversion recovery sequences (PSIR) on cervical cord MRI, J2: T1-weighted postcontrast cervical cord MRI. DIS: dissemination in space. (Adapted with permission from Filippi et al.[68])

event can lead to permanent disability or even death.[36] Although many treatments for MS appear ineffective in NMOSD or myelin oligodendrocyte glycoprotein antibody-associated disease (MOGAD) – and some may even increase NMOSD activity[45,46] – many patients with these conditions are unfortunately first misdiagnosed with MS. In a recent study that included 56 patients from across Latin America with a delayed diagnosis of NMOSD, 66% were diagnosed with MS, making it the most common incorrect diagnosis.[47] A recent survey of 204 patients with MOGAD found that 55% first received an alternate, incorrect diagnosis, with MS being the incorrect diagnosis for 33% of them.[48]

Patients may also suffer unnecessary psychosocial harm as a result of the removal of an incorrect diagnosis of MS. In a survey of MS specialist neurologists, 66% felt that undiagnosing someone with MS was more difficult than making a new diagnosis of MS, with another 28% feeling the two were equally difficult.[38] Sharing this news was so difficult; in fact, that 13% sometimes chose not to disclose the diagnosis, citing risk of psychological harm to the patient. However, withholding this information is usually unethical, and approaches to disclosing a misdiagnosis of MS while minimizing patient harm should be applied (**Box 1**).[49]

Unfortunately patients misdiagnosed with MS have participated in clinical trials for MS therapies.[34,36] Participation in research by a patient with the wrong condition is associated with significant unnecessary risk and can also influence data integrity. This finding raises the question of whether research methodology for MS studies should employ more rigorous confirmation of MS diagnosis in the enrollment process. Similar concerns might be raised about MS patient registries[50,51] used for research studies that rely on self-reported diagnosis of MS.

## PREVENTING DIAGNOSTIC DELAY AND MULTIPLE SCLEROSIS MISDIAGNOSIS NOW AND IN THE FUTURE

Delay in diagnosing MS and misdiagnosing MS in patients without the disease both have serious consequences for affected patients. Remedies for MS diagnostic error include educating neurologists on current diagnostic criteria, effectively disseminating future revisions to the criteria, and incorporating new biomarkers.

The causes of diagnostic delay in patients with MS are complex and multifactorial. Interventions will need to be tailored to the unique host of factors specific to patient populations, geographic regions, physicians, and health care systems that conspire to delay diagnosis. Although the frequent delay of MS diagnosis and its consequences are widely recognized, there remains a dearth of research focused on the causes. Future research focused on the patient diagnostic journey may provide preliminary data to guide subsequent broader public health research, educational initiatives, and interventions focused on improving early diagnosis of MS.

Misapplication of the McDonald criteria (see **Table 1**) in patients with syndromes atypical for MS or lacking objective evidence of a central nervous system (CNS) lesion accompanied by over-reliance on nonspecific MRI findings and misunderstanding of MRI dissemination in space terminology (see **Fig. 1**) appear to contribute to MS misdiagnosis.[36] Common conditions frequently misdiagnosed as MS (eg, cerebrovascular disease and migraine) typically present with symptom characteristics and neurologic examination findings that differ considerably from typical clinical presentations of MS (see **Table 3**). Indeed, recent surveys of neurologists and even MS specialists demonstrated misidentification of MS typical clinical syndromes and misunderstanding of MRI findings specified for fulfillment of the McDonald criteria (see **Fig. 1**).[40,41] Avoiding misdiagnosis of MS can sometimes be challenging, particularly in a patient presenting

**Box 1**
**Suggestions when disclosing a misdiagnosis of multiple sclerosis**

Choose an appropriate time for the discussion. Leave enough time to fully review the misdiagnosis and answer questions.

If the diagnostic error was yours, acknowledge the mistake. If the diagnostic error was not yours, avoid making assumptions regarding another physician's thought process and available information at the time.[69]

Center the discussion around facts of the case. If helpful, review patient's case in regard to diagnostic criteria.[1] Keep in mind that these may have changed since patient was diagnosed.[70]

Avoid jargon. Explain in layperson terms; use visual tools such as MR images or rough sketches as is helpful.

Reassure the patient he or she will not be abandoned. Detail the next steps, tests, and referrals or schedule a follow-up visit to continue the conversation.[69]

with an inflammatory syndrome with clinical and paraclinical features overlapping with MS. Yet data from studies focused on MS misdiagnosis suggest that educational efforts surrounding MS diagnostic criteria may prevent many misdiagnoses. In this context, concerted dissemination and implementation efforts concurrent with future revisions to the McDonald criteria should be considered.

Emerging novel MS diagnostic approaches have shown promise to improve diagnostic accuracy and allow for earlier diagnosis in the future. These include brain imaging, testing cerebrospinal fluid (CSF), and optical imaging. The central vein sign (CVS), the finding of a hypointensity in the center of an MS lesion corresponding to a central venule,[52] appears both sensitive and specific in distinguishing brain MRI of patients with MS from those with its mimics,[53] and has demonstrated accuracy in patients who had been previously misdiagnosed with MS.[54,55] Paramagentic rim lesions (PRLs), a rim of hypointensity around MS lesions on MRI corresponding to iron deposition,[56] have also shown promise, yielding 93% specificity for MS in a recent multicenter study.[57] CSF-specific oligoclonal bands (OCBs) are one of the more sensitive tools for diagnosing MS and are present in over 90% of those with MS.[58] Still, the analysis requires a paired serum sample and is somewhat subjective. Several recent studies demonstrated the increased sensitivity and technical ease of a CSF κFLC (free light chain) assay compared with OCB.[59–64] Optical coherence tomography (OCT) uses light to visualize the retina in 2 dimensions, and is quickly becoming a key tool in MS research and clinical care.[65] Recent studies have demonstrated that OCT can identify findings suggestive of a prior optic neuritis that are difficult to appreciate on standard MRI, an approach that may facilitate earlier diagnosis of MS.[66] Ongoing prospective studies in patients undergoing evaluation for MS[67] are needed to evaluate the potential of these putative biomarkers to aid the diagnosis of MS.

## SUMMARY

Without a highly specific diagnostic biomarker, the diagnostic process for MS leaves room for error. Both delay of a correct diagnosis of MS and a misdiagnosis of MS in patients with other conditions remain a contemporary problem. Limited data make designing interventions challenging; however, these studies suggest that educational efforts surrounding MS clinical presentations and the correct use of MS diagnostic criteria may prevent misdiagnosis. Emerging MS diagnostic biomarkers have shown promise to improve early and accurate diagnosis of MS.

## CLINICS CARE POINTS

- Misdiagnosis and delayed diagnosis of MS are both relatively common.
- Delayed diagnosis impacts prognosis by delaying treatment.
- Misapplication and misunderstanding of the McDonald criteria appear to contribute to MS misdiagnosis.
- Comprehensive educational efforts surrounding MS clinical presentations and the correct use of MS diagnostic criteria may prevent misdiagnoses.

## DISCLOSURE

M. Kaisey has received speaker or consulting compensation from Biogen, Genentech, and Novartis. A.J. Solomon discloses contracted research with Sanofi, Biogen, Novartis, Actelion, and Genentech/Roche; research support from Bristol Myers Squibb; personal compensation for consulting for Genentech, Biogen, Alexion, Celgene, Greenwich Biosciences, Horizon Therapeutics, TG Therapeutics, and Octave Bioscience; and personal compensation for nonpromotional speaking for EMD Serono.

## ACKNOWLEDGMENTS

The authors gratefully acknowledge Dr Shivani Naik for her assistance.

## REFERENCES

1. Thompson AJ, Banwell BL, Barkhof F, et al. Diagnosis of multiple sclerosis: 2017 revisions of the McDonald criteria. Lancet Neurol 2018;17(2):162–73.
2. Giovannoni G, Butzkueven H, Dhib-Jalbut S, et al. Brain health: time matters in multiple sclerosis. Mult Scler Relat Disord 2016;9(Suppl 1):S5–48.
3. Kurtzke JF. Rating neurologic impairment in multiple sclerosis. Neurology 1983; 33(11):1444.
4. Kavaliunas A, Manouchehrinia A, Stawiarz L, et al. Importance of early treatment initiation in the clinical course of multiple sclerosis. Multiple Sclerosis Journal 2016;23(9):1233–40.
5. Goodin DS, Reder AT, Ebers GC, et al. Survival in MS: a randomized cohort study 21 years after the start of the pivotal IFNβ-1b trial. Neurology 2012;78(17):1315–22.
6. Mauvais-Jarvis F, Bairey Merz N, J Barnes P, et al. Sex and gender: modifiers of health, disease, and medicine. Lancet 2020;396(10250):565–82.
7. Lai MC,, Szatmari P. Sex and gender impacts on the behavioural presentation and recognition of autism. Curr Opin Psychiatr 2020;33(2):117–23.
8. Tintore M, Cobo-Calvo A, Carbonell P, et al. Effect of changes in MS diagnostic criteria over 25 years on time to treatment and prognosis in patients with clinically isolated syndrome. Neurology 2021;97(17):e1641–52.
9. Kelly SB, Chaila E, Kinsella K, et al. Multiple sclerosis, from referral to confirmed diagnosis: an audit of clinical practice. Mult Scler 2011;17(8):1017–21.
10. Aires A, Barros A, Machado C, et al. Diagnostic delay of multiple sclerosis in a Portuguese population. Acta Med Port 2019;32(4):289–94.
11. Fernández O, Fernández V, Arbizu T, et al. Characteristics of multiple sclerosis at onset and delay of diagnosis and treatment in Spain (The Novo Study). J Neurol 2010;257(9):1500–7.

12. Anja T, Sørensen PS, Koch-Henriksen N, et al. Comorbidity in multiple sclerosis is associated with diagnostic delays and increased mortality. Neurology 2017; 89(16):1668.
13. Patti F, Chisari CG, Arena S, et al. Factors driving delayed time to multiple sclerosis diagnosis: Results from a population-based study. Mult Scler Relat Disord 2022;57:103361.
14. Kaufmann M, Kuhle J, Puhan MA, et al. Factors associated with time from first-symptoms to diagnosis and treatment initiation of multiple sclerosis in Switzerland. Mult Scler J Exp Transl Clin 2018;4(4). 2055217318814562.
15. Kingwell E, Leung AL, Roger E, et al. Factors associated with delay to medical recognition in two Canadian multiple sclerosis cohorts. J Neurol Sci 2010; 292(1–2):57–62.
16. Khan O, Williams MJ, Amezcua L, et al. Multiple sclerosis in US minority populations. Neurology: Clin Pract 2015;5(2):132.
17. Amezcua L, Lund BT, Weiner LP, et al. Multiple sclerosis in Hispanics: a study of clinical disease expression. Multiple Sclerosis Journal 2011;17(8):1010–6.
18. Stuifbergen A, Becker H, Phillips C, et al. Experiences of African American women with multiple sclerosis. International Journal of MS Care 2020;23(2):59–65.
19. Langer-Gould AM, Grisell Gonzales E, Smith JB, et al. Racial and ethnic disparities in multiple sclerosis prevalence. Neurology 2022;98(18):e1818.
20. Hittle M, Culpepper WJ, Langer-Gould A, et al. Population-based estimates for the prevalence of multiple sclerosis in the United States by race, ethnicity, age, sex, and geographic region. JAMA Neurol 2023;80(7):693–701.
21. Levin N, Mor M, Ben-Hur T. Patterns of misdiagnosis of multiple sclerosis. Isr Med Assoc J 2003;5(7):489–90.
22. Marrie RA, Cutter G, Tyry T, et al. Changes in the ascertainment of multiple sclerosis. Neurology 2005;65(7):1066.
23. Gasperi C, Hapfelmeier A, Daltrozzo T, et al. Systematic assessment of medical diagnoses preceding the first diagnosis of multiple sclerosis. Neurology 2021. https://doi.org/10.1212/WNL.0000000000012074.
24. Solomon AJ, Ascherio A. Early diagnosis of multiple sclerosis. Neurology 2021; 96(24):1111.
25. Willumsen JS, Aarseth JH, Myhr Kjell-Morten, et al. High incidence and prevalence of MS in Møre and Romsdal County, Norway, 1950-2018. Neurol Neuroimmunol Neuroinflamm 2020;7(3):1–10.
26. Kalinowska-Lyszczarz A, Tillema J-M, Tobin WO, et al. Long-term clinical, MRI, and cognitive follow-up in a large cohort of pathologically confirmed, predominantly tumefactive multiple sclerosis. Multiple Sclerosis Journal 2021;28(3):441–52.
27. Schmalstieg WF, Keegan BM, Weinshenker BG. Solitary sclerosis: progressive myelopathy from solitary demyelinating lesion. Neurology 2012;78(8):540–4.
28. Tremlett H,, Marrie RA. The multiple sclerosis prodrome: emerging evidence, challenges, and opportunities. Mult Scler 2021;27(1):6–12.
29. Lebrun-Frénay C, Okuda DT, Siva A, et al. The radiologically isolated syndrome: revised diagnostic criteria. Brain 2023;awad073.
30. Herndon RM, Brooks B. Misdiagnosis of multiple sclerosis. Semin Neurol 1985; 5:94–8.
31. Poser CM. Misdiagnosis of multiple sclerosis and β-interferon. Lancet 1997; 349(9069):1916.
32. Engell T. A clinico-pathoanatomical study of multiple sclerosis diagnosis. Acta Neurol Scand 1988;78(1):39–44.

33. Kaisey M, Solomon AJ, Luu M, et al. Incidence of multiple sclerosis misdiagnosis in referrals to two academic centers. Mult Scler Relat Disord 2019;30:51–6.
34. Midaglia L, Sastre-Garriga J, Pappolla A, et al. The frequency and characteristics of MS misdiagnosis in patients referred to the multiple sclerosis centre of Catalonia. Multiple Sclerosis Journal 2021;27(6):913–21.
35. Gaitán MI, Sanchez M, Farez MF, et al. The frequency and characteristics of multiple sclerosis misdiagnosis in Latin America: a referral center study in Buenos Aires, Argentina. Mult Scler 2022;28(9):1373–81.
36. Solomon AJ, Bourdette DN, Cross AH, et al. The contemporary spectrum of multiple sclerosis misdiagnosis: a multicenter study. Neurology 2016;87(13):1393–9.
37. Abdula A, Kurmanji MT, Mohammed ZA, et al. Revision of multiple sclerosis cases according to new 2017 McDonald Criteria among diagnosed patients in Sulaimani City. Journal of Sulaimani Medical College 2021;11(3):10317.
38. Solomon AJ, Klein EP, Bourdette D. "Undiagnosing" multiple sclerosis: the challenge of misdiagnosis in MS. Neurology 2012;78(24):1986–91.
39. Miller DH, Weinshenker BG, Filippi M, et al. Differential diagnosis of suspected multiple sclerosis: a consensus approach. Mult Scler 2008;14(9):1157–74.
40. Solomon AJ, Pettigrew R, Naismith RT, et al. Challenges in multiple sclerosis diagnosis: misunderstanding and misapplication of the McDonald criteria. Mult Scler 2021;27(2):250–8.
41. Solomon AJ, Kaisey M, Krieger SC, et al. Multiple sclerosis diagnosis: knowledge gaps and opportunities for educational intervention in neurologists in the United States. Multiple Sclerosis Journal 2021;28(8):1248–56.
42. Rommer PS, Zettl UK. Managing the side effects of multiple sclerosis therapy: pharmacotherapy options for patients. Expert Opin Pharmacother 2018;19(5): 483–98.
43. Simoens S. Societal economic burden of multiple sclerosis and cost-effectiveness of disease-modifying therapies. Front Neurol 2022;13:1015256.
44. Sadigh G, Switchenko J, Lava N, et al. Longitudinal changes of financial hardship in patients with multiple sclerosis. Multiple Sclerosis and Related Disorders 2021; 53:103037.
45. Palace J, Leite MI, Nairne A, et al. Interferon beta treatment in neuromyelitis optica: increase in relapses and aquaporin 4 antibody titers. Arch Neurol 2010; 67(8):1016–7.
46. Kitley J, Evangelou N, Küker W, et al. Catastrophic brain relapse in seronegative NMO after a single dose of natalizumab. J Neurol Sci 2014;339(1):223–5.
47. Carnero Contentti E, López PA, Criniti J, et al. Frequency of NMOSD misdiagnosis in a cohort from Latin America: impact and evaluation of different contributors. Mult Scler 2023;29(2):277–86.
48. Santoro JD, Gould J, Panahloo Z, et al. Patient pathway to diagnosis of myelin oligodendrocyte glycoprotein antibody-associated disease (MOGAD): findings from a multinational survey of 204 patients. Neurology and Therapy 2023;12(4): 1081–101.
49. Solomon AJ, Klein E. Disclosing a misdiagnosis of multiple sclerosis: do no harm? Continuum (Minneap Minn) 2013;19(4):1087–91.
50. Vollmer TL, Ni W, Stanton S, et al. The NARCOMS Patient Registry: a resource for investigators. International Journal of MS Care 1999;1(1):28–34.
51. McBurney R, et al. Initial characterization of participants in the iConquerMS Network. In: Proceedings of the Americas Committee for Treatment and Research in Multiple Sclerosis. 2017. p. 23-25.

52. Sati P, Pettigrew R, Naismith RT, et al. The central vein sign and its clinical evaluation for the diagnosis of multiple sclerosis: a consensus statement from the North American Imaging in Multiple Sclerosis Cooperative. Nat Rev Neurol 2016;12(12):714–22.
53. Maggi P, Oh J, Constable RT, et al. Central vein sign differentiates multiple sclerosis from central nervous system inflammatory vasculopathies. Ann Neurol 2018; 83(2):283–94.
54. Solomon AJ, Absinta M, Grammatico M, et al. Diagnostic performance of central vein sign for multiple sclerosis with a simplified three-lesion algorithm. Mult Scler 2018;24(6):750–7.
55. Kaisey M, Watts R, Ontaneda D, et al. Preventing multiple sclerosis misdiagnosis using the "central vein sign": a real-world study. Mult Scler Relat Disord 2021;48:102671.
56. Absinta M, Solomon AJ, Guerrero BL, et al. Seven-tesla phase imaging of acute multiple sclerosis lesions: a new window into the inflammatory process. Ann Neurol 2013;74(5):669–78.
57. Maggi P, Sati P, Gaitán MI, et al. Paramagnetic rim lesions are specific to multiple sclerosis: an international multicenter 3T MRI study. Ann Neurol 2020;88(5):1034–42.
58. Schwenkenbecher P, Sati P, Nair G, et al. The persisting significance of oligoclonal bands in the dawning era of kappa free light chains for the diagnosis of multiple sclerosis. Int J Mol Sci 2018;19. https://doi.org/10.3390/ijms19123796.
59. Saadeh R, Pittock S, Bryant S, et al. CSF kappa free light chains as a potential quantitative alternative to oligoclonal bands in multiple sclerosis (S37. 001). AAN Enterprises; 2019.
60. Saadeh RS, Bryant SC, McKeon A, et al. CSF kappa free light chains: cutoff validation for diagnosing multiple sclerosis. Mayo Clin Proc 2022;97(4):738–51.
61. Gaetani L, Carlo MD, Brachelente G, et al. Cerebrospinal fluid free light chains compared to oligoclonal bands as biomarkers in multiple sclerosis. J Neuroimmunol 2020;339:577108.
62. Altinier S, Puthenparampil M, Zaninotto M, et al. Free light chains in cerebrospinal fluid of multiple sclerosis patients negative for IgG oligoclonal bands. Clin Chim Acta 2019;496:117–20.
63. Christiansen M, Gjelstrup MC, Stilund M, et al. Cerebrospinal fluid free kappa light chains and kappa index perform equal to oligoclonal bands in the diagnosis of multiple sclerosis. Clin Chem Lab Med 2018;57(2):210–20.
64. Gurtner KM, Shosha E, Bryant SC, et al. CSF free light chain identification of demyelinating disease: comparison with oligoclonal banding and other CSF indexes. Clin Chem Lab Med 2018;56(7):1071–80.
65. Graves JS. Optical coherence tomography in multiple sclerosis. Semin Neurol 2019;39(6):711–7.
66. Nolan-Kenney RC, Liu M, Akhand O, et al. Optimal intereye difference thresholds by optical coherence tomography in multiple sclerosis: an international study. Ann Neurol 2019;85(5):618–29.
67. Ontaneda D, Sati P, Raza P, et al. Central vein sign: a diagnostic biomarker in multiple sclerosis (CAVS-MS) study protocol for a prospective multicenter trial. Neuroimage: Clinical 2021;32:102834.
68. Filippi M, Preziosa P, Banwell BL, et al. Assessment of lesions on magnetic resonance imaging in multiple sclerosis: practical guidelines. Brain 2019;142(7):1858–75.
69. Solomon AJ, Klein E. Disclosing a misdiagnosis of multiple sclerosis: do no harm? CONTINUUM: Lifelong Learning in Neurology 2013;19(4):1087–91.
70. Solomon AJ, Arrambide G, Brownlee W, et al. Confirming a historical diagnosis of multiple sclerosis. Neurology: Clin Pract 2022;12(3):263.

# Recent Advances in Diagnostic, Prognostic, and Disease-Monitoring Biomarkers in Multiple Sclerosis

Anibal Chertcoff, MD[a], Raphael Schneider, MD, PhD[a], Christina J. Azevedo, MD, MPH[b], Nancy Sicotte, MD[c], Jiwon Oh, MD, PhD[a,d,*]

**KEYWORDS**

- Multiple sclerosis • Diagnosis • Prognosis • Disease-monitoring • Biomarkers • MRI • Neurofilament light

**KEY POINTS**

- Biomarkers specific to MS pathology could be of substantial clinical utility to improve the specificity and accuracy of diagnostic tools in MS and reduce the rate of misdiagnosis.
- Two emerging MRI diagnostic biomarkers with significant potential for clinical utility are the central vein sign and paramagnetic rim lesions (PRLs).
- MRI measures of whole-brain and substructure atrophy, PRLs, neurofilament light (NfL), and glial fibrillary acidic protein are promising emerging biomarkers to predicting MS outcomes.
- Utilization of serum NfL as a biomarker for disease monitoring and treatment response is likely to become widespread in the near future.
- Emerging progressive disease biology biomarkers include PRLs, slowly expanding lesions, and PET ligands specific for activated microglia.

## INTRODUCTION

Multiple sclerosis (MS) is a chronic inflammatory and neurodegenerative disease of the central nervous system (CNS) and the leading progressive neurologic condition

[a] Division of Neurology, Department of Medicine, St. Michael's Hospital, University of Toronto, 30 Bond Street, PGT 17-742, Toronto, Ontario M5B 1W8, Canada; [b] Department of Neurology, Keck School of Medicine, University of Southern California, HCT 1520 San Pablo Street, Health Sciences Campus, Los Angeles, CA 90033, USA; [c] Department of Neurology, Cedars-Sinai Medical Center, 127 S San Vicente Boulevard, 6th floor, Suite A6600, Los Angeles, CA 90048, USA; [d] Department of Neurology, Johns Hopkins University, Baltimore, MD, USA
* Corresponding author. Department of Medicine (Neurology), St. Michael's Hospital, University of Toronto, 30 Bond Street, PGT 17-742, Toronto, Ontario M5B 1W8, Canada.
*E-mail address:* jiwon.oh@unityhealth.to

Neurol Clin 42 (2024) 15–38
https://doi.org/10.1016/j.ncl.2023.06.008

of young working-age adults, affecting over 2.8 million people worldwide.[1–3] The disease is highly heterogeneous with regard to its clinical presentation, prognosis, and treatment response, and a combination of clinical features, MRI, and cerebrospinal fluid (CSF) analysis is currently used in clinical practice for diagnosis and treatment decisions.[1] However, a need exists for tools that better reflect the pathologic substrates of the disease, which would improve diagnostic accuracy, enable early prediction of disease severity, and allow for improved monitoring of disease progression and response to therapy.

Biomarkers are characteristics that can be objectively measured, serving as indicators of a pathologic process, predicting the incidence of a defined outcome or the response to an intervention.[4,5] Based on their applications, they can be further classified into those that can aid disease detection or identification of disease subtypes (*diagnostic* biomarkers), those useful for predicting the likelihood of a future clinical event or outcome (*prognostic* biomarkers), or those used to assess disease status over time or effect of therapy (*disease-monitoring/treatment-response* biomarkers).[6]

In the last number of years, there have been continuous efforts in the MS field to develop biomarkers to aid in disease diagnosis and early prognosis, evaluation of ongoing inflammatory activity, detection of progressive disease biology, prediction of treatment response, and monitoring of disease-modifying therapy (DMT) safety.[7] In this review, we provide an overview of promising developments of diagnostic, prognostic, and disease-monitoring/treatment-response biomarkers in MS. A summary is provided in **Table 1**.

## CURRENT DIAGNOSTIC BIOMARKERS FOR MULTIPLE SCLEROSIS

Presently, conventional MRI of the brain and spinal cord remains the most valuable biomarker to aid in the diagnosis of MS. MRI criteria to diagnose MS require the presence of focal white matter lesions (WMLs) within the CNS, which should be typical in terms of distribution, morphology, evolution, and signal abnormality on a number of conventional MRI sequences (eg, T2-weighted, T2-FLAIR, and pre- and post-contrast T1-weighted scans).[8] In addition, oligoclonal bands restricted to the CSF still play a valuable role in the diagnosis of MS.[9] Although not exclusive to MS or mandatory for its diagnosis, the evidence of intrathecal antibody production in the proper clinical context can facilitate an MS diagnosis.[8]

The 2017 McDonald criteria for MS diagnosis require the demonstration of disease dissemination in space and time through a combination of clinical symptoms, signs, and paraclinical tests.[8] As these criteria have been designed to diagnose MS in individuals presenting with typical demyelinating syndromes with a high likelihood of MS, their value in helping to distinguish MS from other conditions is limited. When the McDonald criteria are not applied in the appropriate clinical context, the risk for misdiagnosis increases, which remains a relevant issue in MS.[10] Recent multicenter studies have shown that MS misdiagnosis can be seen in up to 20% of cases, even at MS specialty centers, particularly in individuals presenting with atypical clinical or MRI features.[11] Improving the specificity of diagnostic tools would help prevent individuals who do not have MS from being unnecessarily exposed to immunomodulatory/immunosuppressant therapies and would also allow people with MS to receive earlier treatment when appropriate. Therefore, additional diagnostic biomarkers specific to MS pathology would be of substantial clinical utility.[12] The two emerging diagnostic biomarkers that are farthest along in clinical development are the central vein sign (CVS) and paramagnetic rim lesions (PRLs).

**Table 1**
**Current landscape of the most promising developments in diagnostic, prognostic, and disease-monitoring biomarkers in multiple sclerosis**

| Diagnostic Biomarkers | Advantages | Limitations |
|---|---|---|
| Central vein sign | • Highly specific for MS when high proportions of WMLs with the CVS are observed (commonly used threshold is $\geq$ 40%)<br>• Excellent PPV and NPV<br>• Simplified approaches under study | • "40% rule" can be time-consuming<br>• Simplified approaches less specific for MS diagnosis |
| Paramagnetic rim lesions | • Highly specific to MS<br>• Observed in all MS subtypes and RIS but seen in higher numbers in progressive MS subtypes | • Relatively low sensitivity for MS<br>• Lack of consensus on definition, best sequences for visualization and detection with lower field MRI |
| **Prognostic biomarkers** | **Advantages** | **Limitations** |
| MRI measures of atrophy | • Early predictor of long-term disability<br>• Greater atrophy associated with worse relevant clinical outcomes, including global neurologic disability, fatigue, and cognitive disability | • Barriers precluding clinical use: access to appropriate MRI sequences and software, measurement variability, validation of software tools, definition of actionable clinical thresholds, and timing of studies |
| Paramagnetic rim lesions | • Promising role for prediction of disease severity as well as motor and cognitive disability | • Lack of consensus on definition, best sequences for visualization and detection with lower field MRI |
| Neurofilament light chain | • Measurable in CSF and blood<br>• Sensitive to inflammatory-driven neuroaxonal damage<br>• Promising role for prediction of short-term clinical outcomes and MRI disease activity | • Not specific to MS<br>• Role in progressive disease remains unclear<br>• Need to account for comorbidities and age<br>• Harmonization of methods across laboratories needed |
| Glial fibrillary acidic protein | • Measurable in CSF and blood<br>• Likely reflects progressive disease biology<br>• May predict disability independent of acute disease fluctuations | • Not specific to MS<br>• Normative values still need to be established<br>• Weight-, age-, and sex-adjusted reference ranges may be required |

| Disease-monitoring/ treatment-response biomarkers | Advantages | Limitations |
|---|---|---|
| Central vein sign | • May help distinguish etiology of new WMLs in older people with MS (MS vs. co-morbidities) | • Only small studies exist thus far supporting this role and most studies performed in individuals with relapsing MS |
| Neurofilament light chain | • In relapsing MS, potential role for:<br>• Initial treatment selection<br>• Close monitoring of disease activity<br>• Decisions related to treatment escalation, de-escalation, and discontinuation | • Role for disease monitoring in progressive MS remains unclear |
| Paramagnetic rim lesions | • Decrease in PRL formation, or resolution of PRLs, or changes at lesion edge proposed as pharmacologic target for chronic inflammation | • Still in early stages of development |
| Slowly expanding lesions | • Thought to detect a proportion of chronic active lesions<br>• Explored as imaging outcome for progressive disease biology | • Lack of consensus on optimal image processing algorithm, duration over which measurement should occur<br>• Larger longitudinal studies required |
| PET | • Use of radiotracers specific to microglia/macrophages<br>• May allow classification of rim lesions into active and inactive<br>• May also detect meningeal inflammation in vivo | • High cost and low availability<br>• Need for standardization of acquisition procedures<br>• Assessment of risks of serial imaging |

*Abbreviations:* CSF, cerebrospinal fluid, CVS; central vein sign, MS; multiple sclerosis, NPV; negative predictive value, PPV; positive predictive value, PRL; paramagnetic rim lesion, RIS; radiologically isolated syndrome, WMLs; white matter lesions.

## EMERGING DIAGNOSTIC BIOMARKERS FOR MULTIPLE SCLEROSIS

### *Central Vein Sign*

From a histopathological perspective, MS lesions have long been known to form around small central veins.[13] In the perivascular space that surrounds these veins, immunologic events may occur, such as the opening of the blood-brain barrier with the subsequent infiltration of autoreactive immune cells, leading to the formation of demyelinating lesions in the neighboring white matter.[14] The term "central vein sign" has been used to describe a central linear hypointensity visualized within a WML using iron-sensitive MRI sequences, which corresponds to the small vein around which the MS lesion formed.[15] This perivenous distribution of MS lesions has been observed in all MS subtypes (relapsing-remitting MS [RRMS], secondary-progressive MS [SPMS], and primary-progressive MS [PPMS]).[16,17] The CVS has been found in approximately 75% of MS lesions, varying according to the MRI field strength (higher on 7 T vs 1.5 T) and the lesion location (most prevalent in WMLs occurring in the periventricular region).[18,19] Individuals with other non-MS conditions affecting the CNS, including, among others, migraine, cerebral small vessel disease, neuromyelitis optica spectrum disorders, systemic lupus erythematosus, and Susac syndrome, can also present with WMLs showing the CVS, but this is typically seen in a significantly lower proportion.[20] A 2019 meta-analysis found a pooled incidence of observing a central vein in WMLs among non-MS conditions of 33%.[18] Given these differences, the CVS has been proposed as a potential diagnostic biomarker to differentiate MS from other conditions that affect the white matter. In **Fig. 1**, examples of WMLs with and without a central vein are presented in both MS and non-MS conditions.

Different criteria have been proposed to use the CVS as a diagnostic tool in MS. The most common one is the "40% rule," which evaluates the proportion of observed WMLs exhibiting a central vein and uses a cutoff of 40% to distinguish MS from other non-MS conditions.[21] Initial studies have shown that this cutoff provided a positive and negative predictive value for MS of 100%.[22] Limitations for applying this method in clinical practice include the need to examine all WMLs, which can be time-consuming, particularly in individuals with a high lesion load. Alternative simplified approaches that are much more efficient for clinical practice have also been proposed, including "Select6*" (ie, counting six or more CVS-positive WMLs)[23] and even "Select3*" (ie, three or more CVS-positive WMLs).[24] However, these simplified approaches are not as specific as the "40% rule." Large-scale prospective studies to further validate the diagnostic utility of the CVS in typical and atypical clinical syndromes are ongoing, results which will hopefully enable its incorporation into MS clinical practice.[25]

### *Paramagnetic Rim Lesions*

The presence of activated microglia and macrophages at the rim of chronic active or slowly expanding MS lesions can to lead to chronic "smoldering" inflammation, demyelination, and axonal damage and is thought to be an important pathophysiological driver of disease progression in MS.[26,27] A significant proportion of these activated myeloid cells have been found to contain iron, which is thought to be released in response to myelin and oligodendrocyte injury and may be captured on susceptibility-based MRI as a rim of hypointense signal at the lesion edge observed after regression of acute inflammation.[28,29] These lesions, described as "paramagnetic rim lesions" or "iron rim lesions," have been found in all MS types as well as in presymptomatic individuals at risk of developing clinical MS (ie, radiologically isolated syndrome [RIS]).[30] However, they seem to be more frequent in progressive rather than relapsing forms of MS.[31] A multicenter cross-sectional study analyzing 412 scans of

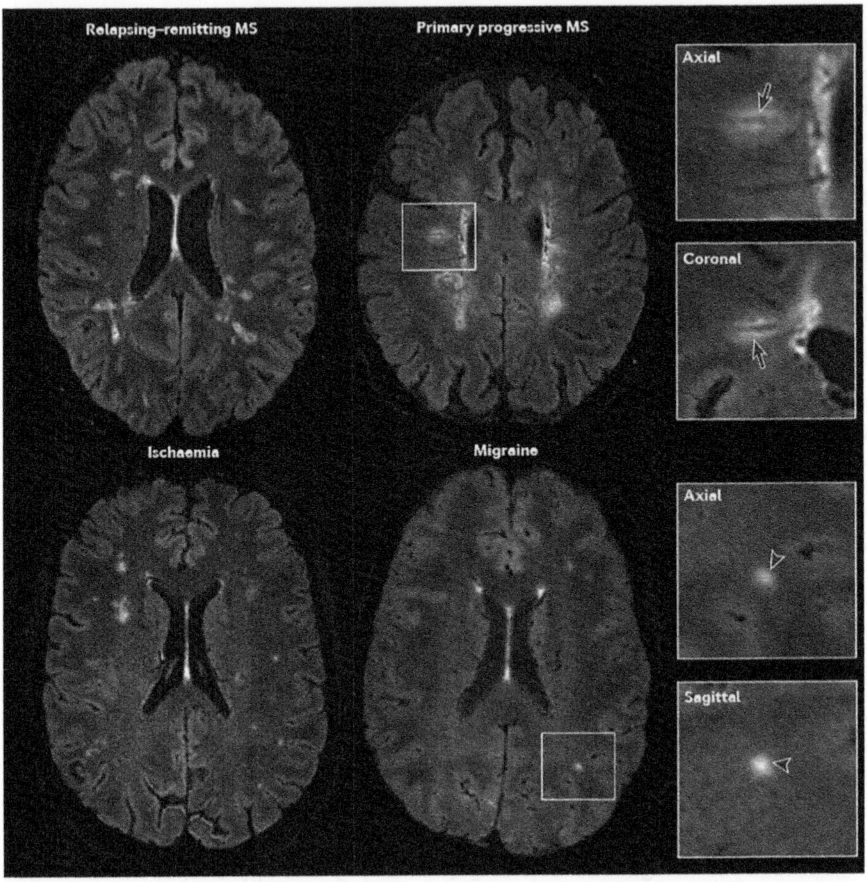


**Fig. 1.** The central vein sign. Most T2-hyperintense lesions observed in individuals with MS harbor a centrally located dark vessel (see *arrows* in boxes). In contrast, no central vein is evident in most lesions from individuals with non-MS conditions (see *arrowheads* in boxes). Images represent 3 T FLAIR* (combined T2*-weighted MRI and fluid-attenuated inversion recovery) sequences obtained at different sites. (*Data from* Sati and colleagues, 2016.[20])

patients with MS versus other non-MS differentials reported PRLs occurring in 52% of the MS cases compared with 7% of those without MS. They also found that the identification of at least one PRL was associated with a high diagnostic specificity for MS (93%) but a relatively low sensitivity (52%). Although the combined detection of PRLs with CVS resulted in an increased specificity (99%), the sensitivity still remained low (59%).[32] An example of a PRL is provided in **Fig. 2**.

Limitations that prevent the translation of PRLs to clinical practice include the lack of a clear consensus on a precise definition of PRLs, determining the most appropriate MRI sequences for optimal visualization,[33] and ensuring its detection at lower field MRI scanners most commonly used in clinical practice.[34]

## CURRENT PROGNOSTIC BIOMARKERS FOR MULTIPLE SCLEROSIS

Accurate prognostication in MS remains a clinical challenge for both short- and long-term clinical outcomes. Presenting symptoms, disease activity/severity, clinical

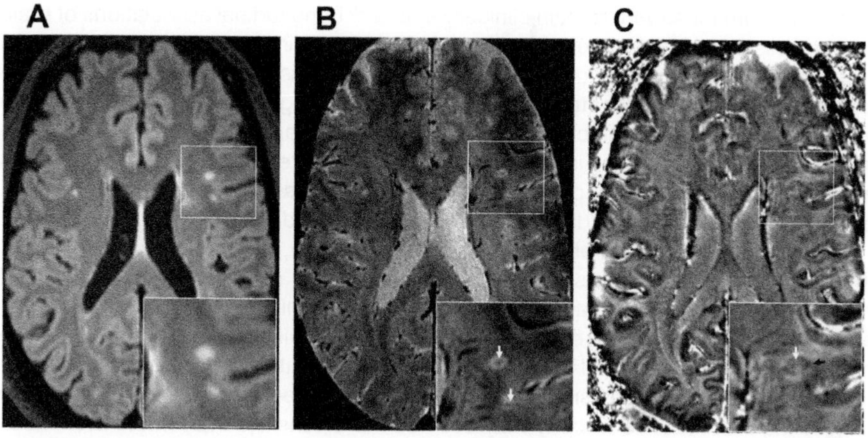


**Fig. 2.** Paramagnetic rim lesions. (*A*) A T2-hyperintense white matter lesion is magnified on a 3D axial FLAIR sequence. (*B*) Central veins are observed within white matter lesions (*white arrows* in the small box) on a 3D axial T2*-weighted segmented echo-planar magnitude image. (*C*) A white matter lesion with a visible central vein (*white arrow*) exhibits a paramagnetic rim (PRL; *black arrow*). (*Data from* Oh and colleagues, 2021.[72])

course, and treatment response vary significantly among patients, with some individuals remaining relatively well for decades with low-/moderate-efficacy therapies, or even without treatment, whereas others progress quickly to develop irreversible sequelae while being partially or completely unresponsive to various high-efficacy therapies.[35] Different prognostic factors are currently used in clinical practice to predict clinical outcomes and to stratify overall disease activity or rate of disability accumulation. These include a combination of demographic, clinical, MRI, and laboratory characteristics, with MRI-based lesion count and location at first presentation being the most prominent,[36] providing a crucial snapshot of current and prior disease activity at a specific point in time.[37] However, MRI techniques currently used in clinical practice have shown only limited sensitivity for predicting disease progression or prognosis,[38] with studies demonstrating high variability when exploring correlations between measures of clinical disability and overall T2-weighted WML load.[39,40]

With the continuing development of new DMTs to treat MS, there is an opportunity to optimize clinical outcomes by tailoring treatments on an individual level. Therefore, developing more reliable biomarkers to accurately predict MS evolution is needed. Recently, several studies investigating both imaging and laboratory biomarkers and their potential to predict disease outcome have been conducted. A selection of those most promising prognostic biomarkers is presented below.

## EMERGING PROGNOSTIC BIOMARKERS FOR MULTIPLE SCLEROSIS

### *MRI Measures of Atrophy (Whole-Brain, Substructure, and Spinal Cord Atrophy)*

Extensive efforts have been made in the field to comprehend and measure how CNS atrophy develops in MS by using different MRI techniques.[41] To this end, numerous cross-sectional[42,43] and longitudinal studies[44,45] have shown the clinical relevance of loss of brain volume as a prognostic measure in MS, including whole- and regional brain atrophy as well as changes in gray matter volumes. For instance, greater brain volume loss has been observed in RRMS patients with confirmed disability progression compared with those who remain clinically stable.[46] Longitudinal associations of brain volume loss have been observed with clinical disability in the longer term, including whole brain, thalamic, and cortical atrophy, which were associated disability progression at 10 years.[47] Another study also found the percentage of change in brain volume to be the most reliable predictor of future neurologic impairment as early as within the first year after disease onset, irrespective of the relapse rate.[48] Moreover, similar results were found regarding the correlation between increased brain volume loss and disability progression, regardless of overall T2-lesion load.[49]

When considering regional measures of brain atrophy, the thalamus has received the most attention due to its crucial role as a key relay center in MS[50] and several studies have demonstrated associations between thalamic atrophy and negative disease outcomes, including disease progression, disability, fatigue, and cognitive dysfunction.[51] A longitudinal study found that thalamic atrophy at baseline was able to predict disability progression for up to 8 years.[52] Moreover, there is also evidence suggesting that thalamic atrophy may even be more sensitive than whole-brain atrophy to predict future disability in MS as a study reported higher odds ratios for disability progression in those with isolated thalamic atrophy compared with those with whole-brain parenchymal atrophy.[53] Similarly, although multiple cross-sectional studies have found an association between whole brain atrophy and cognitive impairment, it seems that cortical gray matter atrophy seems to be the most important MRI predictor of 5-year cognitive decline in patients with MS.[54]

The role of spinal cord atrophy as an MRI biomarker for disability and progressive disease in MS has also been explored,[55] and several studies have even found more robust correlations between spinal cord atrophy and disability compared with measures of brain atrophy.[56–59] Although the upper cervical cord area is typically used to measure spinal cord atrophy in most studies as this region is technically easier to image, there is some discussion about which region of the spinal cord may be most sensitive to predict future disability in MS, particularly concerning higher and lower cervical cord areas.[60–62] A meta-analysis found that the rate of spinal cord atrophy was much higher than that reported in the brain (1.8%/year) and even higher in those with progressive MS (2.1%/year).[63] The rate of spinal cord atrophy seems to be an even better predictor for disability worsening compared with baseline cord measures in longitudinal studies. Individual rates of spinal cord atrophy seem to be highly relevant to disability progression over 2 and 5 years of follow-up.[64,65] Finally, there is also evidence that suggests that the total spinal cord gray matter area might also serve as a sensitive indicator of future disability.[66,67]

Overall, MRI measures of atrophy in the brain and spinal cord seem to be highly predictive of the evolution of MS at the group level, particularly for meaningful outcomes such as disability progression. However, before they can be introduced into everyday clinical practice, there are numerous hurdles that need to be addressed, including access to appropriate technology to generate measures of atrophy, technical issues causing measurement errors (eg, changes in scan parameters, gradient distortions, and intra-scanner variability), confounding factors affecting quantification of volumes (eg, age, sex, lifestyle, and state of hydration), appropriate validation of software tools used for volume measurement,[68] and a lack of clarity as to what clinically actionable cutoff thresholds should be used in specific MS patients and the timing during which these measures should be applied.

### *Paramagnetic Rim Lesions*

In addition to its potential role as a diagnostic biomarker, PRLs have also shown promise as a predictive biomarker in MS. For instance, a study found the presence of PRLs to be associated with various aspects of MS severity, including shorter disease duration, assignment to higher efficacy therapy, and poorer upper extremity dexterity.[69] In addition, PRLs have been linked to earlier motor and cognitive disability and lower brain volume.[70] Furthermore, PRLs have demonstrated their potential as an early predictor of future disability progression in individuals with clinically isolated syndrome (CIS) and early MS, as well as in RIS, where PRLs were found to be the imaging measure most strongly associated with cognitive impairment.[30,71,72] Moreover, a recent study found that the presence of four or more PRLs on baseline MRI was the greatest predictive factor of RIS developing into clinically definite MS over a follow-up period of 6 years.[73] Limitations for implementing PRLs into clinical practice were summarized earlier.

### *Neurofilament Light Chain*

Neurofilament light chain (NfL) is a protein released on neuronal and/or axonal injury into the extracellular space, CSF, and ultimately into the blood. Although serum concentrations of NfL (sNfL) are 40-fold lower than those detected in the CSF, advances in assay technology have allowed for their reliable detection in serum or plasma[74] through single molecule arrays or microfluidics,[75] with blood and CSF levels showing a high correlation.[76] Although NfL has been found to be elevated in the CSF, serum and plasma of individuals with MS, it may also be increased in other conditions affecting the CNS including various neurodegenerative diseases,[77] traumatic brain injury,[78] and even processes affecting the peripheral nervous system.[79] In addition, NfL can also be influenced by other individual characteristics, such as age and concomitant non-neurological comorbidities.[80,81] These features limit the prospect of using NfL as a diagnostic tool in MS,[76] although one study has shown that its use as an additional parameter increased the sensitivity and specificity of the 2017 McDonald criteria to differentiate CIS from RRMS.[82] Nevertheless, the role of NfL as a biomarker for prognostication and disease monitoring/treatment-response has significantly garnered more attention.

Several studies have shown promising results of NfL as a predictor of clinical outcomes and MRI changes in the short-term (relapses, new gadolinium-enhancing or T2-WMLs,[83] cortical lesions,[84] early Expanded Disability Status Scale [EDSS] worsening as well as future brain and cervical spinal atrophy).[85] In this regard, both CSF-NfL (cNfL) and sNfL have shown excellent predictive value in the conversion of RIS or CIS to clinically definite MS.[86–88] Moreover, higher sNfL levels have also been detected for up to 6 years before the clinical onset of MS, suggesting the presence of neuroaxonal damage even during the prodromal phase of the disease.[89] At this point, although sNfL seems to be a sensitive marker of ongoing inflammatory-driven neuroaxonal damage,[82] the role of sNfL in reflecting progressive disease biology remains unclear as correlations between sNfL and clinical/MRI measures of diffuse gradual neurodegenerative damage in the longer run seem to be less evident.[85,88,90–92] For example, contradictory findings have been observed in studies exploring the predictive value of sNfL for conversion SPMS or long-term EDSS scores.[74,92–95] A potential explanation for this may be that its ability to reflect slowly progressing neurodegenerative processes might be masked by its remarkable sensitivity to acute inflammatory neuronal injury secondary to relapse biology, including subclinical MRI activity.[82]

Challenges for implementing sNfL in clinical practice include difficulties with developing normative values, accounting for comorbidities and age,[96,97] and establishing harmonized methods across laboratories.[81,82] Recently, it has been suggested that Z scores should be used when reporting sNfL, which take an individual's age and body mass index (BMI) into consideration.[81,98]

### *Glial Fibrillary Acidic Protein*

Glial fibrillary acidic protein (GFAP) is a cytoskeletal protein of astrocytes that has been regarded as a marker of astrocytic damage[99,100] and reactive astrogliosis.[101,102] Because GFAP is upregulated in many inflammatory and non-inflammatory conditions affecting the CNS,[103–105] its role has been explored as a potential biomarker in MS and other neurologic diseases.[106] Reactive astrocytes are thought to be involved in MS pathology by obstructing remyelination[107] and leading to neuronal and oligodendrocytic death.[108] As these represent hallmark features of progressive MS subtypes and disease progression in MS, GFAP has been explored as a biomarker for prognostication and to monitor disease progression. In keeping with this, serum GFAP (sGFAP) levels were found to be higher in patients with PPMS compared with RRMS,[109] and a correlation between EDSS and GFAP values was found in progressive MS patients but not in those with RRMS.[107,110] Furthermore, sGFAP levels were found to correlate with increased T2-lesion load and decreased white and gray matter volumes in 45 MS patients without a recent relapse (defined as "inactive").[109] Moreover, a recent study that included samples from 257 individuals with MS showed that sGFAP was able to predict 6-month confirmed disability progression only in non-active progressive MS patients but not in those with active-progressive MS. In fact, sGFAP showed highest prognostic value in those with low sNfL, supporting the hypothesis that sGFAP primarily reflects the biology that underlies disease progression.[111] In another recent study, sGFAP was found to predict future progression independent of relapse activity.[112] A very recent study found that sGFAP but not sNfL was correlated with the presence of PRLs in RIS.[113] Other investigators have also found an association between sGFAP levels and higher EDSS scores, longer disease duration, and progressive course.[114] Finally, although NfL levels increase substantially during relapses, several studies have suggested that GFAP levels seem to be less affected by acute disease fluctuations.[111,112]

Of note, normal values for GFAP in blood and CSF still need to be established. GFAP increases with age and some studies have reported levels of sGFAP to be higher in women with MS compared with males.[111,115] Also, individuals with MS and a BMI $\geq$25 kg/m$^2$ were reported to have lower sGFAP concentrations compared with those with lower BMIs.[116] This will need to be taken into account if sGFAP is ever used in clinical practice because weight-, age-, and sex-adjusted reference ranges may be required to interpret sGFAP values.

## CURRENT DISEASE-MONITORING/TREATMENT-RESPONSE BIOMARKERS

MRI is currently the only biomarker used in clinical practice to confidently monitor overall MS disease activity and treatment response. The appearance of new T2 and/or gadolinium-enhancing lesions over time correlates with relapse frequency and is extraordinarily useful to monitor subclinical disease activity in MS.[8] However, these MRI markers mainly detect short-term inflammatory activity.[117,118] Long-term disability in MS seems to better correlate with MRI measures of atrophy, likely linked to neurodegeneration.[119] However, tools for quantification of brain and/or spinal cord atrophy have not yet been widely introduced into clinical practice due to the obstacles and lingering queries outlined above.[120,121]

The current standard of care with respect to evaluating treatment response is to use both clinical and MRI information in individuals with MS. Methods such as NEDA (ie, no evidence of disease activity), which incorporate both clinical data (ie, relapse or disability progression) and MRI findings (ie, new T2-lesions over time), are commonly used in day-to-day practice and clinical trials for monitoring disease activity and assessing treatment response.[122] Moreover, MRI also plays a key role in the early detection of some treatment-related adverse effects (eg, progressive multifocal leukoencephalopathy).[117]

Limitations of conventional MRI in monitoring MS disease activity and treatment response include its weak association with overall clinical status,[123] its lack of sensitivity to all MS-related changes in the brain and spinal cord, including gray matter involvement[124] and diffuse damage in the white matter,[123] and its inadequate capacity to assess the degree of tissue injury as well as its inability to detect changes during late-stage progressive disease.[125] Recently, several studies have been conducted investigating a number of imaging and laboratory markers that aim to better reflect disease activity and treatment effect and hold the promise to fill this void. Following is a selection of a number of promising candidate biomarkers.

## EMERGING DISEASE-MONITORING/TREATMENT-RESPONSE BIOMARKERS

### *Relapse Disease Biology Biomarkers*

#### *Central vein sign*

In addition to its role as a diagnostic biomarker for MS, there may also be a role for the CVS as a biomarker of disease activity/treatment response in the assessment of MS patients experiencing breakthrough radiological disease activity. A 2022 retrospective cohort study characterized the CVS profile of new WMLs in individuals with MS followed for up to 3 years.[126] In people with MS developing new lesions, the majority was CVS+; however, one-third of lesions were not CVS+. This finding suggests that particularly in older people with MS with vascular comorbidities, the decision to change DMT should not be solely made from radiologic breakthrough disease and that the CVS may be of substantial clinical utility to distinguish new T2 lesions related to MS versus other comorbidities, which has significant implications for treatment. Limitations of this study included its small sample size and the fact that it mostly analyzed individuals with RRMS. However, it serves as an initial step to explore the potential role of CVS as a biomarker of disease activity/treatment response and further studies are warranted.

#### *Neurofilament light chain*

The utilization of sNfL as a blood-based biomarker to monitor relapsing MS disease activity and treatment response is likely to become widespread in clinical practice in the near future.[127] Its potential role in assisting therapeutic decisions in individuals with RRMS include aiding in the selection of the initial treatment, assessing subclinical disease activity concurrently with serial MRIs, allowing closer monitoring of clinically active patients and helping in decisions related to treatment escalation, de-escalation, or cessation of DMTs.[82]

Numerous studies have demonstrated that sNfL levels are typically lower in subjects with MS receiving DMTs than in those untreated.[128–130] Furthermore, the initiation of nearly all available DMTs for MS has been associated with a reduction in sNfL concentrations.[129] Retrospective assessments of stored samples from phase 3 clinical trials of different DMTs have also replicated these results.[131,132] In addition, sNfL levels have been found to remain stable in patients who switched from one DMT to another of comparable efficacy but were shown to be significantly lower in those who transitioned to higher efficacy therapies.[130] These findings emphasize the potential role of assessing changes in sNfL levels longitudinally as a component of therapeutic decision-making in individuals with relapsing MS. sNfL has been recently incorporated as a prospectively assessed secondary endpoint in clinical trials (eg, ASCLEPIOS trial; ofatumumab vs teriflunomide).[133]

As sNfL strongly reflects acute inflammatory axonal damage, its role in monitoring progressive disease biology is unclear. Whether sNfL can play a role in monitoring progressive disease biology alone or in combination with other biomarkers that show a stronger association with neurodegeneration (such as GFAP) is an area of active study, for which there is limited evidence at the current time.

### *Non-Relapse/Progressive Disease Biology Biomarkers*

#### *Paramagnetic rim lesions*

The use of PRLs as a disease-monitoring/treatment-response biomarker is beginning to be explored.[33] Recent evidence suggests that although PRLs seem to be stable in the short-to-medium term,[134] the iron rim may vanish over time in some cases.[135,136] This has led to an increasing interest in exploring the potential utility of examining changes at the lesion edge as a pharmacologic target in clinical trials, such as a decrease in PRL formation or faster time to PRL disappearance. As current DMTs for MS have demonstrated poor efficacy in controlling chronic inflammation in PRLs,[70] the development of new drugs that can modulate the inflammatory response within these lesions is an unmet need in clinical practice. For this, PRLs have been included as imaging outcome measures in different phase I/II trials of various drug classes in evaluation for MS, including interleukin-1 receptor antagonists (NCT04025554) and Bruton's tyrosine kinase (BTK) inhibitors,[137] including evobrutinib and tolebrutinib.

#### *Slowly expanding lesions*

Approximately 15% to 30% of MS lesions are chronic active lesions, with even higher proportions observed in individuals with progressive forms of disease.[138–140] These lesions are characterized by a rim of iron-laden activated microglia/macrophages and a slow rate of peripheral ongoing demyelination and axonal loss.[141] Slowly expanding lesions (SELs) are lesions identified through longitudinal analysis of routinely acquired T1 and T2 sequences on clinical MRIs and are thought to capture a proportion of chronic active lesions.[140,142–144] Interestingly, SELs only partially overlap with PRLs, suggesting that similar mechanisms may underlie the formation of PRLs and the expansion of SELs, but that both imaging measures are not necessarily capturing the same lesions (**Fig. 3**).[145,146] Like PRLs, SELs have been explored as an imaging outcome measure of progressive disease biology/disease-monitoring. A study of PPMS patients from the ocrelizumab ORATORIO phase III trial retrospectively assessed the effect of ocrelizumab on SELs. Results showed that patients receiving ocrelizumab, compared with placebo, showed a lower proportion of total preexisting T2-hyperintense lesions identified as SELs, a lower T1-hypointense lesion volume increase in SELs and a significantly reduced decrease in normalized T1 signal intensity in SELs.[144] In addition, T1 lesion volume change in SELs was associated with clinical disability progression in ORATORIO. Another study exploring the effect of natalizumab and fingolimod in preventing SELs occurrence in RRMS patients over a 2-year follow-up period only found a limited impact of these drugs.[147] Results from phase II clinical trials of different BTK inhibitors have shown that SEL volume was lower at 48 weeks with higher doses of evobrutinib in comparison to the placebo/low dose (25 mg) arm.[148] With tolebrutinib, the median total SEL volume at 96 weeks was lowest in the 60 mg arm.[137] SELs will most likely be evaluated as exploratory endpoints of interest in the ongoing phase III BTK inhibitors clinical trials.[149] As with PRLs, consensus definitions, validation of MRI protocols to detect SELs, and larger longitudinal studies are necessary before this biomarker is ready for use in clinical practice.

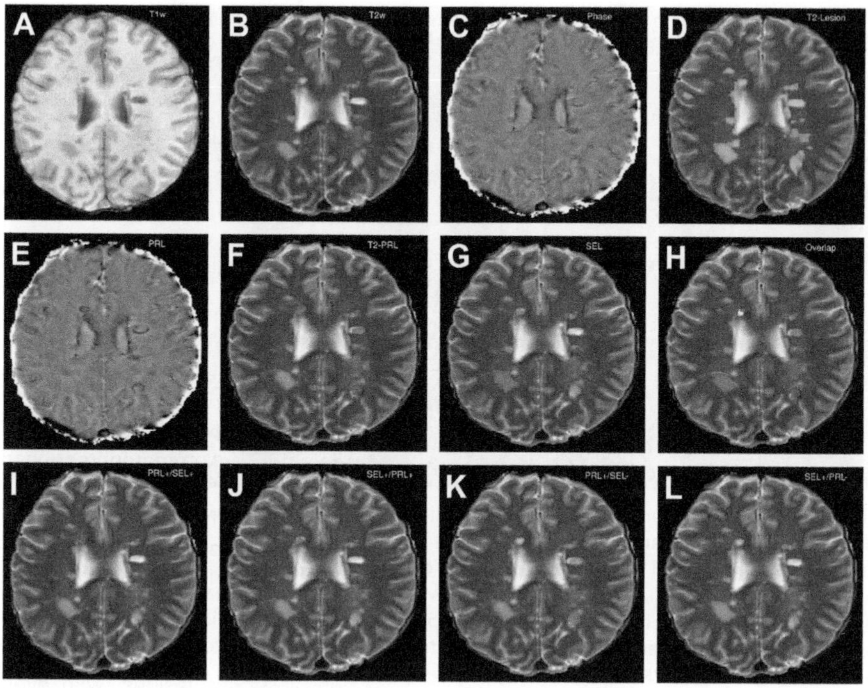


**Fig. 3.** Lesion overlap between slowly expanding and paramagnetic rim lesions. Example of the partial overlap between slowly expanding lesions (SELs) and paramagnetic rim lesions (PRLs) from a 72-week longitudinal MRI analysis of the opicinumab AFFINITY trial. (*A*) T1-weighted image. (*B*) T2-weighted image. (*C*) Filtered SWI-phase image. (*D*) T2-lesion mask. (*E*) PRLs at week 72. (*F*) T2-associated PRLs at week 72. (*G*) SELs detected between baseline and week 72. (*H*) Voxelwise overlap of T2-associated PRLs and SELs (Red = PRLs only, Blue = SELs only, Yellow = both). (*I*) Co-localized PRL+/SEL + mask (dark red). (*J*) Co-localized SEL+/PRL + mask (*dark blue*). (*K*) PRL+/SEL− lesions (light red). (*L*) SEL+/PRL− lesions (*light blue*). (*Data from* Elliot and colleagues.[146])

### *PET*

PET has also been used to study chronic active lesions by using radiotracers specific to microglia/macrophages.[150,151] A cross-sectional study using PET with radioligand binding to the 18 kDa translocator protein (TSPO) was conducted with the objective of characterizing more than 1500 distinct chronic lesions based on their microglial activation status in vivo. Using TSPO-PET, this study found that quantifying innate immune cell activation at the chronic lesion rim is possible, allowing for the classification of lesions into those with an active rim and those with an inactive rim.[152] TSPO-PET has also been recently found to detect in vivo meningeal inflammation in individuals with MS, which is thought to be a crucial mechanism in the pathogenesis of cortical demyelination in MS.[153]

Although these results are encouraging, caution should be exercised before PET can become available to monitor chronic active lesions or meningeal inflammation. The specificity of PET radioligands toward various therapeutic targets still warrants comprehensive validation, and there is a need to optimize and standardize PET acquisition procedures and analyses both cross-sectionally and longitudinally. In addition, the cost of necessary equipment and facilities is a great limiting factor to accessing

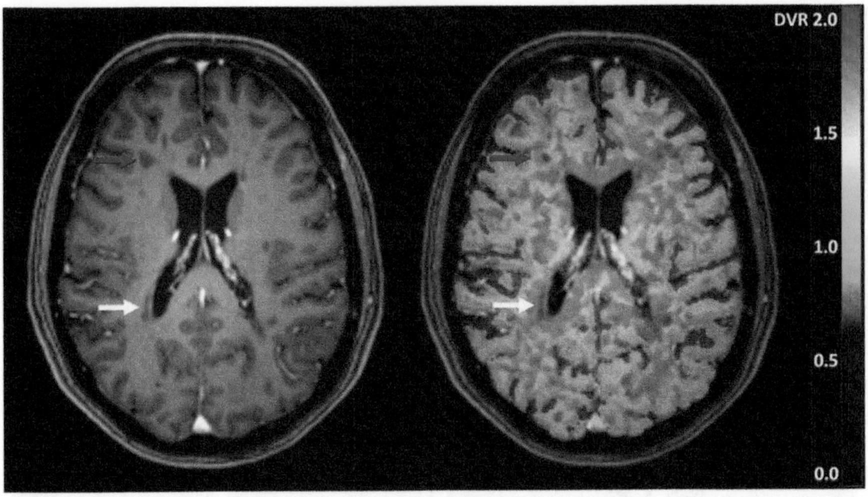


**Fig. 4.** PET for detection of chronic active lesions. On the left, an axial view of a conventional gadolinium-enhanced T1-weighted MRI is shown. On the right, the same MRI is overlaid with a parametric [$^{11}$C]PK11195 image (a common TSPO ligand). The binding intensity of this radioligand is visualized as distribution volume ratio (DVR) in each voxel and denoted by the color scale bar. Increased [$^{11}$C]PK11195 binding is observed in a chronic active T1-hypointense lesion reflecting microglial activation (red *arrows*). A chronic inactive lesion exhibits negligible [$^{11}$C]PK11195 binding (*white arrows*). (*Data from* Airas and colleagues, 2018.[151])

PET, and further research is required to assess the potential risks associated with serial PET imaging.[154]

A representative example of TSPO-PET use for detection of chronic active lesions in MS is provided in **Fig. 4**.

## SUMMARY

In this review, we present several emerging diagnostic, prognostic, and disease-monitoring biomarkers in MS with great promise. Among these, diagnostic biomarkers such as the CVS and PRLs and sNfL for disease-monitoring of relapsing biology seem to be farthest along in clinical development and have a high likelihood of becoming incorporated into clinical practice in the upcoming years. Although other biomarkers discussed have shown potential for clinical utility, they are at an earlier stage and still require further investigation and validation before they can reach clinical application. In addition, access to many of these new biomarkers is a substantial hurdle that may limit widespread use in clinical practice.

There is an urgent need to identify and validate biomarkers that can measure and predict disease progression as well as distinguish between acute axonal damage and relapse biology versus chronic smouldering inflammation and neurodegeneration typical of progressive disease biology. Fortunately, in the last few years, extraordinary developments have been made in investigating biomarkers that likely reflect the latter disease process, including radiological biomarkers such as PRLs, SELs, and PET imaging. Similarly, advances in molecular biomarkers such as GFAP are also encouraging. Ongoing collaborative studies will be important to validate or refute the utility of these emerging measures and offer a promising outlook and hope that many unmet needs will be addressed in the field, particularly with regard to effective treatments for progressive MS.

## AUTHOR CONTRIBUTIONS

All authors participated in the conceptualization and design of the study, performed data analysis, interpreted the results, drafted the manuscript, revised the manuscript critically for intellectual content, approved the final version to be published, and agreed to be accountable for all aspects of the work.

## CLINICS CARE POINTS

- The central vein sign (CVS) is emerging as a useful diagnostic biomarker of MS. The CVS is found in a high proportion of MS white matter lesions. The "40% rule" (ie, detecting ≥40% CVS-positive white matter lesions) has a positive and a negative predictive value of 100% for MS diagnosis but can be time-consuming to implement. The CVS may also be useful in those with established MS to help distinguish new white matter lesions due to MS versus other comorbidities.
- Paramagnetic rim lesions (PRLs) are found in all MS types and radiologically isolated syndrome, although they are more frequent in progressive disease. PRLs have high diagnostic specificity for MS (93%) but lower sensitivity (52%). PRLs have also shown promise as a biomarker in predicting future disability progression in early MS and may also be validated as tools to monitor disease worsening in MS.
- MRI measures of atrophy in the brain and spinal cord have shown to reliably predict future neurologic disability in the long term. However, limitations precluding widespread clinical use include lack of availability of technical requirements to obtain these measures, measurement variability related to technical and physiologic factors, definition of actionable clinical thresholds, and timing of studies. These issues still need to be addressed before these measures can be introduced into everyday clinical practice for MS prognostication.
- The use in clinical practice of neurofilament light chain (NfL) as a blood-based biomarker to predict short-term clinical and MRI outcomes as well as monitor relapsing MS disease activity and treatment response is likely to become widespread in the near future so long as centers can access the technology required to obtain this measure. Its role in progressive disease still remains unclear.
- Glial fibrillary acidic protein (GFAP) has been explored as a biomarker of prognostication and monitoring of disease progression in MS. Early studies suggest that serum GFAP may be particularly useful to predict progression independent of relapse activity, but further studies are required.
- Slowly expanding lesions (SELs) are identified through longitudinal analysis of routinely acquired T1 and T2-sequences and are thought to capture a proportion of chronic active lesions. SELs are being explored as an imaging outcome measure for progressive disease biology in several ongoing clinical trials.
- PET with radioligand binding to the 18 kDa translocator protein (TSPO) can detect innate immune cell activation within chronic active MS lesions, allowing classification of those with an active versus inactive rim. TSPO-PET may also detect in vivo meningeal inflammation, a mechanism linked to cortical demyelination in MS.

## DISCLOSURES

A. Chertcoff receives funding from the MS Society of Canada's endMS Postdoctoral Fellowship. Dr A. Chertcoff has also received support to attend a scientific meeting from Novartis. R. Schneider received research grants from the MS Society of Canada

(#901093), the JP Bickell Foundation, Canada, and the Barrow Neurological Foundation. Dr R. Schneider has received consulting fees from Novartis. Dr R. Schneider has received payment or honoraria for lectures, presentations, speaker's bureaus, manuscript writing or educational events from Biogen-Idec, Sanofi-Genzyme, EMD-Serono, and Roche. Dr R. Schneider has participated on advisory boards for Novartis. Dr R. Schneider has received support to attend a scientific meeting from EMD Serono. Dr C.J. Azevedo has received grant support from the National Multiple Sclerosis Society and National Institutes of Health, consulting fees from Horizon Therapeutics, Genentech, Sanofi Genzyme, TG Therapeutics, EMD Serono, and honoraria for participating in CME activities from Efficient LLC, Spire Learning, and Catamount Medical Education. Dr N. Sicotte has received research funding from the National Institutes of Health, United States (U01NS116776) and the National MS Society, Canada and the Patient-Centered Outcomes Research Institute (PCORI). Dr Oh has received research support from Biogen Idec, Canada, Roche, Switzerland, and EMD Serono, Canada and consulting fees from Biogen-Idec, BMS, Eli-Lilly, EMD-Serono, Novartis, Switzerland, Roche, and Sanofi-Genzyme.

## ACKNOWLEDGMENTS

Funding acknowledgment: Dr Jiwon Oh is supported by the Waugh Family Chair in MS Research and the Barford and Love MS Fund of the St Michael's Hospital Foundation.

## REFERENCES

1. Filippi M, Bar-Or A, Piehl F, et al. Multiple sclerosis [published correction appears in Nat Rev Dis Primers;4:49]. Nat Rev Dis Primers 2018;4:43.
2. Bebo B, Cintina I, LaRocca N, et al. The Economic Burden of Multiple Sclerosis in the United States: Estimate of Direct and Indirect Costs. Neurology 2022;98:e1810–7.
3. Multiple Sclerosis International Federation. Atlas of MS 2020. Accessed May 09, 2023. https://www.atlasofms.org/map/united-kingdom/epidemiology/number-of-people-with-ms.
4. World Health Organization; International Programme on Chemical Safety. Biomarkers in risk assessment: Validity and validation. Geneva, Switzerland: World Health Organization; 2001.
5. BDW Group. Biomarkers and surrogate endpoints: Preferred definitions and conceptual framework. Clin Pharmacol Ther 2001;69:89–95.
6. Califf RM. Biomarker definitions and their applications. Exp Biol Med (Maywood) 2018;243:213–21.
7. Yang J, Hamade M, Wu Q, et al. Current and Future Biomarkers in Multiple Sclerosis. Int J Mol Sci 2022;23:5877.
8. Thompson AJ, Banwell BL, Barkhof F, et al. Diagnosis of multiple sclerosis: 2017 revisions of the McDonald criteria. Lancet Neurol 2018;17:162–73.
9. Arrambide G, Tintore M. CSF examination still has value in the diagnosis of MS - Commentary. Mult Scler 2016;22(8):997–8.
10. Solomon AJ, Naismith RT, Cross AH. Misdiagnosis of multiple sclerosis: Impact of the 2017 McDonald criteria on clinical practice. Neurology 2019;92:26–33.
11. Kaisey M, Solomon AJ, Luu M, et al. Incidence of multiple sclerosis misdiagnosis in referrals to two academic centers. Mult Scler Relat Disord 2019;30:51–6.
12. La Rosa F, Wynen M, Al-Louzi O, et al. Cortical lesions, central vein sign, and paramagnetic rim lesions in multiple sclerosis: Emerging machine learning techniques and future avenues. Neuroimage Clin 2022;36:103205.

13. Charcot JM. Histologie de la Sclérose en Plaques. Paris: Imprimerie L. Pupart-Davyl; 1869.
14. Absinta M, Sati P, Reich DS. Advanced MRI and staging of multiple sclerosis lesions. Nat Rev Neurol 2016;12:358–68.
15. Maggi P, Absinta M, Grammatico M, et al. Central vein sign differentiates Multiple Sclerosis from central nervous system inflammatory vasculopathies. Ann Neurol 2018;83:283–94.
16. Kilsdonk ID, Lopez-Soriano A, Kuijer JP, et al. Morphological features of MS lesions on FLAIR* at 7 T and their relation to patient characteristics. J Neurol 2014; 261:1356–64.
17. Kuchling J, Ramien C, Bozin I, et al. Identical lesion morphology in primary progressive and relapsing-remitting MS–an ultrahigh field MRI study. Mult Scler 2014;20:1866–71.
18. Suh CH, Kim SJ, Jung SC, et al. The "Central Vein Sign" on T2*-weighted Images as a Diagnostic Tool in Multiple Sclerosis: A Systematic Review and Meta-analysis using Individual Patient Data. Sci Rep 2019;9:18188.
19. Tallantyre EC, Brookes MJ, Dixon JE, et al. Demonstrating the perivascular distribution of MS lesions in vivo with 7-Tesla MRI. Neurology 2008;70:2076–8.
20. Sati P, Oh J, Constable RT, et al. The central vein sign and its clinical evaluation for the diagnosis of multiple sclerosis: a consensus statement from the North American Imaging in Multiple Sclerosis Cooperative. Nat Rev Neurol 2016;12: 714–22.
21. Tallantyre EC, Dixon JE, Donaldson I, et al. Ultra-high-field imaging distinguishes MS lesions from asymptomatic white matter lesions. Neurology 2011; 76:534–9.
22. Mistry N, Dixon J, Tallantyre E, et al. Central veins in brain lesions visualized with high-field magnetic resonance imaging: a pathologically specific diagnostic biomarker for inflammatory demyelination in the brain. JAMA Neurol 2013;70: 623–8.
23. Mistry N, Abdel-Fahim R, Samaraweera A, et al. Imaging central veins in brain lesions with 3-T T2*-weighted magnetic resonance imaging differentiates multiple sclerosis from microangiopathic brain lesions. Mult Scler 2016;22:1289–96.
24. Solomon AJ, Watts R, Ontaneda D, et al. Diagnostic performance of central vein sign for multiple sclerosis with a simplified three-lesion algorithm. Mult Scler J. 2018;24:750–7.
25. Ontaneda D, Sati P, Raza P, et al. Central vein sign: A diagnostic biomarker in multiple sclerosis (CAVS-MS) study protocol for a prospective multicenter trial. Neuroimage Clin 2021;32:102834.
26. Absinta M, Sati P, Schindler M, et al. Persistent 7-tesla phase rim predicts poor outcome in new multiple sclerosis patient lesions. J Clin Invest 2016;126: 2597–609.
27. Dal-Bianco A, Grabner G, Kronnerwetter C, et al. Slow expansion of multiple sclerosis iron rim lesions: pathology and 7 T magnetic resonance imaging. Acta Neuropathol 2017;133:25–42.
28. Haacke EM, Makki M, Ge Y, et al. Characterizing iron deposition in multiple sclerosis lesions using susceptibility weighted imaging. J Magn Reson Imaging 2009;29:537–44.
29. Absinta M, Sati P, Fechner A, et al. Identification of Chronic Active Multiple Sclerosis Lesions on 3T MRI. AJNR Am J Neuroradiol 2018;39:1233–8.
30. Suthiphosuwan S, Sati P, Absinta M, et al. Paramagnetic Rim Sign in Radiologically Isolated Syndrome. JAMA Neurol 2020;77:653–5.

31. Calvi A, Haider L, Prados F, et al. In vivo imaging of chronic active lesions in multiple sclerosis. Mult Scler 2022;28:683–90.
32. Maggi P, Sati P, Nair G, et al. Paramagnetic Rim Lesions are Specific to Multiple Sclerosis: An International Multicenter 3T MRI Study. Ann Neurol 2020;88: 1034–42.
33. Kolb H, Al-Louzi O, Beck ES, et al. From pathology to MRI and back: Clinically relevant biomarkers of multiple sclerosis lesions. Neuroimage Clin 2022;36: 103194.
34. Hemond CC, Reich DS, Dundamadappa SK. Paramagnetic rim lesions in multiple sclerosis: comparison of visualization at 1.5-T and 3-T MRI. AJR Am J Roentgenol 2022;219:120–31.
35. Sartori A, Abdoli M, Freedman MS. Can we predict benign multiple sclerosis? Results of a 20-year long-term follow-up study. J Neurol 2017;264:1068–75.
36. Tintore M, Rovira À, Río J, et al. Defining high, medium and low impact prognostic factors for developing multiple sclerosis. Brain 2015;138:1863–74.
37. Bergamaschi R. Prognostic factors in multiple sclerosis. Int Rev Neurobiol 2007; 79:423–47.
38. Rovira À, Wattjes MP, Tintoré M, et al. Evidence-based guidelines: MAGNIMS consensus guidelines on the use of MRI in multiple sclerosis-clinical implementation in the diagnostic process [published correction appears in Nat Rev Neurol. 2015;11:483. Nat Rev Neurol 2015;11:471–82.
39. Zivadinov R, Leist TP. Clinical-magnetic resonance imaging correlations in multiple sclerosis. J Neuroimaging 2005;15:10S–21S.
40. Fisniku LK, Brex PA, Altmann DR, et al. Disability and T2 MRI lesions: A 20-year follow-up of patients with relapse onset of multiple sclerosis. Brain 2008;131: 808–17.
41. Azevedo CJ, Cen SY, Jaberzadeh A, et al. Contribution of normal aging to brain atrophy in MS. Neurol Neuroimmunol Neuroinflamm 2019;6:e616.
42. De Stefano N, Airas L, Grigoriadis N, et al. Clinical relevance of brain volume measures in multiple sclerosis. CNS Drugs 2014;28:147–56.
43. Shiee N, Bazin PL, Zackowski KM, et al. Revisiting brain atrophy and its relationship to disability in multiple sclerosis. PLoS One 2012;7:e37049.
44. Vollmer T, Signorovitch J, Huynh L, et al. The natural history of brain volume loss among patients with multiple sclerosis: a systematic literature review and meta-analysis. J Neurol Sci 2015;357:8–18.
45. Popescu V, Agosta F, Hulst HE, et al. Brain atrophy and lesion load predict long term disability in multiple sclerosis. J Neurol Neurosurg Psychiatry 2013;84: 1082–91.
46. Rudick RA, Fisher E, Lee JC, et al. Use of the brain parenchymal fraction to measure whole brain atrophy in relapsing-remitting MS. Multiple Sclerosis Collaborative Research Group. Neurology 1999;53:1698–704.
47. Zivadinov R, Uher T, Hagemeier J, et al. A serial 10-year follow-up study of brain atrophy and disability progression in RRMS patients. Mult Scler 2016;22: 1709–18.
48. Samann PG, Knop M, Golgor E, et al. Brain volume and diffusion markers as predictors of disability and short-term disease evolution in multiple sclerosis. AJNR Am J Neuroradiol 2012;33:1356–62.
49. Fragoso YD, Wille PR, Abreu M, et al. Correlation of clinical findings and brain volume data in multiple sclerosis. J Clin Neurosci 2017;44:155–7.

50. Azevedo CJ, Cen SY, Khadka S, et al. Thalamic atrophy in multiple sclerosis: A magnetic resonance imaging marker of neurodegeneration throughout disease. Ann Neurol 2018;83:223–34.
51. Schoonheim MM, Pinter D, Prouskas SE, et al. Disability in multiple sclerosis is related to thalamic connectivity and cortical network atrophy. Mult Scler 2022; 28:61–70.
52. Rocca MA, Mesaros S, Pagani E, et al. Thalamic damage and long-term progression of disability in multiple sclerosis. Radiology 2010;257:463–9.
53. Hänninen K, Viitala M, Paavilainen T, et al. Thalamic Atrophy Predicts 5-Year Disability Progression in Multiple Sclerosis. Front Neurol 2020;11:606.
54. Eijlers AJC, van Geest Q, Dekker I, et al. Predicting cognitive decline in multiple sclerosis: a 5-year follow-up study. Brain 2018;141:2605–18.
55. Gass A, Rocca MA, Agosta F, et al. MRI monitoring of pathological changes in the spinal cord in patients with multiple sclerosis. Lancet Neurol 2015;14: 443–54.
56. Lukas C, Knol DL, Sombekke MH, et al. Cervical spinal cord volume loss is related to clinical disability progression in multiple sclerosis. J Neurol Neurosurg Psychiatry 2015;86:410–8.
57. Ciccarelli O, Cohen JA, Reingold SC, et al. Spinal cord involvement in multiple sclerosis and neuromyelitis optica spectrum disorders. Lancet Neurol 2019;18: 185–97.
58. Oh J, Zackowski K, Chen M, et al. Multiparametric MRI correlates of sensorimotor function in the spinal cord in multiple sclerosis. Mult Scler 2013;19: 427–35.
59. Oh J, Saidha S, Chen M, et al. Spinal cord quantitative MRI discriminates between disability levels in multiple sclerosis. Neurology 2013;80:540–7.
60. Bischof A, Papinutto N, Keshavan A, et al. Spinal Cord Atrophy Predicts Progressive Disease in Relapsing Multiple Sclerosis. Ann Neurol 2022;91(2): 268–81.
61. Zeydan B, Gu X, Atkinson EJ, et al. Cervical spinal cord atrophy: an early marker of progressive MS onset. Neurol Neuroimmunol Neuroinflamm 2018;5:e435.
62. Rocca MA, Valsasina P, Meani A, et al. Clinically relevant cranio-caudal patterns of cervical cord atrophy evolution in MS. Neurology 2019;93:e1852–66.
63. Casserly C, Seyman EE, Alcaide-Leon P, et al. Spinal Cord Atrophy in Multiple Sclerosis: A Systematic Review and Meta-Analysis. J Neuroimaging 2018;28: 556–86.
64. Oh J, Chen M, Cybulsky K, et al. Five-year longitudinal changes in quantitative spinal cord MRI in multiple sclerosis. Mult Scler 2021;27:549–58.
65. Tsagkas C, Magon S, Gaetano L, et al. Spinal cord volume loss: A marker of disease progression in multiple sclerosis. Neurology 2018;91(4):e349–58.
66. Schlaeger R, Papinutto N, Panara V, et al. Spinal cord gray matter atrophy correlates with multiple sclerosis disability. Ann Neurol 2014;76:568–80.
67. Schlaeger R, Papinutto N, Zhu AH, et al. Association between thoracic spinal cord gray matter atrophy and disability in multiple sclerosis. JAMA Neurol 2015;72(8):897–904.
68. Sastre-Garriga J, Pareto D, Battaglini M, et al. MAGNIMS consensus recommendations on the use of brain and spinal cord atrophy measures in clinical practice. Nat Rev Neurol 2020;16:171–82.
69. Hemond CC, Baek J, Ionete C, et al. Paramagnetic rim lesions are associated with pathogenic CSF profiles and worse clinical status in multiple sclerosis: A retrospective cross-sectional study. Mult Scler 2022;28:2046–56.

70. Absinta M, Sati P, Masuzzo F, et al. Association of Chronic Active Multiple Sclerosis Lesions With Disability In Vivo [published correction appears in JAMA Neurol. 2019 Dec 1;76(12):1520]. JAMA Neurol 2019;76:1474–83.
71. Blindenbacher N, Brunner E, Asseyer S, et al. Evaluation of the 'ring sign' and the 'core sign' as a magnetic resonance imaging marker of disease activity and progression in clinically isolated syndrome and early multiple sclerosis. Mult Scler J Exp Transl Clin 2020;6(1). 2055217320915480.
72. Oh J, Suthiphosuwan S, Sati P, et al. Cognitive impairment, the central vein sign, and paramagnetic rim lesions in RIS. Mult Scler 2021;27:2199–208.
73. Lim TR, Suthiphosuwan S, Espiritu A, Guenette M, Bharatha A, Sati P, Absinta M, Reich DS, Oh J. Paramagnetic rim lesions predict the development of clinical MS in radiologically isolated syndrome: preliminary results from a prospective cohort study. Oral presentation at: ECTRIMS 2022. October 2022; Amsterdam, The Netherlands. https://journals.sagepub.com/doi/full/10.1177/13524585221123685. Accessed May 05, 2023.
74. Manouchehrinia A, Stridh P, Khademi M, et al. Plasma neurofilament light levels are associated with risk of disability in multiple sclerosis. Neurology 2020;94:e2457–67.
75. Gauthier A, Viel S, Perret M, et al. Comparison of SimoaTM and EllaTM to assess serum neurofilament-light chain in multiple sclerosis. Ann Clin Transl Neurol 2021;8:1141–50.
76. Gaetani L, Blennow K, Calabresi P, et al. Neurofilament light chain as a biomarker in neurological disorders. J Neurol Neurosurg Psychiatry 2019;90:870–81.
77. Bridel C, van Wieringen WN, Zetterberg H, et al. Diagnostic Value of Cerebrospinal Fluid Neurofilament Light Protein in Neurology: A Systematic Review and Meta-analysis. JAMA Neurol 2019;76:1035–48.
78. Gao W, Zhang Z, Lv X, et al. Neurofilament light chain level in traumatic brain injury: A system review and meta-analysis. Medicine (Baltim) 2020;99:e22363.
79. Ciardullo S, Muraca E, Bianconi E, et al. Diabetes Mellitus is Associated With Higher Serum Neurofilament Light Chain Levels in the General US Population. J Clin Endocrinol Metab 2023;108:361–7.
80. Thebault S, Booth RA, Rush CA, et al. Serum Neurofilament Light Chain Measurement in MS: Hurdles to Clinical Translation. Front Neurosci 2021;15:654942.
81. Sotirchos ES, Fitzgerald KC, Singh CM, et al. Associations of sNfL with clinico-radiological measures in a large MS population. Ann Clin Transl Neurol 2023;10:84–97.
82. Bittner S, Oh J, Havrdová EK, et al. The potential of serum neurofilament as biomarker for multiple sclerosis. Brain 2021;144:2954–63.
83. Kuhle J, Barro C, Disanto G, et al. Serum neurofilament light chain in early relapsing remitting MS is increased and correlates with CSF levels and with MRI measures of disease severity. Mult Scler 2016;22:1550–9.
84. Magliozzi R, Howell OW, Nicholas R, et al. Inflammatory intrathecal profiles and cortical damage in multiple sclerosis. Ann Neurol 2018;83:739–55.
85. Barro C, Benkert P, Disanto G, et al. Serum neurofilament as a predictor of disease worsening and brain and spinal cord atrophy in multiple sclerosis. Brain 2018;141:2382–91.
86. van der Vuurst de Vries RM, Wong YYM, Mescheriakova JY, et al. High neurofilament levels are associated with clinically definite multiple sclerosis in children and adults with clinically isolated syndrome. Mult Scler 2019;25:958–67.

87. Rival M, Thouvenot E, Du Trieu de Terdonck L, et al. Neurofilament Light Chain Levels Are Predictive of Clinical Conversion in Radiologically Isolated Syndrome. Neurol Neuroimmunol Neuroinflamm 2022;10:e200044.
88. Dalla Costa G, Martinelli V, Sangalli F, et al. Prognostic value of serum neurofilaments in patients with clinically isolated syndromes. Neurology 2019;92:e733–41.
89. Bjornevik K, Munger KL, Cortese M, et al. Serum Neurofilament Light Chain Levels in Patients With Presymptomatic Multiple Sclerosis. JAMA Neurol 2020; 77:58–64.
90. Chitnis T, Gonzalez C, Healy BC, et al. Neurofilament light chain serum levels correlate with 10-year MRI outcomes in multiple sclerosis. Ann Clin Transl Neurol 2018;5:1478–91.
91. Siller N, Kuhle J, Muthuraman M, et al. Serum neurofilament light chain is a biomarker of acute and chronic neuronal damage in early multiple sclerosis. Mult Scler 2019;25:678–86.
92. Cantó E, Barro C, Zhao C, et al. Association Between Serum Neurofilament Light Chain Levels and Long-term Disease Course Among Patients With Multiple Sclerosis Followed up for 12 Years. JAMA Neurol 2019;76:1359–66.
93. Jakimovski D, Kuhle J, Ramanathan M, et al. Serum neurofilament light chain levels associations with gray matter pathology: a 5-year longitudinal study. Ann Clin Transl Neurol 2019;6:1757–70.
94. Bhan A, Jacobsen C, Myhr KM, et al. Neurofilaments and 10-year follow-up in multiple sclerosis. Mult Scler 2018;24:1301–7.
95. Sellebjerg F, Royen L, Soelberg Sorensen P, et al. Prognostic value of cerebrospinal fluid neurofilament light chain and chitinase-3-like-1 in newly diagnosed patients with multiple sclerosis. Mult Scler 2019;25:1444–51.
96. Khalil M, Pirpamer L, Hofer E, et al. Serum neurofilament light levels in normal aging and their association with morphologic brain changes. Nat Commun 2020;11:812.
97. Khalil M, Teunissen CE, Otto M, et al. Neurofilaments as biomarkers in neurological disorders. Nat Rev Neurol 2018;14:577–89.
98. Benkert P, Meier S, Schaedelin S, et al. Serum neurofilament light chain for individual prognostication of disease activity in people with multiple sclerosis: a retrospective modelling and validation study. Lancet Neurol 2022;21:246–57.
99. Watanabe M, Nakamura Y, Michalak Z, et al. Serum GFAP and neurofilament light as biomarkers of disease activity and disability in NMOSD. Neurology 2019;93:e1299–311.
100. Aktas O, Smith MA, Rees WA, et al. Serum glial fibrillary acidic protein: a neuromyelitis optica spectrum disorder biomarker. Ann Neurol 2021;89:895–910.
101. Sofroniew MV, Vinters HV. Astrocytes: biology and pathology. Acta Neuropathol 2010;119:7–35.
102. Petzold A. Markers for different glial cell responses in multiple sclerosis: clinical and pathological correlations. Brain 2002;125:1462–73.
103. Hol EM, Pekny M. Glial fibrillary acidic protein (GFAP) and the astrocyte intermediate filament system in diseases of the central nervous system. Curr Opin Cell Biol 2015;32:121–30.
104. Bélanger M, Magistretti PJ. The role of astroglia in neuroprotection. Dialogues Clin Neurosci 2009;11:281–95.
105. Yang Z, Wang KK. Glial fibrillary acidic protein: from intermediate filament assembly and gliosis to neurobiomarker. Trends Neurosci 2015;38:364–74.
106. Abdelhak A, Foschi M, Abu-Rumeileh S, et al. Blood GFAP as an emerging biomarker in brain and spinal cord disorders. Nat Rev Neurol 2022;18:158–72.

107. Abdelhak A, Hottenrott T, Morenas-Rodríguez E, et al. Glial activation markers in CSF and serum from patients with primary progressive multiple sclerosis: potential of serum GFAP as disease severity marker? Front Neurol 2019;10:280.
108. Liddelow SA, Guttenplan KA, Clarke LE, et al. Neurotoxic reactive astrocytes are induced by activated microglia. Nature 2017;541:481–7.
109. Ayrignac X, Le Bars E, Duflos C, et al. Serum GFAP in multiple sclerosis: correlation with disease type and MRI markers of disease severity. Sci Rep 2020;10: 10923.
110. Abdelhak A, Huss A, Kassubek J, et al. Serum GFAP as a biomarker for disease severity in multiple sclerosis. Sci Rep 2018;8:14798.
111. Barro C, Healy BC, Liu Y, et al. Serum GFAP and NfL Levels Differentiate Subsequent Progression and Disease Activity in Patients With Progressive Multiple Sclerosis. Neurol Neuroimmunol Neuroinflamm 2022;10:e200052.
112. Meier S, Willemse EAJ, Schaedelin S, et al. Serum Glial Fibrillary Acidic Protein Compared With Neurofilament Light Chain as a Biomarker for Disease Progression in Multiple Sclerosis. JAMA Neurol 2023;80:287–97.
113. Schneider R, Brand-Arzamendi K, Lim TR, Lee LE, Guenette M, Suthiphosuwan S, Bharatha A, Oh J. Plasma glial fibrillary acidic protein levels correlate with unfavourable imaging measures in people with Radiologically Isolated Syndrome. Oral presentation at: ECTRIMS 2022. October 2022; Amsterdam, The Netherlands. https://journals.sagepub.com/doi/full/10.1177/13524585221123685. Accessed May 05, 2023.
114. Högel H, Rissanen E, Barro C, et al. Serum glial fibrillary acidic protein correlates with multiple sclerosis disease severity. Mult Scler 2020;26:210–9.
115. Vågberg M, Norgren N, Dring A, et al. Levels and Age Dependency of Neurofilament Light and Glial Fibrillary Acidic Protein in Healthy Individuals and Their Relation to the Brain Parenchymal Fraction. PLoS One 2015;10:e0135886.
116. Yalachkov Y, Schäfer JH, Jakob J, et al. Effect of Estimated Blood Volume and Body Mass Index on GFAP and NfL Levels in the Serum and CSF of Patients With Multiple Sclerosis. Neurol Neuroimmunol Neuroinflamm 2022;10:e200045.
117. Wattjes MP, Ciccarelli O, Reich DS, et al. 2021 MAGNIMS-CMSC-NAIMS consensus recommendations on the use of MRI in patients with multiple sclerosis. Lancet Neurol 2021;20:653–70.
118. Sormani MP, Bruzzi P. MRI lesions as a surrogate for relapses in multiple sclerosis: a meta-analysis of randomised trials. Lancet Neurol 2013;12:669–76.
119. Filippi M, Preziosa P, Copetti M, et al. Gray matter damage predicts the accumulation of disability 13 years later in MS. Neurology 2013;81:1759–67.
120. Rocca MA, Battaglini M, Benedict RH, et al. Brain MRI atrophy quantification in MS: From methods to clinical application. Neurology 2017;88:403–13.
121. Sormani MP, Arnold DL, De Stefano N. Treatment effect on brain atrophy correlates with treatment effect on disability in multiple sclerosis. Ann Neurol 2014; 75:43–9.
122. Giovannoni G, Turner B, Gnanapavan S, et al. Is it time to target no evident disease activity (NEDA) in multiple sclerosis? Mult Scler Relat Disord 2015;4: 329–33.
123. Seewann A, Vrenken H, van der Valk P, et al. Diffusely abnormal white matter in chronic multiple sclerosis: imaging and histopathologic analysis. Arch Neurol 2009;66:601–9.
124. Ontaneda D, Raza PC, Mahajan KR, et al. Deep grey matter injury in multiple sclerosis: a NAIMS consensus statement. Brain 2021;144:1974–84.

125. Burman J, Zetterberg H, Fransson M, et al. Assessing tissue damage in multiple sclerosis: a biomarker approach. Acta Neurol Scand 2014;130:81–9.
126. Al-Louzi O, Letchuman V, Manukyan S, et al. Central Vein Sign Profile of Newly Developing Lesions in Multiple Sclerosis: A 3-Year Longitudinal Study. Neurol Neuroimmunol Neuroinflamm 2022;9:e1120.
127. Quanterix granted breakthrough device designation from U.S. FDA for NFL test for multiple sclerosis. Quanterix. https://www.quanterix.com/press-releases/quanterix-granted-breakthrough-device-designation-from-us-fda-for-nfl-test-for-multiple-sclerosis/. Published August 16, 2022. Accessed April 26, 2023.
128. Novakova L, Zetterberg H, Sundstrom P, et al. Monitoring disease activity in multiple sclerosis using serum neurofilament light protein. Neurology 2017;89: 2230–7.
129. Bittner S, Steffen F, Uphaus T, et al, KKNMS Consortium. Clinical implications of serum neurofilament in newly diagnosed MS patients: A longitudinal multicentre cohort study. EBioMedicine 2020;56:102807.
130. Sejbaek T, Nielsen HH, Penner N, et al. Dimethyl fumarate decreases neurofilament light chain in CSF and blood of treatment naive relapsing MS patients. J Neurol Neurosurg Psychiatry 2019;90:1324–30.
131. Kuhle J, Kropshofer H, Haering DA, et al. Blood neurofilament light chain as a biomarker of MS disease activity and treatment response. Neurology 2019;92: e1007–15.
132. Kuhle J, Daizadeh N, Benkert P, et al. Sustained reduction of serum neurofilament light chain over 7 years by alemtuzumab in early relapsing–remitting MS. Mult Scler J 2022;28:573573–82.
133. Hauser SL, Bar-Or A, Cohen JA, et al. Ofatumumab versus Teriflunomide in Multiple Sclerosis. N Engl J Med 2020;383:546–57.
134. Zhang S, Nguyen TD, Hurtado Rúa SM, et al. Quantitative susceptibility mapping of time-dependent susceptibility changes in multiple sclerosis lesions. AJNR Am. J. Neuroradiol. 2019;40:987–93.
135. Absinta M, Maric D, Gharagozloo M, et al. A lymphocyte-microglia-astrocyte axis in chronic active multiple sclerosis. Nature 2021;597:709–14.
136. Dal-Bianco A, Grabner G, Kronnerwetter C, et al. Long-term evolution of multiple sclerosis iron rim lesions in 7 T MRI. Brain 2021;144:833–47.
137. Reich DS, Arnold DL, Vermersch P, et al. Safety and efficacy of tolebrutinib, an oral brain-penetrant BTK inhibitor, in relapsing multiple sclerosis: a phase 2b, randomised, double-blind, placebo-controlled trial. Lancet Neurol 2021;20: 729–38.
138. Luchetti S, Fransen NL, van Eden CG, et al. Progressive multiple sclerosis patients show substantial lesion activity that correlates with clinical disease severity and sex: A retrospective autopsy cohort analysis. Acta Neuropathol 2018;135:511–28.
139. Frischer JM, Weigand SD, Guo Y, et al. Clinical and pathological insights into the dynamic nature of the white matter multiple sclerosis plaque. Ann Neurol 2015; 78:710–21.
140. Elliott C, Wolinsky JS, Hauser SL, et al. Slowly expanding/evolving lesions as a magnetic resonance imaging marker of chronic active multiple sclerosis lesions. Mult Scler 2019;25:1915–25.
141. Bagnato F, Hametner S, Yao B, et al. Tracking iron in multiple sclerosis: A combined imaging and histopathological study at 7 tesla. Brain 2011;134:3602–15.

142. Calvi A, Tur C, Chard D, et al. Slowly expanding lesions relate to persisting black-holes and clinical outcomes in relapse-onset multiple sclerosis. Neuroimage Clin 2022;35:103048.
143. Arnold DL, Belachew S, Gafson AR, et al. Slowly expanding lesions are a marker of progressive MS - No. Mult Scler 2021;27:1681–3.
144. Elliott C, Belachew S, Wolinsky JS, et al. Chronic white matter lesion activity predicts clinical progression in primary progressive multiple sclerosis. Brain 2019; 142:2787–99.
145. Calvi A, Carrasco FP, Tur C, et al. Association of slowly expanding lesions on MRI with disability in people with secondary progressive multiple sclerosis. Neurology 2022;98:e1783–93.
146. Elliott C, Rudko DA, Arnold DL, et al. Lesion-level correspondence and longitudinal properties of paramagnetic rim and slowly expanding lesions in multiple sclerosis. Mult Scler 2023;29(6):680–90.
147. Preziosa P, Pagani E, Moiola L, et al. Occurrence and microstructural features of slowly expanding lesions on fingolimod or natalizumab treatment in multiple sclerosis. Mult Scler 2020;27(10):1520–32.
148. Arnold D, Elliott C, Montalban X, et al. Effects of Evobrutinib, a Bruton's Tyrosine Kinase Inhibitor, on Slowly Expanding Lesions: An Emerging Imaging Marker of Chronic Tissue Loss in Multiple Sclerosis (S14.009). Neurology 2022;98:2674.
149. Schneider R, Oh J. Bruton's Tyrosine Kinase Inhibition in Multiple Sclerosis. Curr Neurol Neurosci Rep 2022;22:721–34.
150. Hogel H, Rissanen E, Vuorimaa A, et al. Positron emission tomography imaging in evaluation of MS pathology in vivo. Mult Scler 2018;24:1399–412.
151. Airas L, Nylund M, Rissanen E. Evaluation of Microglial Activation in Multiple Sclerosis Patients Using Positron Emission Tomography. Front Neurol 2018; 9:181.
152. Nylund M, Sucksdorff M, Matilainen M, et al. Phenotyping of multiple sclerosis lesions according to innate immune cell activation using 18 kDa translocator protein-PET. Brain Commun 2021;4:fcab301.
153. Mainero C, Kinkel R, et al. In Vivo And Ex Vivo Characterization Of Meningeal Translocator Protein Expression In Multiple Sclerosis. Poster presentation at: American Academy of Neurology Annual Meeting. April 2023; Boston, MA, United States of America. Available at: https://www.aan.com/MSA/Public/Events/AbstractDetails/52958. Accessed April 26, 2023.
154. Preziosa P, Filippi M, Rocca MA. Chronic active lesions: a new MRI biomarker to monitor treatment effect in multiple sclerosis? Expert Rev Neurother 2021;21: 837–41.

# Pathophysiology, Diagnosis, Treatment and Emerging Neurotherapeutic Targets for Progressive Multiple Sclerosis

## The Age of PIRA

Alise K. Carlson, MD, Robert J. Fox, MD*

**KEYWORDS**

- Multiple sclerosis • Progressive multiple sclerosis • Progression
- Primary progressive multiple sclerosis • Secondary progressive multiple sclerosis

**KEY POINTS**

- Progression of disability is present across all phenotypes of multiple sclerosis from early in the disease process and can be due to either incomplete recovery from clinical relapses or insidious worsening of neurologic function independent of relapses, seen at higher frequencies in patients with progressive multiple sclerosis compared to relapsing-remitting multiple sclerosis.
- Currently, monitoring of disease progression is based entirely on clinical measures as there are no imaging or fluid biomarkers that accurately correlate with progression. Biomarkers to detect the transition from relapsing-remitting multiple sclerosis to secondary progressive multiple sclerosis, and to quantify disease in both primary progressive and secondary progressive multiple sclerosis are needed.
- Effective treatments to slow the relentless course of progressive multiple sclerosis remain elusive. Candidate therapies should target worsening of neuropathological processes, reversing damage, and restoring function.
- Collaborative efforts are likely to accelerate the work needed to better address the unmet needs of this patient population and drive the field forward.

## INTRODUCTION

Multiple sclerosis (MS) is an immune-mediated disorder of the central nervous system (CNS) characterized by chronic inflammation and neurodegeneration, impacting approximately 2.8 million individuals across the globe.[1] Disease state is determined by assessments of disease activity (clinical relapses or imaging activity) and progression (disability worsening/progression independent of relapse activity–known as

Cleveland Clinic Mellen Center, 9500 Euclid Avenue U10, Cleveland, OH 44195, USA
* Corresponding author.
*E-mail address:* foxr@ccf.org

Neurol Clin 42 (2024) 39–54
https://doi.org/10.1016/j.ncl.2023.07.002 

PIRA–over a period of time).[2] Although it is understood that MS is characterized by both inflammation and neurodegeneration from the time of disease onset, the pathological mechanisms underlying the complex relationships leading to clinical evolution remain unclear.

Progressive MS is characterized by a gradually progressive decline in neurologic function, of which two main forms are recognized. In primary progressive multiple sclerosis (PPMS), disease-related disability progresses from the time of symptom onset, and this is diagnosed in approximately 15% of all individuals diagnosed with MS.[3] In secondary progressive multiple sclerosis (SPMS) disease-related disability follows an initial relapsing-remitting (RRMS) course. This form was previously estimated to impact between 50 and 90% of individuals within 25 years of an initial diagnosis of RRMS,[4,5] though this number seems to have decreased in recent years with the development of more effective treatments for RRMS. In combination, progressive forms of MS (PMS) affect more than one million individuals worldwide.[6] Individuals with PPMS tend to be older at the age of diagnosis, and the female predominance seen in RRMS is less apparent.[7] Because progression is insidious over time and clinical relapses are uncommon, diagnosis of PMS can be more challenging than diagnosis of relapsing forms of MS, often delaying diagnosis and treatment.

## PATHOPHYSIOLOGY

Historically, MS subtypes were described as pathologically distinct diseases. However, in recent years increased understanding of underlying pathological mechanisms has shifted this paradigm towards viewing these subtypes as a spectrum of a single disease, where differences are more related to the proportion of features present.

Focal infiltrative inflammation, driven by autoreactive T and B lymphocytes, is common early in the disease and leads to focal areas of demyelination which later form astrocytic scars with variable axon loss and remyelination.[8] When this involves eloquent pathways, clinical relapses may be evident. Neurodegeneration is seen early in the disease course but becomes increasingly common over time. This process appears to be driven by complex relationships between many pathologies including compartmentalized inflammation, iron toxicity, oxidative stress, and mitochondrial dysfunction.[9] It is unknown whether these processes occur dependently or independently of each other and how they differ between individuals.

Other characteristics of progressive MS include slowly expanding lesions (SELs), meningeal inflammation, cortical demyelination, neuronal loss, whole-brain atrophy, diffuse neuroaxonal and myelin injury, disruption of the blood-brain barrier, and deficient remyelination. All these characteristics are more common in progressive MS compared to RRMS.[9] In contrast to acute inflammatory lesions which are common in RRMS, SELs are characterized by a microglial rim, often with iron deposition outside of microglia, and little macrophage recruitment or anti-inflammatory markers.[8] Chronic active lesions are distinct from SELs and are characterized by active migration of leukocytes into brain parenchyma surrounding an inactive core. See **Fig. 1** for examples.

Meningeal inflammation, which was initially thought to be a pathophysiologic feature specific to PMS, occurs in cortical lesions of patients with RRMS to a milder degree.[9] Meningeal aggregates of leukocytes contribute to cortical demyelination and are more prominent in PMS than RRMS.[8]

Neuroaxonal injury and loss are prominent in PMS and may occur independently from demyelination.[9] The presence of pro-inflammatory microglial activation

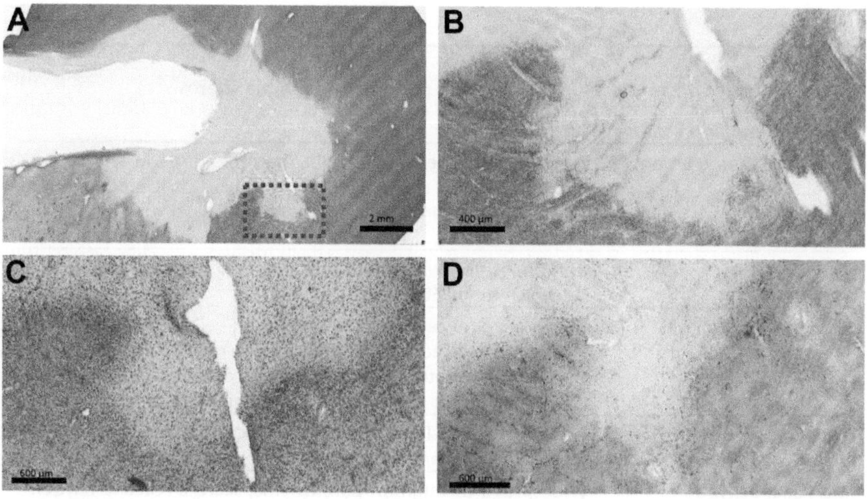

**Fig. 1.** Microscopic lesion pathology in multiple sclerosis. (*A, left upper*) and (*B, right upper*). Proteolipid protein staining for myelin demonstrating a demyelinated chronic active lesion in the periventricular region at low and high field, respectively. (*C, left lower*). MHCII staining for activated microglia/macrophages in the same lesion. (*D, right lower*). Total iron staining (modified Turnbull method) showing increased iron accumulation at the lesion border. MHCII, major histocompatibility complex II. (Methods described in: Mahajan KR, Amin M, Poturalski M, et. al. Juxtacortical susceptibility changes in progressive multifocal leukoencephalopathy at the gray-white matter junction correlates with iron-enriched macrophages. *Mult Scler.* 2021 Dec;27(14):2159-2169. Images courtesy of Kedar Mahajan, MD PhD.)

increases with age and disease duration.[8] Lymphocytes tend to be widely dispersed throughout the CNS parenchyma in PMS, whereas lymphocytes are more often seen aggregated around blood vessels in RRMS.[9] These aggregates show features of tertiary lymph follicles and contain high levels of B lymphocytes.[8] Neuropathological features are summarized in **Table 1**.

Although many potential mechanisms driving progressive MS have been proposed, the true pathophysiology driving insidious disability progression remains unknown. A better understanding of these mechanisms will allow for more accurate identification of therapeutic targets and the development of successful therapies.

## DIAGNOSIS AND TREATMENT

### *Diagnostic approach*

The diagnosis of progressive MS–both PPMS and SPMS–can be challenging. PPMS is diagnosed in individuals with at least 12 months of disability progression in the absence of clinical relapse(s) and at least two of the following three criteria: (1) $\geq$ 1 T2 hyperintense lesions characteristic of MS in $\geq$ 1 region of the brain (periventricular, cortical/juxtacortical, infratentorial); (2) $\geq$ 2 T2 hyperintense lesions in the spinal cord; or (3) presence of cerebrospinal fluid-specific oligoclonal bands.[10] SMPS is diagnosed in individuals with RRMS who have progressive disability worsening in the absence of clinical relapses over 6-12 months (or longer).[11] Importantly, both PPMS and SPMS require the exclusion of alternative conditions that could cause progressive disability worsening, and both are based upon retrospective clinical assessment (history and/or exam).[12,13] See **Fig. 2**.

### *Imaging approach*

Magnetic resonance imaging (MRI) is highly sensitive in detecting the dissemination of white matter lesions in space and time and plays a central role in the diagnosis and

**Table 1**
**Neuropathological features of brain lesions in progressive multiple sclerosis[9]**

| Neuropathological Feature | Description |
|---|---|
| Slowly expanding lesions (SELs) | Typically composed of microglia/macrophages and associated with microglial rims and/or myelin debris; associated with slow radial expansion; more abundant and larger in PMS than in RRMS |
| Microglial rims | Iron deposition within and outside of microglia; often surrounding SELs |
| Leukocyte aggregates | Consisting of B cells, plasma cells, and T cells, located in the meninges or deep sulci; supply soluble mediators of injury that result in neurotoxicity; contribute to cortical and subpial demyelination; more abundant in PMS than RRMS |
| Pre-active lesions | Accumulation of leukocytes in perivascular space (prior to entering the parenchyma); less abundant in PMS than in RRMS |
| Microglial activation | Widespread throughout parenchyma; secrete reactive oxygen species (ROS) and reactive nitrogen species resulting in oxidative stress and direct cell injury; nodules or clusters of microglia may predate plaque formation; correlated with paranodal disruption; more abundant and larger in PMS than in RRMS |
| Active lesions | Leukocytes migrating out of perivascular cuffs; less abundant in PMS than in RRMS; often evolve into chronic active lesions |
| Activated T cells | CD4+ and CD8+ T lymphocytes dispersed throughout the parenchyma |
| Chronic active lesions | Pathologically distinct from SELs |
| Intracortical lesions | Active lesions located in the cortical gray matter |
| Nondescript lesions | Associated with diffuse axonal injury; may occur in many areas of the brain |
| Deficient remyelination | Areas of (typically incomplete/deficient) myelin repair within areas of previously damaged parenchyma; leaves axons deprived of nutrients/loss of trophic support for axon/increased exposure to inflammatory mediators and exposure to ROS; more abundant and larger in PMS than in RRMS |

monitoring of MS. Differentiating between progressive and relapsing forms of MS based on MRI features alone, however, is not yet possible. Similarly, there are no imaging characteristics which definitively differentiate PPMS and SPMS. In recent years, significant efforts have been made to identify and validate imaging features/markers associated with progressive forms of MS, with a specific focus on identifying features which may reflect pathophysiological mechanisms underlying neurodegeneration and may be used to predict disease evolution. These studies suggest that progressive MS probably starts very early during the relapsing phase of the disease.

MRI features more common in PPMS include diffuse signal abnormalities in the spinal cord, spinal cord lesions involving the gray matter and at least two white matter columns in the axial plane, and atrophy of the lower portion of the spinal cord.[14] In contrast, gray matter atrophy of the spinal cord is more common in SPMS than RRMS.[14] Gadolinium-enhancing lesions and spinal cord lesions increase the risk of progression in PPMS. In SPMS features including enhancing lesions, a higher number and volume of brain lesions, and disease activity over time increases the risk of disability progression.[14] In relapse-onset forms of MS, total lesion volume (gray matter

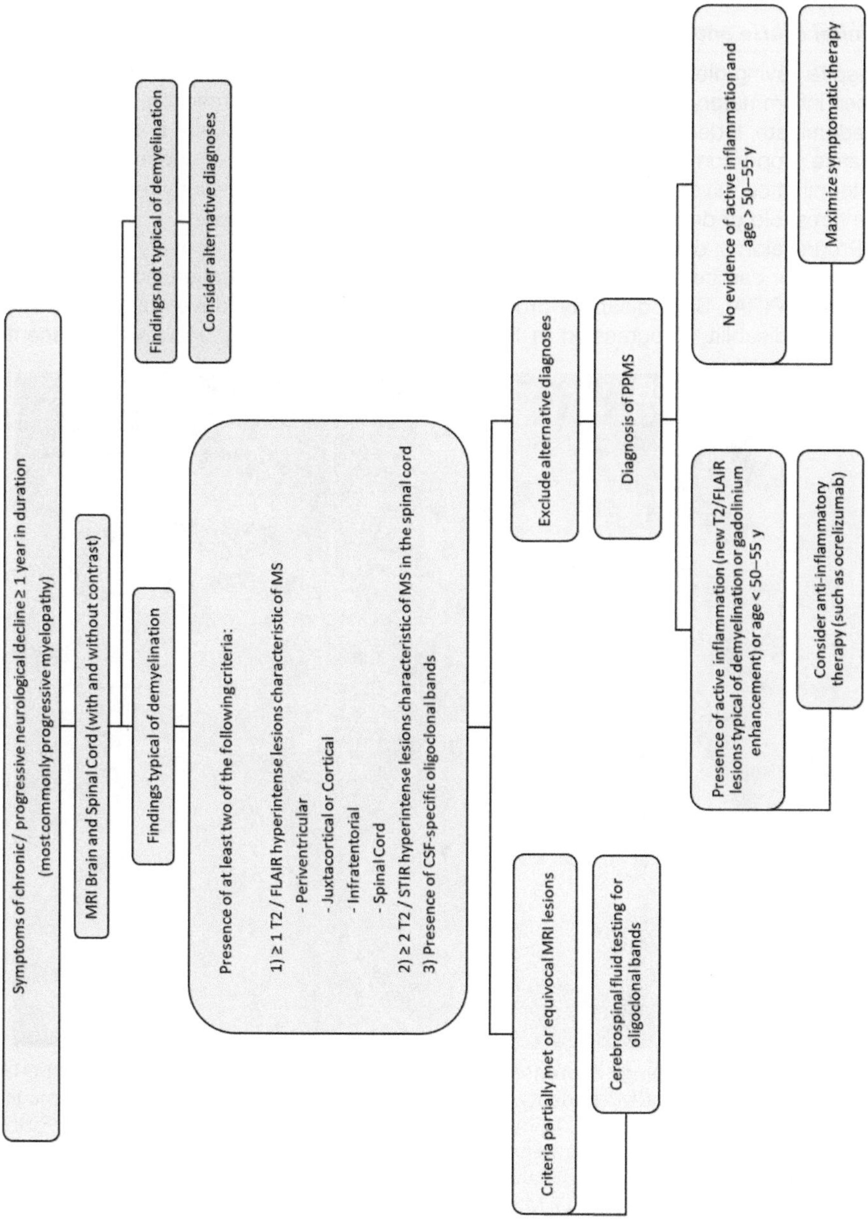


**Fig. 2.** Approach to diagnosis of primary progressive multiple sclerosis.

and cortical), increasing lesion volume, and rate of brain gray matter and deep gray matter atrophy are thought to be predictive of conversion to SPMS.[14] Features consistent with progressive pathology, including presence of paramagnetic rim lesions and SELs, may also be present (**Fig. 3**).

### *Clinical course and monitoring*

Despite having diagnostic criteria as a guide, it is often difficult to clinically determine when inflammatory mechanisms wane, and neurodegenerative mechanisms begin to predominate. Indeed, the two main mechanisms are likely coincident and shift only in relative proportion over time. Clinicians rely heavily on patient reports in making this determination, given the earliest signs and symptoms of progression are often below the threshold of detection with a routine neurological examination.

Progression of disability in MS can be either from incomplete recovery from clinical relapses or can be due to insidious worsening of neurologic function independent of relapses (PIRA). Slow disability progression in RRMS is often driven by the former, whereas disability progression in PMS is driven by the latter. However, a recent

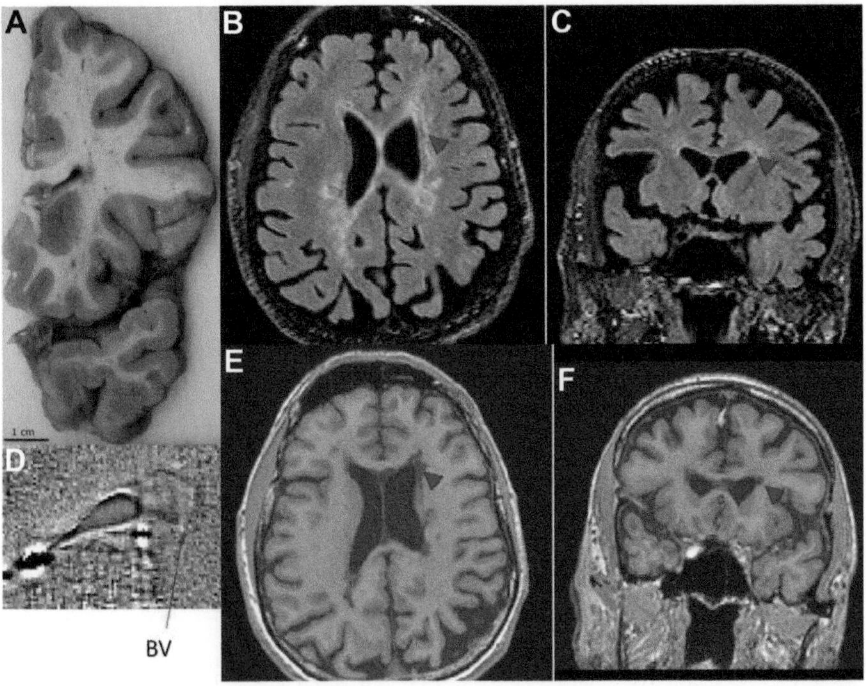


**Fig. 3.** MRI lesion pathology in progressive multiple sclerosis. (*A, left upper*) Hemispheric 1-cm fixed coronal slice of MS patient. (*B, center upper*). Post-mortem 3T axial FLAIR image demonstrating a periventricular T2-hyperintense lesion (*red arrow*). (*C, right upper*) Post-mortem 3T coronal FLAIR image demonstrating the same periventricular T2-hyperintense lesion (*red arrow*). (*D, left lower*). Paramagnetic rim and central vessel on SWI-phase imaging at lesion border, shown on 7T MRI following fixation of coronal tissue slice. (*E, center lower*). Post-mortem 3T axial T1 image demonstrating a T1 black hole, corresponding to lesion in B (red arrow). (*F, right lower*). Post-mortem 3T coronal T1 image demonstrating a T1 black hole, corresponding to lesion in C (*red arrow*). (*Adapted from* a case reported in: Mey GM, Mahajan KR, DeSilva TM. Neurodegeneration in multiple sclerosis. *WIREs Mech Dis.* 2023 Jan;15(1):e1583. Images courtesy of Kedar Mahajan, MD PhD.)

analysis of a large clinical dataset revealed that PIRA was seen across all phenotypes in adult patients with MS form early in the disease process, though at higher frequencies in patients with PMS compared to RRMS.[15]

Currently, monitoring of disease progression is based entirely on clinical measures since there are no imaging or fluid biomarkers that accurately correlate with progression. The traditional and most frequently utilized tool in both routine clinical care and clinical trials is the Expanded Disability Status Scale (EDSS).[16] Other measures used to monitor disability progression include the timed 25-foot walk (25FW), 9-hole peg test (9HPT), cognitive tool symbol digit modality test (SDMT), and low contrast visual acuity test (LC-VA), which together comprise the modern MS Functional Composite.[17] The MS performance Test (MSPT) is an iPad-based adaptation of the MS Functional Composite and consists of four modules that parallel the components of the MS Functional Composite: including a Walking Speed Test (WST), Manual Dexterity Test (MDT), Processing Speed Test (PST), and Contrast Sensitivity Test (CST).[18] Patient reported outcome measures (PROMs) such as the Patient Reported Outcomes Measurement Information System (PROMIS) and Quality of Life in Neurological Disorders (NEURO-QoL) are used to monitor patient perceptions of functional status and overall quality of life.[19,20] These measures may be used in combination with the tools mentioned above to detect gradual worsening beyond the clinical threshold of detection. Of note, there are no established cut-offs to determine clinical worsening based on the measures/tools mentioned above. See **Table 2** for commonly accepted definitions of clinical worsening.

Biomarkers to detect the transition from RRMS to SPMS and to quantify disease in both PPMS and SPMS remain elusive and continue to be a primary area of research focus. Serum neurofilament light chain (sNfL), a structural protein comprising up to 85% of CNS cytoskeleton proteins,[21] has been extensively evaluated as a biomarker in MS. sNfL is strongly associated with recent neuroaxonal injury driven by inflammation,[22] and anti-inflammatory disease-modifying therapies reduce sNfL in relapsing MS.[23,24] However, recent studies have demonstrated that sNfL does not provide additional prognostic value beyond a marker of focal inflammation, and at times provides misleading results where disability progression occurred in the context of decreasing sNfL levels and vice versa.[25–27] Post-hoc analysis of sNfL levels in the SPRINT-MS[28] trial and MS-STAT[29] trial showed no association of sNfL levels with treatment–even though each trial showed that treatment slows the progression of brain atrophy. Additional biomarkers such as glial fibrillary acid protein (GFAP) are currently under study.

### *Treatment approach*

Despite significant progress in the development of treatments for RRMS, the armamentarium of treatments directed toward pathophysiologic mechanisms underlying

**Table 2**
**Definitions of clinical worsening for disability monitoring tools**

| Clinical Measure/Tool | Definition of Clinical Worsening |
|---|---|
| Expanded Disability Status Scale (EDSS) | Worsening of 1 point from baseline score of 5.5 or less, and worsening of 0.5 points from baseline score of 5.5 or greater[16] |
| Low Contrast Visual Acuity Test (LC-VA) | 7-point change[52] |
| Timed 25-Foot Walk (WST) | 20% worsening[53] |
| 9-Hole Peg Test (9HPT) | 20% worsening[54] |
| Symbol Digit Modality test (SDMT) | 4-point change[55] |
| MS performance Test (MSPT) | 20% worsening[18] |

MS progression remains limited.[30] Therapies effective in RRMS often fail to yield similar results in PMS, likely because their primary therapeutic effect is by decreasing focal inflammation.

To date, there have been only two approved disease-modifying therapies (DMTs) for the treatment of PPMS; mitoxantrone and ocrelizumab, whereas over 18 unique DMTs are available to treat relapsing forms of MS. Due to its unfavorable side effect profile, mitoxantrone has limited use in modern practice. Furthermore, mitoxantrone likely doesn't impact the true pathophysiology of progressive MS, and therefore will not be discussed in detail herein.

Evaluation of rituximab compared to placebo did not demonstrate improvement in time to confirmed disability progression, though subgroup analyses suggested that younger patients with greater degrees of inflammation may benefit.[31] Ocrelizumab was shown to have benefit on sustained disability progression compared to placebo over 120 weeks in a cohort of 732 patients with PPMS in the ORATORIO trial.[23,32] However, further analysis of this trial found that this benefit was attenuated in older patients and in patients without active inflammation at the beginning of the trial (absence of gadolinium-enhancing MRI lesions).[23,33] Research evaluating the treatment effect on older, more disabled patients with PPMS is ongoing (ORATORIO-hand trial).

Other DMTs have been investigated for the treatment of PPMS, though none have been proven to be effective. The PROMISE trial, a study of 943 patients evaluating glatiramer acetate compared to placebo, demonstrated no benefit in slowing of disability progression over 3 years.[34] The treatment effect of fingolimod compared to placebo on sustained disability progression was evaluated in 823 PPMS patients (INFORMS trial) and did not demonstrate benefit over 3 years on disability progression.[35]

Several DMTs were also studied in SPMS. Siponimod was evaluated in the EXPAND trial, which demonstrated benefit in a cohort of 1651 individuals compared to placebo.[23] Importantly, the effect was attenuated in patients who were older, were more disabled, had less active inflammation, and had longer duration of disease (response appeared to be driven by patients who were younger, had relapses or gadolinium-enhancing lesions in the two years prior to the study, and had lower EDSS).[24] The ASCEND trial, evaluating the treatment effect of natalizumab on a composite measure of progression confirmed at six months compared to placebo in 889 patients, demonstrated no overall benefit.[26] However, a post-hoc subgroup analysis showed that benefit was seen with upper extremity function (based on 9HPT).[26]

Other therapies studied for use in PMS include MD1003 (a high-dose preparation of biotin) and masitinib. MD1003 was evaluated in a one-year trial evaluating sustained improvement in 154 patients and suggested a possible benefit: 12.6% of treatment patients had sustained improvement while none of the placebo group showed improvement.[36] A follow-up study in 642 patients with PMS over 20 months did not demonstrate a benefit of MD1003 on sustained disability improvement,[37] and thus this therapy has been abandoned in MS. A recent phase 2 study of masitinib demonstrated modest benefit on sustained EDSS improvement (using average EDSS across the patient cohort) compared to placebo,[38] with a confirmatory phase 3 trial currently underway.

### *Symptom management approach*

Due to the limited therapeutic repertoire, the main management of progressive MS has historically focused on symptom management and maximization of function.[39] Individuals with progressive MS can experience a multitude of symptoms which may negatively impact quality of life in multiple domains. Fatigue, cognitive impairment, mobility and upper extremity impairment, and pain are the most frequently reported (and often most debilitating) symptoms in this patient population, impacting up to 95% of individuals.[40] Population-based studies have demonstrated that patients with progressive forms of MS suffer from significantly higher socioeconomic burden, including direct and indirect health care costs, and quality of life compared to those with RRMS.[41,42]

A recent publication from the International Progressive MS Alliance invoked a coordinated call to action urging the prioritization of research focusing on effective symptom management and rehabilitation strategies for individuals with progressive forms of MS.[40] Several pharmacologic therapies have been tried or are currently under investigation for symptom management and rehabilitation in PMS, including amantadine, dronabinol, modafinil, nabiximols, amantadine, dalfampridine, mitoquinone, estriol, ACTH, mixed-amphetamine salts, carbidopa, and intranasal insulin.[6] Rehabilitation strategies including functional electrical stimulation, use of robotics, transcranial stimulation, behavioral activation, and exercise/yoga are non-pharmaceutical approaches under investigation.[6]

## EMERGING THERAPEUTIC TARGETS

Comprehensive therapies which are successful in the prevention of disability worsening, reversal of damage, and the restoration of function remain a major unmet need in progressive MS.[43] Multiple PMS treatments are in clinical development, aiming to target the pathophysiological features present at the progressive stage of disease. Goals of these treatments include addressing compartmentalized immune mechanisms, neuroprotection, and myelin repair, which may be accomplished through successful drug entry to the CNS (ability to cross the blood–brain barrier), ablation of free radical stress and mitochondrial injury (antioxidant effects), neutralization of compartmentalized lymphocytes (either via antagonism or depletion within the CNS), promotion of remyelination to locally protect axons, inhibition of microglial reactivity, and exertion of direct neuroprotective effects on axons and neurons.[9]

Newer therapeutic candidates include Bruton's tyrosine kinase (BTK) inhibitors, ibudilast, alpha lipoic acid (ALA), bile acids, and erythropoietin. Various stem cell therapies (hematopoietic stem cell transplant, adipose stem cells, human neural stem cells, autologous mesenchymal stromal cells, mesenchymal stem cells, and tolerogenic dendritic cells) are also under investigation. Re-purposing of established therapeutic agents and add-on therapeutics for use in the treatment of PMS have also been evaluated and include simvastatin, niacin, metformin, and hydroxychloroquine.[9] See **Table 3** for a summary of ongoing phase 3 clinical trials in progressive MS.

### *Bruton's Tyrosine Kinase Inhibitors*

BTK inhibitors, including fenebrutinib and tolebrutinib, are currently being evaluated in phase 3 progressive MS clinical trials. Additional BTK inhibitor trials are also ongoing in relapsing MS. These therapies portend benefit by regulating the development of B cells and activation of T cells, alleviating oxidative stress in immune cells, and mediating the activity of stimulated microglia and their production of pro-inflammatory cytokines.[9] Due to their unique mechanism of action with respect to B cells (inhibition of B cell function without depletion), this class of therapies may have a more favorable risk profile compared to other currently available high efficacy therapies, to which phase 3 trial data will provide further insight.

### *Ibudilast*

Ibudilast, a phosphodiesterase and macrophage inhibitory factor (MIF) inhibitor, blocks pro-inflammatory cytokine production and neuronal damage by activated microglia, as well as the infiltration of peripheral T and B lymphocytes into the

**Table 3**
**Phase 3 clinical trials for the treatment of progressive multiple sclerosis**

| Trial Name | Study Therapy | Comparator | MS Phenotype | Target Enrollment | Age | EDSS | Primary Outcome |
|---|---|---|---|---|---|---|---|
| O'HAND | Ocrelizumab | Placebo | PPMS | 1000 | 18–65 yrs | 3.0–8.0 | 12 wk confirmed 20% increase 9HPT |
| ChariotMS | Cladribine | Placebo | "Advanced" MS | 200 | ≥18 yrs | 6.5–8.5 | Change in 9HPT speed; % with stable 9HPT |
| FENtrepid | Fenebrutinib | Ocrelizumab | PPMS | 946 | 18–65 yrs | 3–6.5 | Confirmed composite disability progression |
| PERSEUS | Tolebrutinib | Placebo | PPMS | 990 | 18–55 yrs | 2.0–6.5 | 6m confirmed EDSS progression |
| HERCULES | Tolebrutinib | Placebo | SPMS | 1290 | 18–60 yrs | 3.0–6.0 | 6m confirmed EDSS progression |
| | Masitinib | Placebo | PPMS, non-active SPMS | 800 | 18–65 yrs | 3.0–6.0 | Confirmed EDSS progression |
| MS-STAT-2 | Simvastatin | Placebo | SPMS | 964 | 25–65 yrs | 4.0–6.5 | 6m confirmed EDSS progression |

CNS.[9] In a phase 2 trial evaluating ibudilast in PMS (SPRINT-MS), whole brain atrophy was reduced by 48% compared to placebo over 96 weeks, along with benefits on magnetization transfer ratio (MTR) and cortical atrophy.[44] However, there was no significant effect on new or enlarging lesions.[45] Post hoc analysis found that the treatment effect was driven primarily by the PPMS cohort, possibly due to faster rates of atrophy progression in the PPMS placebo group.[46] Despite these promising results, no further trials of ibudilast in progressive MS are ongoing.

### *Alpha Lipoic Acid*

ALA is a potent antioxidant which exerts its biological effect by chelating iron and scavenging reactive oxygen species (ROS) and reactive nitrogen species, as well as by reducing the transmigration of leukocytes into the CNS, reducing the aggregation of lymphocytes, and inhibiting microglial activation.[9] A 2-year single-center trial evaluating the use of ALA versus placebo in SPMS patients showed a slowing in the progression of brain atrophy.[47] A phase 2 trial of a larger PMS cohort is ongoing.

### *Statins*

Simvastatin and lovastatin (lipophilic statins) have been shown to induce a shift in T-cell differentiation to an anti-inflammatory state, inhibit microglial activation and secretion of ROS, inhibit pro-oxidative NADPH oxidase, protect against glutamate excitotoxicity, improve the survival and proliferation of oligodendrocyte precursor cells, and improve remyelination in mouse models of MS.[9] The MS-STAT trial, a phase 2 trial evaluating simvastatin in SPMS, showed a reduction in annualized brain atrophy and EDSS scores compared to placebo.[27] A phase 3 trial of simvastatin is currently underway.

### *Hydroxychloroquine*

Hydroxychloroquine has an extensive track record of use in other immunological conditions including rheumatoid arthritis and systemic lupus erythematosus. This antimalarial therapy exerts is therapeutic effect by inhibiting microglial and B-cell activity.[9] Non-futility was demonstrated for use in PPMS in a phase 2 trial[48] with a Simon 2-stage approach, which generates estimates based on proportions of patients expected to experience worsening over a pre-specified time period. Unlike traditional phase 2 trials, which use a biomarker to identify potentially promising therapies, the Simon 2-stage approach only identifies those that are futile and should be abandoned. Thus, there is greater uncertainty carrying a therapy that passed through Simon 2-stage trial testing into phase 3 trials.

## DISCUSSION

To date, studies evaluating DMT efficacy have focused primarily on patients with relapsing forms of disease. Despite recent advancements in the treatment of relapsing forms of MS, effective therapies targeting progressive neuropathology remain a significant unmet need. Available therapies are effective in targeting focal inflammation, and therefore clinical relapses and relapse-associated worsening (including when sometimes seen in progressive MS), but do not address the concomitant neurodegenerative processes which drive PIRA. Although features unique to progressive neuropathology have been identified, much remains unknown, and effective targets for both remyelination and direct neuronal protection are needed. Further elucidation of these pathological mechanisms will likely reveal novel therapeutic targets for the treatment of PMS. Importantly, the pathologies of progressive MS are likely present during the earlier, relapsing phase of MS, and thus the potential applicability of treatments targeting progression may be quite broad.

Trials investigating neuroprotective agents may benefit from being used in combination with concomitant anti-inflammatory therapies which target focal inflammation. This approach was used recently in the SPRINT-MS,[44] SYNERGY,[49] AFFINITY,[50] and alpha lipoic acid trials.[51] The same outcome measures used to assess disease progression in RRMS may not be sufficient in PMS. Furthermore, trials must be powered to detect differences in outcomes to a degree sufficient to support approval by regulatory agencies. The ideal outcome measure remains to be established. Trials utilizing composite outcome measures, such as the INFORMS trial, have higher percentages of participants reaching the primary endpoints compared to trials with a single-scale outcome.[34] Therefore, it seems logical that composite outcomes (combining clinical tools such as the T25FW, 9HPT, SDMT, LC-VA, or MSPT with EDSS) may facilitate more efficient clinical trials in which a greater number of participants meet (and thus contribute to) the primary endpoint. Additionally, it remains unclear as to whether outcome measures should focus primarily on slowing disability progression or on improvement.

Collaborative efforts are likely to accelerate this process. The International Progressive MS Alliance is an example of such a collaborative effort, comprised of global MS organizations, researchers, health care professionals, pharmaceutical industry, companies, foundations, donors, and people affected by progressive MS, working together to address the unmet needs of people with progressive MS. Together, the group aims to better address study design, define sensitive and responsive outcomes, and develop effective therapies for people with PMS. This type of approach is likely to better address the unmet needs of this patient population and drive the field forward.

## SUMMARY

Progressive forms of MS affect more than one million individuals worldwide. Improved understanding of mechanisms underlying MS progression, identification and validation of biomarkers, identification of novel therapeutic targets, and improved trial design are needed to further propel progress in the management of individuals with progressive forms of MS. Effective therapies targeting progressive mechanisms in MS remains a significant unmet need, though there are several encouraging potential therapeutics on the horizon. The future of progressive MS is indeed bright.

## CLINICS CARE POINTS

- PPMS may be diagnosed in individuals with at least 12 months of disability progression in the absence of clinical relapse(s) in the presence of at least two of the following three criteria: (1) $\geq$ 1 T2 hyperintense lesions characteristic of MS in $\geq$ 1 region of the brain (periventricular, cortical/juxtacortical, infratentorial); (2) $\geq$ 2 T2 hyperintense lesions in the spinal cord; or (3) presence of cerebrospinal fluid-specific oligoclonal bands.
- SMPS may be diagnosed in individuals retrospectively based on the assessment of progressive disability worsening in the absence of clinical relapses over the course of 6-12 months (or longer).
- Current MS disease-modifying therapies predominantly work on focal, infiltrative inflammation that is typical of relapsing MS and has little impact (if any) on the underlying mechanisms of progressive MS.
- Individuals with progressive MS experience a multitude of symptoms which may negatively impact quality of life in multiple domains, of which fatigue, cognitive impairment, mobility and upper extremity impairment, and pain are the most frequently reported.

## DISCLOSURE

A.K. Carlson: Dr Carlson has received fellowship funding (Grant 16696-P-FEL) from Biogen and institutional clinical training award (ICT-1805-31154) from National MS Society. R.J. Fox: Dr Fox has received personal consulting fees from AB Science, Biogen, Celgene, EMD Serono, Genentech, Genzyme, Greenwich Biosciences, Immunic, Janssen, Novartis, Sanofi, Siemens, and TG Therapeutics, has served on advisory committees for AB Science, Biogen, Genzyme, Immunic, Janssen, Novartis, Sanofi, and TG Therapeutics, and has received clinical trial contract and research grant funding from Biogen, United States, Novartis, Switzerland, and Sanofi, Paris, France.

## REFERENCES


1. Walton C, King R, Rechtman L, et al. Rising prevalence of multiple sclerosis worldwide: Insights from the Atlas of MS, third edition. Mult Scler 2020;26(14): 1816–21.
2. Lublin FD, Coetzee T, Cohen JA, et al. International Advisory Committee on Clinical Trials in MS. The 2013 clinical course descriptors for multiple sclerosis: a clarification. Neurology 2020;94(24):1088–92, published correction appears in Neurology. 2022 Feb 1;98(5):215.
3. McGinley MP, Goldschmidt CH, Rae-Grant AD. Diagnosis and treatment of multiple sclerosis: a review. JAMA 2021;325:765–79.
4. Barzegar M, Najdaghi S, Afshari-Safavi A, et al. Early predictors of conversion to secondary progressive multiple sclerosis. Mult Scler Relat Disord 2021;54: 103115.
5. Scalfari A, Neuhaus A, Degenhardt A, et al. The natural history of multiple sclerosis: a geographically based study 10: relapses and long-term disability. Brain 2010;133(Pt 7):1914–29.
6. Thompson AJ, Carroll W, Ciccarelli O, et al. Charting a global research strategy for progressive MS-An international progressive MS Alliance proposal. Mult Scler 2022;28(1):16–28.
7. Miller DH, Leary SM. Primary-progressive multiple sclerosis. Lancet Neurol 2007; 6(10):903–12, published correction appears in Lancet Neurol. 2009 Aug;8(8):699.
8. Lassmann H. Targets of therapy in progressive MS. Mult Scler 2017;23(12): 1593–9.
9. Yong HYF, Yong VW. Mechanism-based criteria to improve therapeutic outcomes in progressive multiple sclerosis. Nat Rev Neurol 2022;18(1):40–55.
10. Thompson AJ, Banwell BL, Barkhof F, et al. Diagnosis of multiple sclerosis: 2017 revisions of the McDonald criteria. Lancet Neurol 2018 Feb;17(2):162–73. Epub 2017 Dec 21.
11. Lorscheider J, Buzzard K, Jokubaitis V, et al, MSBase Study Group. Defining secondary progressive multiple sclerosis. Brain 2016;139(pt 9):2395–405.
12. Solomon A. J. Diagnosis, differential diagnosis, and misdiagnosis of multiple sclerosis. Continuum 2019;25(3):611–35.
13. Katz Sand I, Krieger S, Farrell C, et al. Diagnostic uncertainty during the transition to secondary progressive multiple sclerosis. Mult Scler 2014;20(12):1654–7.
14. Filippi M, Preziosa P, Barkhof F, et al. Diagnosis of progressive multiple sclerosis from the imaging perspective: a review. JAMA Neurol 2021;78(3):351–64.
15. Lublin FD, Häring DA, Ganjgahi H, et al. How patients with multiple sclerosis acquire disability. Brain 2022 Sep 14;145(9):3147–61.
16. Kurtzke JF. Rating neurologic impairment in multiple sclerosis: an expanded disability status scale (EDSS). Neurology 1983;33(11):1444–52.

17. Meyer-Moock S, Feng YS, Maeurer M, et al. Systematic literature review and validity evaluation of the Expanded Disability Status Scale (EDSS) and the Multiple Sclerosis Functional Composite (MSFC) in patients with multiple sclerosis. BMC Neurol 2014;14:58.
18. Rudick RA, Miller D, Bethoux F, et al. The Multiple Sclerosis Performance Test (MSPT): an iPad-based disability assessment tool. J Vis Exp 2014;88:e51318.
19. Cella D, Riley W, Stone A, et al. The patient-reported outcomes measurement information system (PROMIS) developed and tested its first wave of adult self-reported health outcome item banks: 2005-2008. J Clin Epidemiol 2010;63(11):1179–94.
20. Cella D, Lai JS, Nowinski CJ, et al. Neuro-QOL: Brief measures of health-related quality of life for clinical research in neurology. Neurology 2012;78(23):1860–7.
21. Khalil M, Teunissen CE, Otto M, et al. Neurofilaments as biomarkers in neurological disorders. Nat Rev Neurol 2018;14(10):577–89.
22. Williams T, Zetterberg H, Chataway J. Neurofilaments in progressive multiple sclerosis: a systematic review. J Neurol 2021;268:3212–22.
23. Montalban X, Hauser SL, Kappos L, et al. Ocrelizumab versus placebo in primary progressive multiple sclerosis. N Engl J Med 2017;376(3):209–20.
24. Kappos L, Bar-Or A, Cree BAC, et al. Siponimod versus placebo in secondary progressive multiple sclerosis (EXPAND): a double-blind, randomised, phase 3 study. Lancet 2018;391(10127):1263–73, published correction appears in Lancet. 2018 Nov 17;392(10160):2170.
25. Gafson AR, Jiang X, Shen C, et al. Serum neurofilament light and multiple sclerosis progression independent of acute inflammation. JAMA Netw Open 2022;5(2):e2147588.
26. Kapoor R, Ho PR, Campbell N, et al. Effect of natalizumab on disease progression in secondary progressive multiple sclerosis (ASCEND): a phase 3, randomised, double-blind, placebo-controlled trial with an open-label extension. Lancet Neurol 2018;17(5):405–15.
27. Chataway J, Schuerer N, Alsanousi A, et al. Effect of high-dose simvastatin on brain atrophy and disability in secondary progressive multiple sclerosis (MS-STAT): a randomised, placebo-controlled, phase 2 trial. Lancet 2014;383(9936):2213–21.
28. Fox RJ, Raska P, Barro C, et al. Neurofilament light chain in a phase 2 clinical trial of ibudilast in progressive multiple sclerosis. Mult Scler 2021;27(13):2014–22.
29. Williams TE, Holdsworth KP, Nicholas JM, et al. Assessing neurofilaments as biomarkers of neuroprotection in progressive multiple sclerosis. Neurol Neuroimmunol Neuroinflamm 2022;9:e1130.
30. Amin M, Hersh CM. Updates and advances in multiple sclerosis neurotherapeutics. Neurodegener Dis Manag 2023;13(1):47–70.
31. Hawker K, O'Connor P, Freedman MS, et al. Rituximab in patients with primary progressive multiple sclerosis: results of a randomized double-blind placebo-controlled multicenter trial. Ann Neurol 2009;66(4):460–71.
32. Fox EJ, Markowitz C, Applebee A, et al. Ocrelizumab reduces progression of upper extremity impairment in patients with primary progressive multiple sclerosis: findings from the phase III randomized ORATORIO trial. Mult Scler 2018;24(14):1862–70.
33. Wolinsky JS, Montalban X, Hauser SL, et al. Evaluation of no evidence of progression or active disease (NEPAD) in patients with primary progressive multiple sclerosis in the ORATORIO trial. Ann Neurol 2018;84(4):527–36.

34. Wolinsky JS, Narayana PA, O'Connor P, et al. Glatiramer acetate in primary progressive multiple sclerosis: results of a multinational, multicenter, double-blind, placebo-controlled trial. Ann Neurol 2007;61(1):14–24.
35. Lublin F, Miller DH, Freedman MS, et al. Oral fingolimod in primary progressive multiple sclerosis (INFORMS): a phase 3, randomised, double-blind, placebo-controlled trial. Lancet 2016;387(10023):1075–84, published correction appears in Lancet. 2017 Jan 21;389(10066):254.
36. Tourbah A, Lebrun-Frenay C, Edan G, et al. MD1003 (high-dose biotin) for the treatment of progressive multiple sclerosis: A randomised, double-blind, placebo-controlled study. Mult Scler 2016;22(13):1719–31.
37. Cree BAC, Cutter G, Wolinsky JS, et al. Safety and efficacy of MD1003 (high-dose biotin) in patients with progressive multiple sclerosis (SPI2): a randomised, double-blind, placebo-controlled, phase 3 trial. Lancet Neurol 2020;19(12):988–97.
38. Vermersch P, Brieva-Ruiz L, Fox RJ, et al. Efficacy and safety of masitinib in progressive forms of multiple sclerosis: a randomized, phase 3, clinical trial. Neurol Neuroimmunol Neuroinflamm 2022;9(3):e1148.
39. Feinstein A, Freeman J, Lo AC. Treatment of progressive multiple sclerosis: what works, what does not, and what is needed. Lancet Neurol 2015;14(2):194–207.
40. Zackowski KM, Freeman J, Brichetto G, et al. Prioritizing progressive MS rehabilitation research: a call from the international progressive MS alliance. Mult Scler 2021;27(7):989–1001.
41. Blinkenberg M, Kjellberg J, Ibsen R, et al. Increased socioeconomic burden in patients with primary progressive multiple sclerosis: a Danish nationwide population-based study. Mult Scler Relat Disord 2020;46:102567.
42. Purmonen T, Hakkarainen T, Tervomaa M, et al. Impact of multiple sclerosis phenotypes on burden of disease in Finland. J Med Econ 2020;23(2):156–65.
43. Ontaneda D, Thompson AJ, Fox RJ, et al. Progressive multiple sclerosis: prospects for disease therapy, repair, and restoration of function. Lancet 2017;389(10076):1357–66.
44. Fox RJ, Coffey CS, Conwit R, et al. Phase 2 trial of ibudilast in progressive multiple sclerosis. N Engl J Med 2018;379(9):846–55.
45. Naismith RT, Bermel RA, Coffey CS, et al. Effects of Ibudilast on MRI Measures in the Phase 2 SPRINT-MS Study. Neurology 2021;96(4):e491–500.
46. Goodman AD, Fedler JK, Yankey J, et al. Response to ibudilast treatment according to progressive multiple sclerosis disease phenotype. Ann Clin Transl Neurol 2021;8(1):111–8.
47. Spain R, Powers K, Murchison C, et al. Lipoic acid in secondary progressive MS: a randomized controlled pilot trial. Neurol Neuroimmunol Neuroinflamm 2017;4(5):e374.
48. Koch MW, Kaur S, Sage K, et al. Hydroxychloroquine for primary progressive multiple sclerosis. Ann Neurol 2021;90(6):940–8.
49. Cadavid D, Mellion M, Hupperts R, et al. Safety and efficacy of opicinumab in patients with relapsing multiple sclerosis (SYNERGY): a randomised, placebo-controlled, phase 2 trial. Lancet Neurol 2019;18:845–56.
50. Bing Z, Peter C, Gavin G, et al. Phase 2 AFFINITY trial evaluates opicinumab in a targeted population of patients with relapsing multiple sclerosis: rationale, design and baseline characteristics (P3.2-072). Neurology 2019;92(15 Supplement). P3.2-072.

51. VA Office of Research and Development. Lipoic Acid for the Treatment of Progressive Multiple Sclerosis. clinicaltrials.gov, 2023. Available at: https://clinicaltrials.gov/ct2/show/NCT03161028. (accessed April 6, 2023).
52. Balcer LJ, Raynowska J, Nolan R, et al. Validity of low-contrast letter acuity as a visual performance outcome measure for multiple sclerosis. Mult Scler 2017;23(5):734–47.
53. Motl RW, Cohen JA, Benedict R, et al. Validity of the timed 25-foot walk as an ambulatory performance outcome measure for multiple sclerosis. Mult Scler 2017;23(5):704–10.
54. Feys P, Lamers I, Francis G, et al. The nine-hole peg test as a manual dexterity performance measure for multiple sclerosis. Mult Scler 2017;23(5):711–20.
55. Benedict RH, DeLuca J, Phillips G, et al. Validity of the symbol digit modalities test as a cognition performance outcome measure for multiple sclerosis. Mult Scler 2017;23(5):721–33.

# Relationship Between Multiple Sclerosis, Gut Dysbiosis, and Inflammation

## Considerations for Treatment

Larissa Jank, MD, Pavan Bhargava, MD*

**KEYWORDS**

• Gut dysbiosis • Microbiome • Multiple sclerosis • Neuroinflammation
• Bacterial-derived metabolites • Gut-brain axis • Diet

**KEY POINTS**

- Multiple sclerosis is associated with gut dysbiosis.
- Gut dysbiosis promotes disease pathology by promoting local inflammation in the gut, as well as systemic immune activation and neuroinflammation.
- Beneficial effects of the microbiome can be harnessed in therapeutic interventions by normalizing the gut microbiome composition and promoting its immune regulatory function.
- There is a great need for randomized controlled clinical trials assessing the efficacy of these interventions in people with multiple sclerosis.

## INTRODUCTION

The gut microbiome is a mixture of bacteria, fungi, and viruses that inhabit the intestinal lumen. In healthy individuals the colonizing microbes and host mutually benefit each other. The host provides the microbes with nutrients and a stable environment. Commensals (1) supply essential nutrients through the catabolism of dietary substances, (2) protect the gut from infection by competing with pathobionts, and (3) help develop and maintain immune homeostasis by inducing tolerance. A disturbance of these functions due to the loss of a substantial amount of commensal microbes and reduction in diversity or pathobiont overpopulation is referred to as gut dysbiosis.

Multiple sclerosis (MS) is a chronic immune-mediated demyelinating disease characterized by demyelinating lesions in the central nervous system (CNS), accompanied by peripheral immune activation and compartmentalized CNS inflammation. The underlying causes of disease onset and progression are not fully understood but likely

Division of Neuroimmunology and Neurological Infections, Department of Neurology, Johns Hopkins University School of Medicine, 600 N. Wolfe Street, Meyer 6-144, Baltimore, MD 21287, USA
* Corresponding author.
*E-mail address:* pbharga2@jhmi.edu

Neurol Clin 42 (2024) 55–76
https://doi.org/10.1016/j.ncl.2023.07.005
neurologic.theclinics.com

include a multitude of environmental factors as well as genetic predisposition. These causes either directly lead to dysregulation of the immune system and inflammatory demyelination or indirectly contribute to disease by lowering the threshold for autoimmunity, neuroinflammation, and neurodegeneration.

The gut microbiome, as a key regulator of immune functions throughout life largely affected by environmental factors, has gained increasing attention in MS research. Indeed, many reports show pathologic changes in the gut microbiome composition and a compromised intestinal barrier function in people with MS (pwMS).

The causes of gut dysbiosis in MS are most likely individual-dependent and multifactorial. Possible contributors currently discussed in the literature include diet, immune status, disease-modifying therapies (DMTs), host genetic factors,[1] host age (in particular associations with puberty[2] and inflammaging/immunosenescence[3,4]), sex,[5] and environmental factors.[6]

This review examines the changes in the gut microbiome in pwMS, the relevance of gut dysbiosis, the mechanism through which this gut dysbiosis promotes inflammation, and how resolving gut dysbiosis or its consequences may be an avenue for treatment.

## CHARACTERIZATION OF GUT DYSBIOSIS IN PEOPLE WITH MULTIPLE SCLEROSIS

Physiologically approximately 90% of the human gut microbiota species belong to the phyla of Firmicutes and Bacteroidota.[7] Other species are from the phyla Actinobacteria, Proteobacteria, Fusobacteria, and Verrucomicrobia. Most studies characterize changes in the gut microbiome of pwMS by assessing changes in the fecal microbiota composition (for a meta-analysis of reported changes see[8]).

Genera consistently altered across several studies in pwMS compared with healthy controls include the following: (1) from the phylum Firmicutes (Clostridial clusters IV and XIVa),[9,10] *Roseburia*,[10–12] *Lachnospira*,[12–14] and *Faecalibacterium*[9,11,14,15]; (2) from the phylum Bacteroidota *Prevotella*[9,13,16–18] and *Parabacteroides*,[16,18,19] which were generally reduced in pwMS. In addition, generally increased in pwMS are (3) from the phylum Verrucomicrobia *Akkermansia*[10,13,17–20] and (4) from Firmicutes *Streptococcus*.[9,10,12,14] Interestingly, the only study using biopsies from the small intestine to assess the gut microbiome confirmed a decrease in *Prevotella* and an increase in *Streptococcus* in patients with higher disease activity compared with patients with no disease activity and healthy controls.[21] The diversity of microbes in the microbiome of individual samples, known as the alpha diversity, has also been investigated in pwMS. A few studies reported a reduced alpha diversity in pwMS,[11,22] but generally the current literature suggests that there is no significant difference in the microbial diversity of pwMS.

Overall, despite some concurring changes, there is a lack of consensus on altered microbe profiles associated with disease. Possible explanations for divergent results are (1) differences in the selection of bacteria through methodological differences in sample collection, processing, or analysis; (2) differences in control group selection (eg, household controls, monozygotic twins, or unrelated age-matched controls); and (3) different types of pathologic gut microbiome changes depending on study population demographics, location, disease subtype, and treatment.

Further, the variable results could also be an indication that changes in fecal microbiome composition may not be a sufficient readout to assess gut dysbiosis. Instead, parameters evaluating the functions of the microbiome, in particular metabolic functions, might show clearer differences. To this end, several recent studies have taken a combined approach of investigating both the microbiome composition and changes in gut-derived circulating metabolites, revealing significant changes in circulating, exclusively gut-derived metabolites such as aromatic amino acids and short-chain fatty acids (SCFA).[15,23] Interestingly, these metabolites are among the most strongly dysregulated metabolites in pwMS in global unbiased metabolic screenings,[23–25] supporting a clear association between gut dysbiosis and MS.

## EVIDENCE FOR THE RELEVANCE OF GUT DYSBIOSIS FROM MOUSE MODELS OF MULTIPLE SCLEROSIS

Some of the most compelling evidence for the importance of the gut microbiome in disease development comes from animal studies. Here, in contrast to human studies, one can more easily demonstrate not only correlation but also causality.

Germ-free (GF) or specific pathogen-free (SPF) mice have been a key tool in investigating the link between the gut microbiome and CNS autoimmunity in mouse models of MS. One of the first studies established this association 2 decades ago in transgenic mice that have a T-cell receptor engineered to exclusively recognize myelin basic protein and develop spontaneous relapsing-remitting experimental autoimmune encephalomyelitis (EAE). These mice were found to be protected from the disease if kept under SPF conditions.[26] Further GF mice with a T-cell receptor specific for myelin oligodendrocyte glycoprotein did not develop spontaneous EAE until commensal flora was reintroduced into their gut; this was confirmed in GF mice immunized with myelin oligodendrocyte glycoprotein and an adjuvant (classic EAE model), which developed less severe EAE compared with regularly housed mice.[27]

At the cellular level, GF mice show aberrant proinflammatory immune responses involved in MS disease pathology. The polarization of T cells into pathogenic T helper 17 and 1 cells (TH17 and TH1) in the gut is impaired, favoring tolerogenic regulatory T cells (Tregs)[27] and antiinflammatory TH2 responses.[28] GF mice have fewer intestinal plasma cells[29] and reduced immunoglobulin (Ig) G production.[30] Macrophages of GF mice show aberrant phagocytosis and lysosomal enzyme induction in response to inflammatory activation.[31]

Overall, this suggests that the gut microbiome is required or at least plays an integral role in mounting and sustaining autoimmune responses. However, it must be noted that GF mice have an altered immune system from birth, possibly inherently changing their susceptibility to autoimmune diseases irrespective of the gut microbiome status in adulthood.

To this end, another approach has been depletion of the gut microbiota with antibiotics including ampicillin, vancomycin, neomycin, and metronidazole. This reduces disease severity and delays onset in various animal models of MS, including conventional EAE, relapsing-remitting EAE, and a virus-induced EAE model.[32–34]

Further experiments highlighting the importance of gut dysbiosis in MS pathology involve human microbiota-xenotransplantation mouse models, where the human fecal microbiome is transferred into GF mice.[35] Berer and colleagues transferred fecal microbiota from monozygotic twins, of which only one sibling had MS, into transgenic mice with a T-cell receptor engineered to exclusively recognize a myelin protein. They found that mice that obtained the MS microbiome developed signs of EAE more frequently than mice that received the non-MS twin control microbiome.[20]

## MECHANISM THROUGH WHICH GUT DYSBIOSIS CONTRIBUTES TO DISEASE PATHOLOGY

Possible mechanisms (**Fig. 1**) include (1) increased gut permeability that leads to elevated levels of circulating proinflammatory pathogen-associated molecular patterns (PAMPs), (2) reduced production of tolerogenic PAMPs, (3) molecular mimicry,

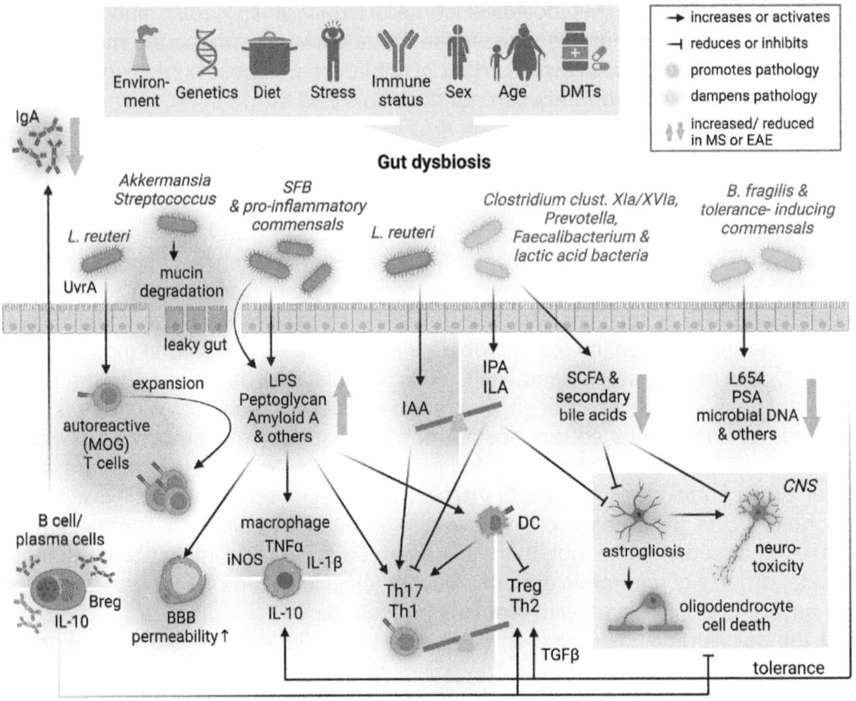


**Fig. 1.** Mechanisms through which the gut microbiome contributes to MS disease pathology include (1) modulation of gut microbe–reactive IgA-producing plasma cells that home to the brain, (2) induction of autoreactive T cells, (3) induction of innate and adaptive immune responses through PAMPs, (4) alteration of gut microbial tryptophan, short-chain fatty acid, and secondary bile acid metabolism, and (5) reduction of immune regulatory factors. These mechanisms lead to an increase in disease-promoting TH17 T cells, the induction of proinflammatory innate immune cells, increased BBB permeability, and aggravated compartmentalized CNS inflammation. Created with BioRender.com. B fragilis, *Bacillus fragilis*; BBB, blood-brain barrier; Breg, regulatory B cell; CNS, central nervous system; DC, dendritic cell; EAE, experimental autoimmune encephalomyelitis; IAA, indole acetate; ILA, indole lactate; iNOS, inducible nitric oxidase; IPA, indole propionate; L reuteri, *Lactobacillus reuteri;* L654, Lipid 654; LPS, lipopolysaccharide; PSA, polysaccharide A; SFB, segmented filamentous bacteria; Th1, Th17, or Th2, T helper 1, 7, or 2 cells; Treg, regulatory T cell.

(4) a metabolic shift of the gut microbiota from the production of anti- to proinflammatory metabolites, and (5) changed IgA responses.

### *Leaky Gut and Circulating Proinflammatory Pathogen-Associated Molecular Patterns in Multiple Sclerosis*

PwMS have enhanced gut permeability, often referred to as the "leaky gut."[36,37] PwMS have higher circulating levels of markers of enterocyte damage, ileal bile acid–binding protein, and D-lactate.[38] Interestingly, there is also a positive correlation between zonulin, a negative regulator of intestinal tight junctions, and disease progression in progressive MS (PMS) and blood-brain barrier (BBB) permeability in relapsing-remitting MS (RRMS).[38] The cause of leaky gut in pwMS is unclear. One explanation could be the increase of barrier dysfunction, promoting commensals including *Akkermansia* and *Streptococcus*, both known mucin degraders.[39]

Alternatively, inflammatory processes in pwMS may lead to barrier dysfunction or a modulation of the gut microbiome favoring gut leakiness. Some evidence for this can be found in preclinical studies: mice with EAE develop barrier dysfunction.[40]

Consequences of the leaky gut are the entry of PAMPs into the circulation and ultimately the CNS. PwMS have higher circulating levels of lipopolysaccharide,[41] a PAMP from gram-negative bacterial cell walls, and its binding protein.[42] Further, RNAs of numerous gut microbes are elevated in MS brain biopsies.[43] The host immune system recognizes these PAMPs with pattern recognition receptors (PRRs), such as Toll-like receptors (TLRs), and mounts an immune response against them. There is evidence of this via the presence of antigen-presenting cells containing peptidoglycan, another gut bacterium–derived PAMP, and peptidoglycan-specific plasma cells in the CNS of pwMS.[44] Further downstream, these changes in basal immune activation by the gut microbiota in pwMS might affect innate immune responses as well as adaptive immune responses. Yet, based on the literature, it is currently unclear if circulating PAMPs from the gut contribute to inflammatory pathways and ultimately disease pathology in pwMS.

Further evidence for the proinflammatory effects of commensals in MS can be found in studies with segmented filamentous bacteria (SFB), a nonculturable Clostridia-related species. SFB protects its host from intestinal pathogens by inducing an inflammatory and antimicrobial response under physiologic conditions but has also been shown to induce autoimmunity in mice.[45] Recolonization of GF mice with SFB alone was enough to restore their susceptibility to EAE.[27] Mechanistically, SFB elevates circulating levels of the acute phase protein serum amyloid A, which among other receptors binds to PRRs; this promotes the differentiation of various T helper cells including TH17, TH1, and Tregs.[46,47] Further the flagellins of SFB can directly bind to TLR5 on lamina propria dendritic cells (DCs), inducing TH1/TH17 polarization.[48,49] Although SFB colonization is diminished in humans by the age of 3 years,[50] similar processes might be induced by other bacterial species in pwMS.

## *Reduced Production of Tolerogenic Pathogen-Associated Molecular Patterns*

Besides inducing proinflammatory processes, the gut microbiome and its PAMPs can also induce tolerance and antiinflammatory pathways through TLRs. These protective mechanisms of the microbiome could be hampered in pwMS.

### *Polysaccharide A and other Toll-like receptor 2 ligands*

One of the most extensively studied protective PAMPs in preclinical models of MS is polysaccharide A (PSA) from *Bacteroides fragilis*. PSA reduces EAE severity following disease induction and suppresses disease incidence when given prophylactically.[51,52] PSA both indirectly, through DCs, and directly promotes the expansion of CD39+ Tregs[51–53]; this is at least partially mediated through TLR2.[51,53] To our knowledge, there are no studies linking PSA or *B fragilis* to human disease.

Another tolerance inducing gut microbial PAMP is lipid 654 (L654). Circulating L654 is reduced in pwMS.[54] In preclinical studies, low-dose exposure to this PAMP caused TLR2-induced tolerance and ameliorated adoptive transfer EAE.[55] Using a synthetic TLR2 ligand, another group was able to confirm the protective effect of low-dose TLR2 ligand-induced tolerance induction in the cuprizone model of toxic demyelination.[56]

Further possible tolerogenic TLR2 ligands reduced in pwMS could be factors derived from *Clostridium* and *Lactobacillus* species and *Faecalibacterium prausnitzii*, which all induce antiinflammatory effects via TLR2[57–59] and are reduced in pwMS.

#### *Microbial DNA and other Toll-like receptor 9 ligands*

Another group of gut-derived ligands shown to induce tolerance are TLR9 ligands. TLR9 is an intracellular PRR that recognizes unmethylated cytosine-phosphate-guanine motifs, which are primarily present in microbes. In animals, ligation of TLR9 by gut-derived factors delay EAE onset and reduces EAE severity. Mechanistically, TLR9 induces immune suppressive function in plasmacytoid DCs, induces Tregs, and reduces brain-infiltrating TH1/TH17 cells.[60,61] To our knowledge there are currently no studies that have investigated TLR9 ligand levels in pwMS, but a change in TLR9 responses in pwMS has been reported.[62] To this end, reduced tolerogenic TLR9-mediated microbiome-host interactions in pwMS could be another mechanism through which the gut microbiome contributes to MS disease pathology.

Arguing against the relevance of TLR2- and 9-induced tolerance in EAE and MS are reports showing that global and cell-specific depletion of these receptors reduces EAE severity.[63–65]

### *Gut Microbiome Molecular Mimicry*

Another mechanism through which the gut microbiome might contribute to induction of autoimmunity is through cross-reactive T cells that recognize both microbial factors and CNS molecules, a phenomenon referred to as molecular mimicry.

*Lactobacillus reuteri* contains several epitopes, including a UvrA, that show cross-reactivity with MOG-specific T cells, mildly activating and expanding these cells. Interestingly, in vivo *L reuteri* monocolonization did not affect EAE onset or severity, but a second hit, in the form of a proinflammatory commensal such as SFB, expanded the autoreactive TH17 cells and worsened disease severity.[33] Similar molecular mimicry mechanisms in EAE have been shown with other, not gut-specific, microbial proteins.[66] Although these microbes are also present in humans, it is unclear whether gut microbiome cross-reactivity–induced autoimmunity plays a role in MS.

### *Gut-Derived Metabolites in Multiple Sclerosis*

Physiologically, a key function of the gut microbiome is to catabolize dietary substances into metabolites essential for the human body. Many of these metabolites such as SCFA, secondary bile acids (2°BAs), and indole derivatives of tryptophan cannot be produced by the host. In pwMS gut dysbiosis induces changes in these metabolic pathways and thereby might contribute to peripheral and CNS immune dysfunction.

#### *Short-chain fatty acids*

SCFA are produced from dietary fibers by the gut microbiota. The most abundant SCFA produced are acetate, propionate, and butyrate. Numerous bacteria can produce these SCFA including Clostridium clusters IV and XIVa, *Bacteroides* species, and *Akkermansia*.

Circulating SCFA levels are reduced in pwMS, with particularly low levels in RRMS when compared with SPMS.[10,19,67] Numerous SCFA-producing gut microbial species including the Clostridium clusters IV and XIVa and *Bacteroides* are reduced in pwMS, although some SCFA-producing bacteria such as *Akkermansia* are elevated.[9,10,13,17,18]

Preclinical studies show that supplementation with acetate, propionate, or butyrate or a mix of several SCFAs reduced EAE severity.[68,69] Further, in a clinical trial propionate supplementation in pwMS restored the Treg to TH17/TH1 balance.[19] Mechanistically, preclinical studies suggest that SCFAs have several more effects on neuroinflammation. With respect to T cells, in EAE SCFA do not only increase the number of Tregs in the spinal cord but also increase infiltrating TH17 and TH1 cells,[68,69] suggesting that SCFA affects CD4 polarization in general, and their overall effect might vary depending on the SCFA type or contextual cues. Further, SCFA dampen the compartmentalized neuroinflammation by reducing BBB permeability,[70] promoting remyelination[71] (most likely through indirect effects on oligodendrocyte lineage cells), and limiting astrogliosis, promoting the release of neurotrophic and oligodendrocyte precursor cell (OPC) survival-enhancing factors from astrocytes.[72,73] Several of these effects have been shown to be mediated via G protein–coupled receptors 43 and 41.

***Secondary bile acids***

2°BAs are exclusively produced by the gut microbiota by modifying primary bile acids from the liver through processes including deconjugation, dehydroxylation, and reconjugation. The bacteria involved include *Bacteroides*, *Lactobacillus*, *Bifidobacterium*, and Clostridium cluster XIVa species, which are reduced in pwMS. Levels of circulating 2°BAs are altered in pwMS[74] and EAE.[75] In preclinical studies supplementation with the 2°BA tauroursodeoxycholic acid (TUDCA) reduced EAE severity.[74] Hence, 2°BAs have been suggested as another gut-derived metabolite linking the gut microbiome to MS disease pathology.

On a cellular level, TUDCA shifts microglia and astrocytes from a proinflammatory neurotoxic phenotype to an antiinflammatory phenotype, reducing oligodendrocyte cell death.[74,76] TUDCA shows no effect on T-cell polarization nor activation in vitro.[74] Similar to TUDCA, the 2°BA ursodeoxycholic acid (UDCA) has been reported to dampen TLR4-induced proinflammatory activation of microglia[77] and lithocholic acid (LCA) of circulating monocytes.[78] In part, these effects were shown to be dependent on Takeda G protein–coupled receptor 5, which has been shown to be expressed on macrophages and astrocytes in demyelinating lesions in pwMS.[74]

***Indole metabolites of tryptophan***

Tryptophan is an essential amino acid present in foods, including dairy, fish, and poultry. It can be absorbed and catabolized by the human body along the kynurenine pathway (which is not discussed in this review). Alternatively, tryptophan can be catabolized into indole metabolites by the gut microbiome. GF mice show strongly reduced levels of the indole metabolites of tryptophan in the circulation and CNS.[79]

In pwMS these metabolites are dysregulated. Two independent multi-omics studies investigating the circulating metabolome in MS found indole lactate (ILA) to be one of the most strongly reduced metabolites in pwMS, with particularly low levels in PMS.[23,24] In pediatric MS circulating ILA levels predicted disease onset and indole propionate (IPA) levels inversely correlated with disability.[80] ILA-producing gut microbes were reduced in pwMS.[23]

This suggests that reduced gut-derived indole metabolites may contribute to MS disease pathology. Indeed, IPA, indole, indoxyl-3-sulfate (I3S), and indole-3-aldehyde supplementation dampens EAE disease severity when administered therapeutically.[81] Surprisingly, indole acetate[82] and prophylactic I3S[83] have been shown to exacerbate EAE. In preclinical studies both the protective and detrimental effects of indole metabolites were linked to aryl hydrocarbon receptor (AhR), suggesting that ligation of the receptor might cause ligand-dependent or context-dependent differential downstream effects. Whether the cellular targets and AhR dependency described in the preclinical models will hold true for the indole metabolites dysregulated in pwMS is unknown.

## *Immunoglobulin A and Regulatory B Cells*

IgA plays an important role in gut microbiome-immune system crosstalk. The gut microbials induce IgA production, and IgA in turn regulates the function and composition of the gut microbiome.[84]

Increased intrathecal oligoclonal bands are a diagnostic marker for MS, and B-cell depletion is a well-established treatment, suggesting pathologic functions of B cells and Igs in MS. Indeed, cerebrospinal fluid microbiome-reactive IgA and IgA plasma cells are particularly highly elevated in the CSF of patients with MS compared with other neurologic diseases[85] and predict cortical atrophy and disability in RRMS.[86] Yet these elevated IgA molecules exclusively recognize their gut microbial antigens and show no reactivity for CNS proteins.[87] The microbiome-reactive IgA-producing B cells could have protective effects through the production of interleukin-10 (IL-10) and might be elevated in a compensatory fashion, as shown in preclinical studies[88] and supported by the presence of IgA and IL-10 double-positive cells in the CNS of pwMS.[87,89]

## TARGETING THE GUT MICROBIOME FOR TREATMENT

Therapeutic interventions targeting MS-associated gut dysbiosis include antibiotics, fecal microbiota transplantation (FMT), supplementation of gut microbiota–derived metabolites, probiotics, prebiotics, and dietary changes (**Table 1**).

### *Antibiotics*

There are numerous studies in different mouse models of MS showing delayed disease onset and reduced severity with a vancomycin, ampicillin, neomycin, and metronidazole mix.[32–34] Based on these preclinical studies, there is an ongoing randomized placebo-controlled phase 1 trial investigating vancomycin as a possible modulator of the gut-brain axis in MS. Readouts of this trial include changes in the gut microbiome, peripheral immune cell profiling, and assessment of brain MRI lesions (NCT05539729).

Besides this ongoing study, there have been studies showing some beneficial effects of second-generation tetracycline antibiotics, doxycycline[90] (NCT00246324) and minocycline[91] (NCT00666887), in pwMS, although they are not thought to target the gut microbiome. Short-term ($\sim$6 months) intake of minocycline reduced the risk of a clinically isolated syndrome converting to MS in a phase 3 trial[91] and reduced disease activity on MRI in pwMS in a small pilot trial,[92] but the benefits are unclear or lost when minocycline is taken long-term (2 years).[91] Doxycycline in combination with interferon $\beta$ (IFN$\beta$), a well-established DMT, has been shown to be safe, to reduce MRI disease activity and disability in a single-group assignment phase 4 trial.[90] Tetracycline antibiotics are thought to induce their antiinflammatory effects directly in the periphery, so changes in the gut microbiome were not included as a readout in these studies.

### *Fecal Microbiota Transplantation*

FMT involves the depletion of the recipient's microbiota using antibiotics followed by the transfer of the microbiota from a healthy donor through nasogastric or duodenal tube, colonoscopy, rectal enema, or oral ingestion of capsules. Preclinical studies investigating FMT from healthy mice into EAE mice show amelioration of disease. FMT promoted an increase of beneficial microbes, stabilized the BBB, reduced reactive gliosis, and had neuroprotective effects.[93,94]

To this end, there are several ongoing clinical trials investigating FMT in pwMS. A pilot randomized controlled trial of FMT via rectal enema (NCT03183869) showed that FMT reduced intestinal permeability and had beneficial effects on gut microbiota composition.[95] Further, anecdotal evidence for the beneficial effects of FMT can be found in case reports describing long-term stabilization of disease, accompanied by sustained effects on the microbiota composition and SCFA metabolism.[96,97]

**Table 1**
**Gut microbiome–targeted interventions currently under clinical investigation and their advantages and disadvantages**

| Gut Microbiome–Targeted Interventions | Clinical Evidence | FDA Approval | Advantages | Disadvantages |
|---|---|---|---|---|
| Vancomycin (antibiotic) | Phase 1 ongoing | For other conditions | • Easy oral intake<br>• Well established | • Unclear efficacy to date<br>• Possible colonization with opportunistic bacteria for example, *C. difficile* after oral vancomycin<br>• Reduced microbial production of anti-inflammatory metabolites: Reduced 2°BA synthesis after oral vancomycin |
| FMT | Phase 1 and 2 ongoing | For other conditions | • Restoration of numerous gut microbial functions<br>• Established | • Unclear long-term efficacy to date<br>• More elaborate interventions with peri-procedural risks (but can be taken as orally)<br>• Risks associated with antibiotic pre-treatment |
| Gut microbiome metabolites | *2°BA:* phase 1/2 with TUDCA ongoing<br>*SCFA:* pilot trial, no RCTs<br>*Indoles:* no | *2°BA:* TUDCA for ALS<br>*SCFA:* NA[a]<br>*Indoles:* no | • Easy oral intake<br>• Possibly good safety profile because physiologically present<br>• Possible personalized medicine approach[b] | • Unclear efficacy to date<br>• New therapeutics so some metabolites are not produced at a pharmaceutical grade (only in combination products)<br>• More studies required to understand effects (including possible off-target effects) |
| Probiotics | Completed/more ongoing (phase NA[a]) | NA[a] | • Easy oral intake<br>• Good safety profile | • Unclear long-term efficacy to date |

(*continued on next page*)

**Table 1**
***(continued)***

| Gut Microbiome–Targeted Interventions | Clinical Evidence | FDA Approval | Advantages | Disadvantages |
| --- | --- | --- | --- | --- |
| Prebiotics: dietary fiber | Completed/more ongoing (phase NA[a]) | NA[a] | • Easy oral intake<br>• Good safety profile | • Might have limited effect alone (often combined with probiotic)<br>• Long-term intake required<br>• Possibly age dependent efficacy (vit. D) |
| Diets | Completed/more ongoing (phase NA) | NA | • Good safety profile<br>• Improvement of general health and MS-associated comorbidities<br>• Leads to increased exercise that improves outcome | • Elaborate interventions ideally executed by a team including a dietician<br>• Requires compliant patient<br>• May be limited by socioeconomic and cultural factors<br>• Currently no recommended diet for MS patients (cost not covered in the United States) |

*Abbreviations: C difficile*; *C difficile*; FDA, Food and Drug Administration; FMT, fecal microbiota transplant; 2°BA, secondary bile acids; NA, not applicable; SCFA, short-chain fatty acid; TUDCA, tauroursodeoxycholic acid.

[a] Recognized as dietary supplements.

[b] Patients with low circulating metabolite levels are selected for treatment.

There are numerous ongoing randomized controlled clinical trials investigating FMT in pwMS, many of which include analysis of the gut microbiome composition and function as a readout (NCT04014413, NCT04203017, NCT03594487, NCT04150549, and NCT04096443).

Risks of FMT include risks associated with antibiotic pretreatment such as unwanted recolonization with pathobionts and risks associated with transplantation, especially if it is carried out as an endoscopic intervention. Further the long-term benefits of FMTs are unclear because some factors contributing to gut dysbiosis, such as dietary habits, age, and DMTs, might cause an eventual return to the original state of gut dysbiosis, making repeated FMTs necessary.

## SUPPLEMENTATION OF GUT-DERIVED METABOLITES

Gut-derived metabolites with antiinflammatory properties including SCFA, secondary bile acids, and indole derivatives of tryptophan are reduced in pwMS.[19,24,74] Supplementing these to restore their homeostatic, antiinflammatory effects could be a potential therapeutic strategy in pwMS.

As outlined in detail earlier in preclinical studies using the EAE model supplementation with SCFAs, the secondary bile acid TUDCA and indole metabolites reduce disease severity. This approach is now also explored in clinical trials. In a proof-of-concept trial, 2 weeks of propionate supplementation restored the Treg to TH1/17 balance, and long-term intake of at least 1 year reduced relapse rates and stabilized disability.[19] Further, supplementation of TUDCA is currently being explored in a randomized placebo-controlled phase 1/2 trial (NCT03423121).

### *Probiotics*

Another approach to target MS-associated gut dysbiosis is through probiotics, gut microbes with known beneficial effects. In preclinical studies, supplementation with *Lactobacilli*, *Bifidobacterium*, and *Prevotella* species, which are reduced in pwMS, ameliorates EAE by increasing the Treg to TH17/TH1 ratio in the periphery and the CNS.[98–101]

Clinical trials have focused on probiotics containing a mix of different *Lactobacilli* and *Bifidobacterium* species. After 2 to 3 months, probiotics reduce the inflammatory activation in circulating monocytes and improve disability, depression, and general health in pwMS.[102,103]

### *Dietary Supplements and Prebiotics*

Supplements investigated in clinical trials include dietary fiber, vitamins, and omega-3 fatty acids. All have been shown to alter the gut microbiome in a beneficial manner[104–106] and are therefore considered prebiotics.

#### *Dietary fiber*

In EAE, dietary fibers delay onset and reduce disease severity, promoting beneficial changes in microbiota composition and metabolic pathways depending on the nature of the fiber. Guar gum for instance increases SCFAs and reduces TH1 polarization,[107] whereas cellulose increases LCFA in the gut and induces TH2s.[105]

In humans the effect of daily high-fiber supplements for 8 weeks is currently being investigated in a randomized placebo-controlled phase 1 and 2 trial (NCT04574024). Several other ongoing randomized clinical trials combine probiotics and fiber prebiotics containing inulin and oligofructose (NCT04038541 and NCT05779449). In all these trials the effect of the intervention on the gut microbiome will be assessed.

### *Vitamin D*

Low circulating levels of vitamin D are associated with an increased risk of developing MS and affect disease activity.[108] Interestingly vitamin D also affects the gut microbiome and intestinal barrier function.[106] In animal models of MS, vitamin D supplementation reduces disease severity,[109,110] although the effect depends on the developmental stage.[111] Yet in humans, the findings of numerous clinical studies are contradictory. The current Cochrane systematic review concludes that there is no benefit of vitamin D supplementation in pwMS.[111–114]

### *Omega-3 fatty acids*

Omega-3 fatty acids have a beneficial impact on the diversity, metabolic pathways, and composition of the gut microbiome (increase of Lachnospiraceae, which are reduced in pwMS).[112] In animal studies, supplementation of omega-3 fatty acids suppresses EAE by attenuating DC maturation and TH1/TH17 differentiation and promotes remyelination in rats. In small clinical studies omega 3 was shown to have beneficial effects in pwMS.[113–115] However, in a randomized, placebo-controlled phase 2 and 3 trial (NCT00360906) daily omega-3 fatty acid supplementation for 6 months had no beneficial effects on disease activity.[116] In this trial, effects on the gut microbiome were not investigated.

## *Diets*

### *Intermittent fasting and calorie restriction*

In preclinical studies, fasting and calorie-restricting diets reduced disease severity in both EAE and cuprizone-induced toxic demyelination models. The fasting diet reduced inflammation, through increased circulating corticosteroid levels, reduced axonal injury, and promoted remyelination.[117–120]

Randomized controlled clinical trials investigated the effect of different calorie restricting/fasting diets in pwMS, including a 7-day prolonged fasting diet (NCT01538355), a continuous moderate calorie restriction diet and an intermittent calorie restriction diet (NCT02647502), and alternate day fasting diet (NCT02411838). Overall, intermittent fasting diets were associated with improved patient perceived physical and mental health and weight loss.[119,121] All studies reported effects on T cells, including a reduction of circulating leukocytes during fasting periods,[119] reduction in the ratio of memory to naïve T cells,[122] and an increase in the ratio of Tregs to TH17 cells in the gut.[120] In NCT02411838, the intervention increased gut microbiota families that are reduced in MS, enhanced gut microbiota diversity, and affected microbial metabolic pathways.[120]

Intermittent fasting diets in pwMS are being further investigated in 3 randomized controlled trials (NCT04042415, NCT03508414, and NCT03539094).

### *Ketogenic diets*

Ketogenic diets involve significantly reduced carbohydrates, moderate protein, and high fat intake that induce a shift from glucose to lipids as a source of energy, mimicking fasting-like states and inducing ketosis. In mice, a ketogenic diet reduced EAE disease severity, with reduced inflammation, attenuated oxidative stress responses, and improved motor and cognitive function.[123]

A randomized pilot trial of an adapted ketogenic diet (NCT01538355) showed a biphasic effect of the diet with initial reduction, followed by a significant increase in gut microbial mass and diversity after 5 months on the diet.[11],[124] Further ketogenic diets had antiinflammatory and neuroprotective effects in pwMS as evident by reduced levels of enzymes producing proinflammatory eicosanoids[125] and serum neurofilament light chain,[126] respectively.[127] The effects of ketogenic diets on clinical parameters and the gut microbiome in pwMS are being further investigated (NCT03508414).

***High vegetable diets***
Another dietary approach investigated in pwMS is plant-based diets. In a 1-year non-randomized pilot trial, a high vegetable diet with low protein intake reduced the relapse rate and disability in RRMS compared with a control western diet, characterized by regular consumption of red meat and high fat, sugar, and salt intake. The diet had beneficial effects on the gut microbiome, increasing *Lachnospiraceae* colonization, and decreased circulating TH17 cells.[12] However, in a 1-year randomized controlled clinical trial of a plant-based diet with very low fat intake in RRMS, there was no significant effects of the diet on disability and MRI activity compared with a control group with no dietary changes. However, the patients showed significant weight loss, reduced dyslipidemia, reduced insulin levels, and an improvement of patient-reported fatigue.[2]

***Limitations of diets***
Dietary interventions are usually long-term treatments, ideally accomplished by a multidisciplinary team. They can be a profound change in the patient's lifestyle and be limited by socioeconomic and cultural factors, making adherence difficult for some patients. Nonetheless, successful dietary changes can have wide-reaching secondary effects on disease by inducing weight loss, affecting comorbidities driving systemic inflammation, and often enhancing patient's exercise behaviors.

Despite these promising prospects, there is no recommended diet for pwMS, and our knowledge of how diets affect disease pathology is limited; this is partially because it is hard to correlate disease parameters or gut microbiome changes to diet alone, as they are often accompanied by the confounding secondary effects mentioned earlier that also independently affect disease and the gut microbiome.

## ***The Effects of Disease-Modifying Therapies on the Gut Microbiome***

Another important aspect to consider in pwMS is the impact of currently prescribed DMTs on the gut microbiome. Studies have described both beneficial and detrimental effects.

DMTs with primarily beneficial effects include IFNβ, dimethyl fumarate (DMF), and ocrelizumab. In pwMS IFNβ treatment normalizes MS-associated changes in *Prevotella* colonization.[128] Similarly, DMF increases *Faecalibacterium*,[124] *Roseburia*,[127] and *Bacteroides*[129] species,[130] which are reduced in pwMS. However, DMF also further reduces the abundance of bacteria already reduced in pwMS.[129] There are several ongoing studies further investigating the effects of DMF on the microbiome (NCT02736279 and NCT03092544) that might lead to more definitive conclusions. In a small longitudinal study, ocrelizumab, a monoclonal anti-CD20 antibody, increased alpha-diversity and strongly reduced the abundance of proinflammatory opportunistic bacteria. However, the investigators also reported a mild decrease in SCFA-producing bacteria already reduced in pwMS, associated with probiotic effects.[131] In another study, anti-CD20 therapies induced *Faecalibacterium* species, which are reduced in pwMS.[127]

Glatiramer acetate (GA) and alemtuzumab are 2 DMTs with reported negative effects on the microbiota. GA is a synthetic polymer with structural similarities to MBP with immunomodulatory effects in pwMS. It further decreases the abundance of *Lachnospiraceae* and *Veillonellaceae* species, which are already reduced in pwMS.[129,131] The detrimental effects of GA on the gut microbiome might partially be explained by its antimicrobial effects on gram-negative bacteria.[132] The effects of alemtuzumab, an anti-CD52 monoclonal antibody depleting lymphocytes, on the gut microbiome in pwMS is not yet known, but in cynomolgus monkeys, alemtuzumab treatment reduced *Lactobacillus* species and increased gut opportunistic microbes.[130]

## SUMMARY

Although the cause of MS is yet unclear, environmental factors are thought to play an important role. One major interaction of the immune system with the environment is through the gut microbiome. Indeed, gut dysbiosis in both clinical and preclinical studies may cause increased susceptibility to and promote ongoing neuroinflammation. The gut microbiome-immune system interaction is not, however, unidirectional. MS and its currently available treatments, DMTs, also affect the microbiome in return.

The microbiome also has numerous functions that dampen MS disease processes. It induces tolerance by promoting antiinflammatory functions of the innate and adaptive immune system directly or indirectly through metabolites and dampens compartmentalized neuroinflammation. Some of these processes are elevated in a compensatory fashion, whereas others that are reduced can possibly be harnessed in gut microbiome–targeted interventions. As our understanding of MS and the gut microbiome evolve, it is hoped that we will be able to develop more targeted and possibly personalized therapies tailored to restore specific microbiome functions and make them an integral part of MS care.

## CLINICS CARE POINTS

- While it is clear that gut microbiota dysbiosis exists in MS there are no proven interventions to reverse this phenomenon.
- While several interventions potentially impact the gut microbiome there is a lack of large randomized placebo-controlled trials upon which to base clinical recommendations.
- Since MS-specific datsa are lacking we generally tend to recommend interventions that have shown benefit in overal systemic health, such as improving diet quality and patterns, for people with MS.

## DISCLOSURE

The authors have nothing to disclose.

## FUNDING

This work was supported in part by a postdoctoral fellowship from the National Multiple Sclerosis Society to LJ and a Harry Weaver Neuroscience Scholar Award from the National Multiple Sclerosis Society to PB.

## REFERENCES

1. Maglione A, Zuccalà M, Tosi M, et al. Host Genetics and Gut Microbiome: Perspectives for Multiple Sclerosis. Genes 2021;12:1181.

2. Yadav SK, Boppana S, Ito N, et al. Gut dysbiosis breaks immunological tolerance toward the central nervous system during young adulthood. Proc Natl Acad Sci U S A 2017;114(44):E9318–27.
3. Bosco N, Noti M. The aging gut microbiome and its impact on host immunity. Gene Immun 2021;22(5):289–303.
4. Fransen F, van Beek AA, Borghuis T, et al. Aged Gut Microbiota Contributes to Systemical Inflammaging after Transfer to Germ-Free Mice. Front Immunol 2017; 8(NOV). https://doi.org/10.3389/FIMMU.2017.01385.
5. Cox LM, Abou-El-Hassan H, Maghzi AH, et al. The sex-specific interaction of the microbiome in neurodegenerative diseases. Brain Res 2019;1724:146385.
6. Khan MF, Wang H. Environmental Exposures and Autoimmune Diseases: Contribution of Gut Microbiome. Front Immunol 2020;10:501043.
7. Eckburg PB, Bik EM, Bernstein CN, et al. Diversity of the human intestinal microbial flora. Science 2005;308(5728):1635–8.
8. Ordoñez-Rodriguez A, Roman P, Rueda-Ruzafa L, et al. Changes in Gut Microbiota and Multiple Sclerosis: A Systematic Review. Int J Environ Res Public Health 2023;20(5). https://doi.org/10.3390/IJERPH20054624.
9. Miyake S, Kim S, Suda W, et al. Dysbiosis in the Gut Microbiota of Patients with Multiple Sclerosis, with a Striking Depletion of Species Belonging to Clostridia XIVa and IV Clusters. PLoS One 2015;10(9):e0137429.
10. Takewaki D, Suda W, Sato W, et al. Alterations of the gut ecological and functional microenvironment in different stages of multiple sclerosis. Proc Natl Acad Sci U S A 2020;117(36):22402–12.
11. Swidsinski A, Dörffel Y, Loening-Baucke V, et al. Reduced Mass and Diversity of the Colonic Microbiome in Patients with Multiple Sclerosis and Their Improvement with Ketogenic Diet. Front Microbiol 2017;8(JUN). https://doi.org/10.3389/FMICB.2017.01141.
12. Saresella M, Mendozzi L, Rossi V, et al. Immunological and clinical effect of diet modulation of the gut microbiome in multiple sclerosis patients: A pilot study. Front Immunol 2017;8(OCT):1391.
13. Ventura RE, Iizumi T, Battaglia T, et al. Gut microbiome of treatment-naïve MS patients of different ethnicities early in disease course. Sci Rep 2019;9(1):1–10.
14. Forbes JD, Chen CY, Knox NC, et al. A comparative study of the gut microbiota in immune-mediated inflammatory diseases-does a common dysbiosis exist? Microbiome 2018;6(1). https://doi.org/10.1186/S40168-018-0603-4.
15. Cantoni C, Lin Q, Dorsett Y, et al. Alterations of host-gut microbiome interactions in multiple sclerosis. EBioMedicine 2022;76. https://doi.org/10.1016/J.EBIOM.2021.103798.
16. Chen J, Chia N, Kalari KR, et al. Multiple sclerosis patients have a distinct gut microbiota compared to healthy controls. Sci Rep 2016;6. https://doi.org/10.1038/SREP28484.
17. Jangi S, Gandhi R, Cox LM, et al. Alterations of the human gut microbiome in multiple sclerosis. Nat Commun 2016;7(1):1–11.
18. Cekanaviciute E, Yoo BB, Runia TF, et al. Gut bacteria from multiple sclerosis patients modulate human T cells and exacerbate symptoms in mouse models. Proc Natl Acad Sci U S A 2017;114(40):10713–8.
19. Duscha A, Gisevius B, Hirschberg S, et al. Propionic Acid Shapes the Multiple Sclerosis Disease Course by an Immunomodulatory Mechanism. Cell 2020; 180(6):1067–80.e16.

20. Berer K, Gerdes LA, Cekanaviciute E, et al. Gut microbiota from multiple sclerosis patients enables spontaneous autoimmune encephalomyelitis in mice. Proc Natl Acad Sci U S A 2017;114(40):10719–24.
21. Cosorich I, Dalla-Costa G, Sorini C, et al. High frequency of intestinal TH17 cells correlates with microbiota alterations and disease activity in multiple sclerosis. Sci Adv 2017;3(7). https://doi.org/10.1126/SCIADV.1700492.
22. Choileáin SN, Kleinewietfeld M, Raddassi K, et al. CXCR3+ T cells in multiple sclerosis correlate with reduced diversity of the gut microbiome. J Transl Autoimmun 2020;3. https://doi.org/10.1016/J.JTAUTO.2019.100032.
23. Levi I, Gurevich M, Perlman G, et al. Potential role of indolelactate and butyrate in multiple sclerosis revealed by integrated microbiome-metabolome analysis. Cell Rep Med 2021;2(4). https://doi.org/10.1016/J.XCRM.2021.100246.
24. Fitzgerald KC, Smith MD, Kim S, et al. Multi-omic evaluation of metabolic alterations in multiple sclerosis identifies shifts in aromatic amino acid metabolism. Cell Rep Med 2021;2(10). https://doi.org/10.1016/J.XCRM.2021.100424.
25. Ntranos A, Park HJ, Wentling M, et al. Bacterial neurotoxic metabolites in multiple sclerosis cerebrospinal fluid and plasma. Brain 2022;145(2):569–83.
26. Goverman J, Woods A, Larson L, et al. Transgenic mice that express a myelin basic protein-specific T cell receptor develop spontaneous autoimmunity. Cell 1993;72(4):551–60.
27. Lee YK, Menezes JS, Umesaki Y, et al. Proinflammatory T-cell responses to gut microbiota promote experimental autoimmune encephalomyelitis. Proc Natl Acad Sci U S A 2011;108(Suppl 1):4615–22.
28. Mazmanian SK, Cui HL, Tzianabos AO, et al. An immunomodulatory molecule of symbiotic bacteria directs maturation of the host immune system. Cell 2005; 122(1):107–18.
29. Hapfelmeier S, Lawson MAE, Slack E, et al. Reversible microbial colonization of germ-free mice reveals the dynamics of IgA immune responses. Science 2010; 328(5986):1705–9.
30. Zeng MY, Cisalpino D, Varadarajan S, et al. Gut Microbiota-Induced Immunoglobulin G Controls Systemic Infection by Symbiotic Bacteria and Pathogens. Immunity 2016;44(3):647–58.
31. Mørland B, Midtvedt T. Phagocytosis, peritoneal influx, and enzyme activities in peritoneal macrophages from germfree, conventional, and ex-germfree mice. Infect Immun 1984;44(3):750–2.
32. Mestre L, Carrillo-Salinas FJ, Mecha M, et al. Manipulation of Gut Microbiota Influences Immune Responses, Axon Preservation, and Motor Disability in a Model of Progressive Multiple Sclerosis. Front Immunol 2019;10(JUN). https://doi.org/10.3389/FIMMU.2019.01374.
33. Miyauchi E, Kim SW, Suda W, et al. Gut microorganisms act together to exacerbate inflammation in spinal cords. Nature 2020;585(7823):102–6.
34. Ochoa-Repáraz J, Mielcarz DW, Ditrio LE, et al. Role of gut commensal microflora in the development of experimental autoimmune encephalomyelitis. J Immunol 2009;183(10):6041–50.
35. Arrieta MC, Walter J, Finlay BB. Human Microbiota-Associated Mice: A Model with Challenges. Cell Host Microbe 2016;19(5):575–8.
36. Buscarinu MC, Cerasoli B, Annibali V, et al. Altered intestinal permeability in patients with relapsing-remitting multiple sclerosis: A pilot study. Mult Scler 2017; 23(3):442–6.

37. Yacyshyn B, Meddings J, Sadowski D, et al. Multiple sclerosis patients have peripheral blood CD45RO+ B cells and increased intestinal permeability. Dig Dis Sci 1996;41(12):2493–8.
38. Camara-Lemarroy CR, Silva C, Greenfield J, et al. Biomarkers of intestinal barrier function in multiple sclerosis are associated with disease activity. Mult Scler 2020;26(11):1340–50.
39. Glover JS, Ticer TD, Engevik MA. Characterizing the mucin-degrading capacity of the human gut microbiota. Sci Rep 2022;12(1). https://doi.org/10.1038/S41598-022-11819-Z.
40. Nouri M, Bredberg A, Weström B, et al. Intestinal barrier dysfunction develops at the onset of experimental autoimmune encephalomyelitis, and can be induced by adoptive transfer of auto-reactive T cells. PLoS One 2014;9(9). https://doi.org/10.1371/JOURNAL.PONE.0106335.
41. Teixeira B, Bittencourt VCB, Ferreira TB, et al. Low sensitivity to glucocorticoid inhibition of in vitro Th17-related cytokine production in multiple sclerosis patients is related to elevated plasma lipopolysaccharide levels. Clin Immunol 2013;148(2):209–18.
42. Escribano BM, Medina-Fernández FJ, Aguilar-Luque M, et al. Lipopolysaccharide Binding Protein and Oxidative Stress in a Multiple Sclerosis Model. Neurotherapeutics 2017;14(1):199–211.
43. Kriesel JD, Bhetariya P, Wang ZM, et al. Spectrum of Microbial Sequences and a Bacterial Cell Wall Antigen in Primary Demyelination Brain Specimens Obtained from Living Patients. Sci Rep 2019;9(1). https://doi.org/10.1038/S41598-018-38198-8.
44. Schrijver IA, Van Meurs M, Melief MJ, et al. Bacterial peptidoglycan and immune reactivity in the central nervous system in multiple sclerosis. Brain 2001;124(Pt 8):1544–54.
45. Ivanov II, Frutos R de L, Manel N, et al. Specific Microbiota Direct the Differentiation of IL-17-Producing T-Helper Cells in the Mucosa of the Small Intestine. Cell Host Microbe 2008;4(4):337–49.
46. Ivanov II, Atarashi K, Manel N, et al. Induction of intestinal Th17 cells by segmented filamentous bacteria. Cell 2009;139(3):485–98.
47. Gaboriau-Routhiau V, Rakotobe S, Lécuyer E, et al. The Key Role of Segmented Filamentous Bacteria in the Coordinated Maturation of Gut Helper T Cell Responses. Immunity 2009;31(4):677–89.
48. Kuwahara T, Ogura Y, Oshima K, et al. The lifestyle of the segmented filamentous bacterium: a non-culturable gut-associated immunostimulating microbe inferred by whole-genome sequencing. DNA Res 2011;18(4):291–303.
49. Uematsu S, Fujimoto K, Jang MH, et al. Regulation of humoral and cellular gut immunity by lamina propria dendritic cells expressing Toll-like receptor 5. Nat Immunol 2008;9(7):769–76.
50. Yin Y, Wang Y, Zhu L, et al. Comparative analysis of the distribution of segmented filamentous bacteria in humans, mice and chickens. ISME J 2013;7(3):615–21.
51. Wang Y, Telesford KM, Ochoa-Repáraz J, et al. An intestinal commensal symbiosis factor controls neuroinflammation via TLR2-mediated CD39 signalling. Nat Commun 2014;5. https://doi.org/10.1038/NCOMMS5432.
52. Ochoa-Repáraz J, Mielcarz DW, Ditrio LE, et al. Central nervous system demyelinating disease protection by the human commensal Bacteroides fragilis depends on polysaccharide A expression. J Immunol 2010;185(7):4101–8.

53. Round JL, Lee SM, Li J, et al. The Toll-like receptor 2 pathway establishes colonization by a commensal of the human microbiota. Science 2011;332(6032):974–7.
54. Farrokhi V, Nemati R, Nichols FC, et al. Bacterial lipodipeptide, Lipid 654, is a microbiome-associated biomarker for multiple sclerosis. Clin Transl Immunology 2013;2(11):e8.
55. Anstadt EJ, Fujiwara M, Wasko N, et al. TLR Tolerance as a Treatment for Central Nervous System Autoimmunity. J Immunol 2016;197(6):2110–8.
56. Wasko NJ, Kulak MH, Paul D, et al. Systemic TLR2 tolerance enhances central nervous system remyelination. J Neuroinflammation 2019;16(1):1–15.
57. Hayashi A, Sato T, Kamada N, et al. A single strain of Clostridium butyricum induces intestinal IL-10-producing macrophages to suppress acute experimental colitis in mice. Cell Host Microbe 2013;13(6):711–22.
58. Ren C, Zhang Q, De Haan BJ, et al. Identification of TLR2/TLR6 signalling lactic acid bacteria for supporting immune regulation. Sci Rep 2016;6. https://doi.org/10.1038/SREP34561.
59. Alameddine J, Godefroy E, Papargyris L, et al. Faecalibacterium prausnitzii Skews Human DC to Prime IL10-Producing T Cells Through TLR2/6/JNK Signaling and IL-10, IL-27, CD39, and IDO-1 Induction. Front Immunol 2019;10(FEB). https://doi.org/10.3389/FIMMU.2019.00143.
60. Crooks J, Gargaro M, Vacca C, et al. CpG Type A Induction of an Early Protective Environment in Experimental Multiple Sclerosis. Mediators Inflamm 2017;2017. https://doi.org/10.1155/2017/1380615.
61. Letscher H, Agbogan VA, Korniotis S, et al. Toll-like receptor-9 stimulated plasmacytoid dendritic cell precursors suppress autoimmune neuroinflammation in a murine model of multiple sclerosis. Sci Rep 2021;11(1). https://doi.org/10.1038/S41598-021-84023-0.
62. Hirotani M, Niino M, Fukazawa T, et al. Decreased IL-10 production mediated by Toll-like receptor 9 in B cells in multiple sclerosis. J Neuroimmunol 2010;221(1–2):95–100.
63. Miranda-Hernandez S, Gerlach N, Fletcher JM, et al. Role for MyD88, TLR2 and TLR9 but not TLR1, TLR4 or TLR6 in experimental autoimmune encephalomyelitis. J Immunol 2011;187(2):791–804.
64. Reynolds JM, Pappu BP, Peng J, et al. Toll-like receptor 2 signaling in CD4(+) T lymphocytes promotes T helper 17 responses and regulates the pathogenesis of autoimmune disease. Immunity 2010;32(5):692–702.
65. Prinz M, Garbe F, Schmidt H, et al. Innate immunity mediated by TLR9 modulates pathogenicity in an animal model of multiple sclerosis. J Clin Invest 2006;116(2):456.
66. Ercolini AM, Miller SD. Molecular Mimics Can Induce Novel Self Peptide-Reactive CD4+ T Cell Clonotypes in Autoimmune Disease. J Immunol 2007;179(10):6604–12.
67. Saresella M, Mendozzi L, Rossi V, et al. Immunological and Clinical Effect of Diet Modulation of the Gut Microbiome in Multiple Sclerosis Patients: A Pilot Study. Front Immunol 2017;8(OCT). https://doi.org/10.3389/FIMMU.2017.01391.
68. Mizuno M, Noto D, Kaga N, et al. The dual role of short fatty acid chains in the pathogenesis of autoimmune disease models. PLoS One 2017;12(2). https://doi.org/10.1371/JOURNAL.PONE.0173032.
69. Park J, Wang Q, Wu Q, et al. Bidirectional regulatory potentials of short-chain fatty acids and their G-protein-coupled receptors in autoimmune neuroinflammation. Sci Rep 2019;9(1). https://doi.org/10.1038/S41598-019-45311-Y.

70. Braniste V, Al-Asmakh M, Kowal C, et al. The gut microbiota influences blood-brain barrier permeability in mice. Sci Transl Med 2014;6(263). https://doi.org/10.1126/SCITRANSLMED.3009759.
71. Chen T, Noto D, Hoshino Y, et al. Butyrate suppresses demyelination and enhances remyelination. J Neuroinflammation 2019;16(1). https://doi.org/10.1186/S12974-019-1552-Y.
72. Gao Y, Xie D, Wang Y, et al. Short-Chain Fatty Acids Reduce Oligodendrocyte Precursor Cells Loss by Inhibiting the Activation of Astrocytes via the SGK1/IL-6 Signalling Pathway. Neurochem Res 2022;47(11):3476–89.
73. Spichak S, Donoso F, Moloney GM, et al. Microbially-derived short-chain fatty acids impact astrocyte gene expression in a sex-specific manner. Brain Behav Immun Health 2021;16. https://doi.org/10.1016/J.BBIH.2021.100318.
74. Bhargava P, Smith MD, Mische L, et al. Bile acid metabolism is altered in multiple sclerosis and supplementation ameliorates neuroinflammation. J Clin Invest 2020;130(7):3467–82.
75. Mangalam AK, Poisson L, Nemutlu E, et al. Profile of Circulatory Metabolites in a Relapsing-remitting Animal Model of Multiple Sclerosis using Global Metabolomics. J Clin Cell Immunol 2013;4(03). https://doi.org/10.4172/2155-9899.1000150.
76. Yanguas-Casás N, Barreda-Manso MA, Nieto-Sampedro M, et al. Tauroursodeoxycholic acid reduces glial cell activation in an animal model of acute neuroinflammation. J Neuroinflammation 2014;11. https://doi.org/10.1186/1742-2094-11-50.
77. Joo SS, Kang HC, Won TJ, et al. Ursodeoxycholic acid inhibits pro-inflammatory repertoires, IL-1 beta and nitric oxide in rat microglia. Arch Pharm Res (Seoul) 2003;26(12):1067–73.
78. Hu J, Zhang Y, Yi S, et al. Lithocholic acid inhibits dendritic cell activation by reducing intracellular glutathione via TGR5 signaling. Int J Biol Sci 2022;18(11):4545–59.
79. Lai Y, Liu CW, Yang Y, et al. High-coverage metabolomics uncovers microbiota-driven biochemical landscape of interorgan transport and gut-brain communication in mice. Nat Commun 2021;12(1). https://doi.org/10.1038/S41467-021-26209-8.
80. Nourbakhsh B, Bhargava P, Tremlett H, et al. Altered tryptophan metabolism is associated with pediatric multiple sclerosis risk and course. Ann Clin Transl Neurol 2018;5(10):1211–21.
81. Rothhammer V, Mascanfroni ID, Bunse L, et al. Type I interferons and microbial metabolites of tryptophan modulate astrocyte activity and central nervous system inflammation via the aryl hydrocarbon receptor. Nat Med 2016;22(6):586–97.
82. Montgomery TL, Eckstrom K, Lile KH, et al. Lactobacillus reuteri tryptophan metabolism promotes host susceptibility to CNS autoimmunity. Microbiome 2022;10(1):1–27.
83. Hwang SJ, Hwang YJ, Yun MO, et al. Indoxyl 3-sulfate stimulates Th17 differentiation enhancing phosphorylation of c-Src and STAT3 to worsen experimental autoimmune encephalomyelitis. Toxicol Lett 2013;220(2):109–17.
84. Nakajima A, Vogelzang A, Maruya M, et al. IgA regulates the composition and metabolic function of gut microbiota by promoting symbiosis between bacteria. J Exp Med 2018;215(8):2019–34.

85. Ú Muñoz, Sebal C, Escudero E, et al. High prevalence of intrathecal IgA synthesis in multiple sclerosis patients. Sci Rep 2022;12(1). https://doi.org/10.1038/S41598-022-08099-Y.
86. Kroth J, Ciolac D, Fleischer V, et al. Increased cerebrospinal fluid albumin and immunoglobulin A fractions forecast cortical atrophy and longitudinal functional deterioration in relapsing-remitting multiple sclerosis. Mult Scler 2019;25(3):338–43.
87. Pröbstel AK, Zhou X, Baumann R, et al. Gut microbiota-specific IgA+ B cells traffic to the CNS in active multiple sclerosis. Sci Immunol 2020;5(53). https://doi.org/10.1126/SCIIMMUNOL.ABC7191.
88. Rojas OL, Pröbstel AK, Porfilio EA, et al. Recirculating Intestinal IgA-Producing Cells Regulate Neuroinflammation via IL-10. Cell 2019;176(3):610–24.e18.
89. Machado-Santos J, Saji E, Tröscher AR, et al. The compartmentalized inflammatory response in the multiple sclerosis brain is composed of tissue-resident CD8+ T lymphocytes and B cells. Brain 2018;141(7):2066–82.
90. Minagar A, Alexander JS, Schwendimann RN, et al. Combination therapy with interferon beta-1a and doxycycline in multiple sclerosis: an open-label trial. Arch Neurol 2008;65(2):199–204.
91. Metz LM, Li DKB, Traboulsee AL, et al. Trial of Minocycline in a Clinically Isolated Syndrome of Multiple Sclerosis. N Engl J Med 2017;376(22):2122–33.
92. Metz LM, Zhang Y, Yeung M, et al. Minocycline reduces gadolinium-enhancing magnetic resonance imaging lesions in multiple sclerosis. Ann Neurol 2004;55(5):756.
93. Wang S, Chen H, Wen X, et al. The Efficacy of Fecal Microbiota Transplantation in Experimental Autoimmune Encephalomyelitis: Transcriptome and Gut Microbiota Profiling. J Immunol Res 2021;2021. https://doi.org/10.1155/2021/4400428.
94. Li K, Wei S, Hu L, et al. Protection of Fecal Microbiota Transplantation in a Mouse Model of Multiple Sclerosis. Mediators Inflamm 2020;2020. https://doi.org/10.1155/2020/2058272.
95. Al KF, Craven LJ, Gibbons S, et al. Fecal microbiota transplantation is safe and tolerable in patients with multiple sclerosis: A pilot randomized controlled trial. Mult Scler J Exp Transl Clin 2022;8(2). https://doi.org/10.1177/20552173221086662.
96. Engen PA, Zaferiou A, Rasmussen H, et al. Single-Arm, Non-randomized, Time Series, Single-Subject Study of Fecal Microbiota Transplantation in Multiple Sclerosis. Front Neurol 2020;11. https://doi.org/10.3389/FNEUR.2020.00978.
97. Makkawi S, Camara-Lemarroy C, Metz L. Fecal microbiota transplantation associated with 10 years of stability in a patient with SPMS. Neurol Neuroimmunol Neuroinflamm 2018;5(4):459.
98. He B, Hoang TK, Tian X, et al. Lactobacillus reuteri Reduces the Severity of Experimental Autoimmune Encephalomyelitis in Mice by Modulating Gut Microbiota. Front Immunol 2019;10(MAR). https://doi.org/10.3389/FIMMU.2019.00385.
99. Mangalam A, Shahi SK, Luckey D, et al. Human Gut-Derived Commensal Bacteria Suppress CNS Inflammatory and Demyelinating Disease. Cell Rep 2017;20(6):1269–77.
100. Lavasani S, Dzhambazov B, Nouri M, et al. A novel probiotic mixture exerts a therapeutic effect on experimental autoimmune encephalomyelitis mediated by IL-10 producing regulatory T cells. PLoS One 2010;5(2). https://doi.org/10.1371/JOURNAL.PONE.0009009.

101. Salehipour Z, Haghmorad D, Sankian M, et al. Bifidobacterium animalis in combination with human origin of Lactobacillus plantarum ameliorate neuroinflammation in experimental model of multiple sclerosis by altering CD4+ T cell subset balance. Biomed Pharmacother 2017;95:1535–48.
102. Kouchaki E, Tamtaji OR, Salami M, et al. Clinical and metabolic response to probiotic supplementation in patients with multiple sclerosis: A randomized, double-blind, placebo-controlled trial. Clin Nutr 2017;36(5):1245–9.
103. Tankou SK, Regev K, Healy BC, et al. Investigation of probiotics in multiple sclerosis. Mult Scler 2018;24(1):58–63.
104. Vijay A, Astbury S, Le Roy C, et al. The prebiotic effects of omega-3 fatty acid supplementation: A six-week randomised intervention trial. Gut Microb 2021; 13(1):1–11.
105. Berer K, Martínez I, Walker A, et al. Dietary non-fermentable fiber prevents autoimmune neurological disease by changing gut metabolic and immune status. Sci Rep 2018;8(1). https://doi.org/10.1038/S41598-018-28839-3.
106. Luthold RV, Fernandes GR, Franco-de-Moraes AC, et al. Gut microbiota interactions with the immunomodulatory role of vitamin D in normal individuals. Metabolism 2017;69:76–86.
107. Fettig NM, Robinson HG, Allanach JR, et al. Inhibition of Th1 activation and differentiation by dietary guar gum ameliorates experimental autoimmune encephalomyelitis. Cell Rep 2022;40(11). https://doi.org/10.1016/J.CELREP.2022.111328.
108. Sintzel MB, Rametta M, Reder AT. Vitamin D and Multiple Sclerosis: A Comprehensive Review. Neurol Ther 2018;7(1):59–85.
109. Chiuso-Minicucci F, Ishikawa LLW, Mimura LAN, et al. Treatment with Vitamin D/MOG Association Suppresses Experimental Autoimmune Encephalomyelitis. PLoS One 2015;10(5). https://doi.org/10.1371/JOURNAL.PONE.0125836.
110. Mimura LAN, de Campos Fraga-Silva TF, de Oliveira LRC, et al. Preclinical Therapy with Vitamin D3 in Experimental Encephalomyelitis: Efficacy and Comparison with Paricalcitol. Int J Mol Sci 2021;22(4):1–21.
111. Adzemovic MZ, Zeitelhofer M, Hochmeister S, et al. Efficacy of vitamin D in treating multiple sclerosis-like neuroinflammation depends on developmental stage. Exp Neurol 2013;249:39–48.
112. Menni C, Zierer J, Pallister T, et al. Omega-3 fatty acids correlate with gut microbiome diversity and production of N-carbamylglutamate in middle aged and elderly women. Sci Rep 2017;7(1):1–11.
113. Bates D, Cartlidge NEF, French JM, et al. A double-blind controlled trial of long chain n-3 polyunsaturated fatty acids in the treatment of multiple sclerosis. J Neurol Neurosurg Psychiatry 1989;52(1):18–22.
114. Weinstock-Guttman B, Baier M, Park Y, et al. Low fat dietary intervention with omega-3 fatty acid supplementation in multiple sclerosis patients. Prostaglandins Leukot Essent Fatty Acids 2005;73(5):397–404.
115. Hoare S, Lithander F, Van Der Mei I, et al. Higher intake of omega-3 polyunsaturated fatty acids is associated with a decreased risk of a first clinical diagnosis of central nervous system demyelination: Results from the Ausimmune Study. Mult Scler 2016;22(7):884–92.
116. Torkildsen Ø, Wergeland S, Bakke S, et al. ω-3 fatty acid treatment in multiple sclerosis (OFAMS Study): a randomized, double-blind, placebo-controlled trial. Arch Neurol 2012;69(8):1044–51.
117. Bai M, Wang Y, Han R, et al. Intermittent caloric restriction with a modified fasting-mimicking diet ameliorates autoimmunity and promotes recovery in a

mouse model of multiple sclerosis. J Nutr Biochem 2021;87. https://doi.org/10.1016/J.JNUTBIO.2020.108493.
118. Piccio L, Stark JL, Cross AH. Chronic calorie restriction attenuates experimental autoimmune encephalomyelitis. J Leukoc Biol 2008;84(4):940–8.
119. Choi IY, Piccio L, Childress P, et al. A Diet Mimicking Fasting Promotes Regeneration and Reduces Autoimmunity and Multiple Sclerosis Symptoms. Cell Rep 2016;15(10):2136–46.
120. Cignarella F, Cantoni C, Ghezzi L, et al. Intermittent Fasting Confers Protection in CNS Autoimmunity by Altering the Gut Microbiota. Cell Metab 2018;27(6):1222–35.e6.
121. Fitzgerald KC, Vizthum D, Henry-Barron B, et al. Effect of intermittent vs. daily calorie restriction on changes in weight and patient-reported outcomes in people with multiple sclerosis. Mult Scler Relat Disord 2018;23:33–9.
122. Fitzgerald KC, Bhargava P, Smith MD, et al. Intermittent calorie restriction alters T cell subsets and metabolic markers in people with multiple sclerosis. EBioMedicine 2022;82.
123. Kim DY, Hao J, Liu R, et al. Inflammation-mediated memory dysfunction and effects of a ketogenic diet in a murine model of multiple sclerosis. PLoS One 2012;7(5). https://doi.org/10.1371/JOURNAL.PONE.0035476.
124. Storm-Larsen C, Myhr KM, Farbu E, et al. Gut microbiota composition during a 12-week intervention with delayed-release dimethyl fumarate in multiple sclerosis - a pilot trial. Mult Scler J Exp Transl Clin 2019;5(4). https://doi.org/10.1177/2055217319888767.
125. Bock M, Karber M, Kuhn H. Ketogenic diets attenuate cyclooxygenase and lipoxygenase gene expression in multiple sclerosis. EBioMedicine 2018;36:293–303.
126. Bock M, Steffen F, Zipp F, et al. Impact of Dietary Intervention on Serum Neurofilament Light Chain in Multiple Sclerosis. Neurology(R) neuroimmunology & neuroinflammation. 2021;9(1). https://doi.org/10.1212/NXI.0000000000001102.
127. Cox LM, Maghzi AH, Liu S, et al. Gut Microbiome in Progressive Multiple Sclerosis. Ann Neurol 2021;89(6):1195–211.
128. Castillo-Álvarez F, Pérez-Matute P, Oteo JA, et al. The influence of interferon β-1b on gut microbiota composition in patients with multiple sclerosis. Neurologia 2021;36(7):495–503.
129. Katz Sand I, Zhu Y, Ntranos A, et al. Disease-modifying therapies alter gut microbial composition in MS. Neurology(R) neuroimmunology & neuroinflammation. 2018;6(1). https://doi.org/10.1212/NXI.0000000000000517.
130. Li QR, Wang CY, Tang C, et al. Reciprocal interaction between intestinal microbiota and mucosal lymphocyte in cynomolgus monkeys after alemtuzumab treatment. Am J Transplant 2013;13(4):899–910.
131. Troci A, Zimmermann O, Esser D, et al. B-cell-depletion reverses dysbiosis of the microbiome in multiple sclerosis patients. Sci Rep 2022;12(1). https://doi.org/10.1038/S41598-022-07336-8.
132. Christiansen SH, Murphy RA, Juul-Madsen K, et al. The Immunomodulatory Drug Glatiramer Acetate is Also an Effective Antimicrobial Agent that Kills Gram-negative Bacteria. Sci Rep 2017;7(1). https://doi.org/10.1038/S41598-017-15969-3.

# Updates in NMOSD and MOGAD Diagnosis and Treatment

## A Tale of Two Central Nervous System Autoimmune Inflammatory Disorders

Laura Cacciaguerra, MD, PhD[a], Eoin P. Flanagan, MB, BCh[a,b,*]

**KEYWORDS**

• AQP4-IgG • MOG-IgG • Diagnosis • Treatment
• myelin oligodendrocyte glycoprotein • MOG • aquaporin-4
• neuromyelitis optica spectrum disorder

**KEY POINTS**

- The recognition of aquaporin-4-IgG positive neuromyelitis optica spectrum disorder (AQP4+NMOSD) and myelin-oligodendrocyte glycoprotein antibody-associated disease (MOGAD) as distinct disorders led to separate diagnostic criteria for each.
- AQP4-IgG is highly specific for NMOSD diagnosis at any titer. In contrast, caution is needed with low-titer myelin-oligodendrocyte glycoprotein-IgG (MOG-IgG), which can be encountered with other diseases.
- Recognition of the MRI features of AQP4+NMOSD and MOGAD is helpful because there are important discriminators between each other and multiple sclerosis.
- Maintenance treatment should be started after the first attack in AQP4+NMOSD but is generally not started until the second attack in MOGAD given the latter can have a monophasic course in more than half of cases.
- Studies elucidating the pathophysiology of AQP4+NMOSD led to the development of proven targeted treatments in AQP4+NMOSD, and similar analyses in MOGAD are underway in an attempt to develop attack-prevention treatments in that disease.

## INTRODUCTION

Aquaporin-4-IgG positive neuromyelitis optica spectrum disorder (AQP4+NMOSD) and myelin-oligodendrocytes glycoprotein antibody-associated disease (MOGAD)

[a] Department of Neurology, Mayo Clinic Center for Multiple Sclerosis and Autoimmune Neurology, Mayo Clinic, Rochester, MN, USA; [b] Laboratory Medicine and Pathology, Mayo Clinic, Rochester, MN, USA
* Corresponding author. Department of Neurology, 200 1st street SW, 55905, Rochester, MN, USA
*E-mail address:* Flanagan.Eoin@mayo.edu

Neurol Clin 42 (2024) 77–114
https://doi.org/10.1016/j.ncl.2023.06.009 **neurologic.theclinics.com**

are recently identified antibody-mediated autoimmune disorders of the central nervous system (CNS).[1,2]

Biomarkers of these diseases are antibodies targeting the aquaporin-4 (AQP4) water channel on the astrocyte end-feet in AQP4+NMOSD[3] and myelin-oligodendrocyte glycoprotein (MOG) on the outermost myelin sheath layer in MOGAD.[4]

For a long time, the clinical and radiological overlaps have hampered the recognition of these two diseases as separate entities. Initially, these disorders were considered variants of multiple sclerosis (MS), given their similar predilection for the optic nerve and spinal cord. Later, after the discovery of the AQP4-IgG, it was recognized that some patients with an NMOSD phenotype were negative for AQP4-IgG. After the discovery of MOG-IgG, it became apparent that some of these AQP4-IgG seronegative NMOSD cases were positive for MOG-IgG. However, the phenotype of MOGAD is much broader than that of NMOSD and only a minority of patients with MOGAD fulfilled NMOSD criteria.[5] Moreover, recent investigations have highlighted substantial prognostic differences in terms of relapse-risk and disability accrual during the disease course, supporting a separate pathophysiology for each. There are also important differences in demographic, clinical, radiologic, and pathologic features that resulted in the need for separate criteria for MOGAD from NMOSD. This ultimately led to the publication of separate diagnostic criteria for MOGAD in 2023 to capture these patients and no longer label them as seronegative NMOSD.[1]

### *Epidemiology of AQP4+NMOSD and MOGAD*

AQP4+NMOSD and MOGAD are rare disorders. The estimated annual incidence of AQP4+NMOSD is 0.4 to 7.3/million people[6,7]; it is largely unknown in MOGAD, although a few European studies estimated it at 1.6 to 3.4/million people.[8,9] AQP4+NMOSD mainly affects middle-aged women (40–60 years, 9:1 female to male ratio)[6,7] with a predilection for Afro-Caribbean or Asian individuals.[6,7] MOGAD incidence has a biphasic behavior, with a peak of incidence in children (reported up to 3 times higher)[9] and later in young adults (20–30 years).[10–12] No clear sex preference or high-risk ethnicities have been identified in MOGAD thus far.

### *Pathophysiology of AQP4+NMOSD and MOGAD*

Similar to most autoimmune disorders, the first step of the pathophysiological cascade is represented by an unknown mechanism of loss of self-tolerance, which occurs in the periphery. B cells differentiate into antibody-producing plasmablasts that secrete the pathological autoantibodies that eventually enter the CNS.[13,14] Antibody production and entry into the CNS may be facilitated by high levels of a proinflammatory cytokine called interleukin-6 (IL-6), which increases blood–brain barrier permeability and promotes differentiation of B cells into plasmablasts to enhance antibody-production.[15] Alternatively, CNS regions free of the blood–brain barrier, such as the area postrema, may be another route of entry, especially in AQP4+NMOSD. However, intrathecal MOG-IgG production is reported in MOGAD but not AQP4+NMOSD.[16–20]

Other major differences in pathophysiology emerge once the respective antibodies reach the CNS. AQP4-IgGs bind to the water channel on astrocytes at the blood–brain barrier.[3] The binding between the antibody and its target activates the classical pathway of the complement cascade, with primary damage to the astrocytes through the formation of the membrane attack complex and antibody-dependent cellular cytotoxicity.[13] Meanwhile, secondary products of complement activation, such as the C5a anaphylatoxin, act as a chemoattractant for granulocytes, which are locally recruited and cause secondary axonal loss and eventually demyelination in bystander tissue.[13]

This pathogenesis is supported by pathology findings in AQP4+NMOSD showing: (1) antibody and complement deposition, (2) astrocyte damage or loss (even outside of lesioned tissue) with reduced AQP4 expression, (3) granulocyte infiltration, and (4) secondary demyelination and axonal loss in the white matter and gray matter.[21]

The mechanism of CNS damage has yet to be fully elucidated in MOGAD. One reason is that human MOG-IgG do not usually cross-react with rodent MOG, making studies of animal models more challenging. The selective loss of MOG is also inconsistent in human pathology samples,[22,23] raising doubts on the pathogenicity of MOG-IgG. However, MOG-IgG pathogenicity was supported by using the small proportion of MOG-IgG that does cross-react to MOG rodent epitopes, showing that intrathecal MOG-IgG induces a similar disease to humans in murine models.[24]

According to the most recent hypothesis, in the CNS the binding between MOG-IgG and myelin may lead to increased local production of IL-6 and B-cell activating factor (BAFF), with recruitment of CD4+ T cells and macrophages that will ultimately damage neurons and oligodendrocytes.[14] Complement may also contribute to MOGAD pathophysiology, as supported by preclinical models,[25] evidence of complement deposition with antibody-dependent cellular phagocytosis on pathology samples[22,23,26] and higher activation of both the classic and alternative complement pathways in patients than healthy individuals.[27] However, complement activation seems less effective with MOG-IgG than AQP4-IgG, possibly because most patients have bivalent binding MOG-IgG, which are known to be less effective in complement activation.[28] In addition, MOG-IgGs were able to induce demyelination also by activating the neonatal Fc-receptor pathway, which enhanced the activation and tissue infiltration by T cells in animal models.[29] The involvement of CD4+ T cells represents one of the main differences with MS, where CD8+ T cells are usually predominant on pathology samples.[22]

Cytokine profiling is similar in AQP4+NMOSD and MOGAD but different to MS, showing upregulation of T helper 17-related and some T helper 1-related molecules.[30]

Differences and similarities in AQP4+NMOSD and MOGAD pathophysiology are summarized in **Table 1** and graphically shown in **Fig. 1**.

## AQP4+NMOSD AND MOGAD DIAGNOSIS

### *Summary of Core Clinical Manifestations*

AQP4+NMOSD and MOGAD share several core clinical features, namely the presence of optic neuritis and myelitis, and are discussed below:

- *Optic neuritis* is associated with variable degrees of visual loss, eye pain worsened by eye movements, and dyschromatopsia. At disease onset, it is the most common presentation in adult MOGAD (50%–65%)[14] and relatively common in AQP4+NMOSD (35%).[31] It can occur in isolation, in association with myelitis, or in the context of acute disseminated encephalomyelitis (ADEM).[1,2] In contrast to MS, bilateral simultaneous involvement of the optic nerves is common in both AQP4+NMOSD (17%–82%)[32,33] and MOGAD (50%–84%).[33,34] Visual loss at nadir is usually severe with a median visual acuity of hand movement in AQP4+NMOSD and between hand movements and count fingers in MOGAD.[35,36] Clues suggesting a diagnosis of MOGAD may be the presence of eye pain before the onset of visual loss (often mistaken for headache, especially in children)[37] and evidence of optic disc edema at fundoscopy (86%–90%)[11,36] that is often moderate to severe and sometimes accompanied by peripapillary hemorrhages.[36] At follow-up, recovery is usually complete or almost complete

**Table 1**
**Differences and similarities in AQP4+NMOSD and MOGAD pathophysiology**

| | AQP4+NMOSD | MOGAD |
|---|---|---|
| Targets | | |
| Antigen | AQP4 | MOG |
| Cell | Astrocyte | Oligodendrocyte |
| Site of antibody production | | |
| Periphery | Yes | Yes |
| CNS | No | Yes |
| Cytokines | | |
| IL-6 | Yes | Yes |
| IL-10 | Yes | Yes |
| IL-17a | Yes | Yes |
| G-CSF | Yes | Yes |
| TNF-alfa | Yes | Yes |
| BAFF/APRIL | Yes | Yes |
| Effectors of damage | | |
| Complement | Yes | Yes, but less prominent |
| Cell infiltrates | Granulocytes | CD4+T cells, macrophages/microglia |
| Outcomes | | |
| Neuronal loss | Yes | Yes, but less severe |
| Astrocytic damage | Yes | No |
| Oligodendrocyte damage | Not prominent | Yes |
| Demyelination | Yes | Yes |
| Damage Biomarkers | | |
| Neurofilament light chain | High (during attacks) | High (during attacks) |
| GFAP | High | Normal |
| Myelin basic protein | Normal | High |

*Abbreviations:* APRIL, a proliferation-inducing ligand; AQP4, aquaporin-4; AQP4+NMOSD, aquaporin-4-IgG positive neuromyelitis optica spectrum disorder; BAFF, B-cell activating factor; CD4, cluster of differentiation 4; G-CSF, granulocytes colony-stimulating factor; GFAP, glial fibrillary acidic protein; IL, interleukin; MOG, myelin oligodendrocyte glycoprotein; MOGAD, myelin oligodendrocyte glycoprotein antibody-associated disease; TNF-alfa, tumor necrosis factor-alfa.

in MOGAD (visual acuity of 20/30 or 20/25),[35,36] whereas recovery can be partial or absent in AQP4+NMOSD (median visual acuity of count fingers).[35] Residual permanent blindness in at least one eye (ie, visual acuity of ≤20/200) is rare in MOGAD (6%–12%)[35,36] and relatively common in AQP4+NMOSD (60%–69%).[32,35] However, a proportion of patients with MOGAD (16%)[36] may develop a steroid-dependent chronic form of optic neuropathy, which relapses at steroid-withdrawal or tapering (chronic relapsing inflammatory optic neuropathy).

- *Myelitis*: these episodes are characterized by acute/subacute onset of motor, sensory, and autonomic symptoms indicating an involvement of the spinal cord, including but not limited to para/tetraparesis or plegia, sensory level across the trunk, Lhermitte's phenomenon, sphincteric urgency or retention, and sexual dysfunction. Myelitis is the most common presentation in patients with

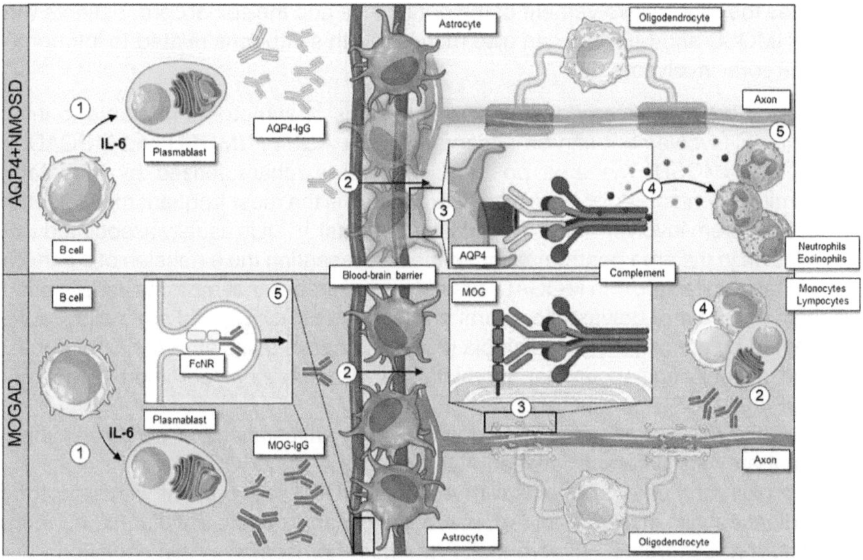


**Fig. 1. AQP4+NMOSD and MOGAD pathogenesis.** AQP4+NMOSD: 1. IL-6 promotes the differentiation of B cells into AQP4-IgG secreting plasmablasts; 2. AQP4-IgGs reach the blood stream and cross the blood–brain barrier; 3. AQP4-IgGs bind to AQP4 on astrocytes and activate the complement cascade through the classical pathway leading to astrocyte damage; 4. The release of anaphylatoxins after complement activation recruit granulocytes, which will ultimately damage neurons and eventually, although not primarily, oligodendrocytes (5). MOGAD: 1. IL-6 promotes the differentiation of B cells into MOG-IgG secreting plasmablasts; 2. MOG-IgGs reach the blood stream and cross the blood–brain barrier but recent evidence suggest they might also be produced intrathecally; 3. MOG-IgGs bind to MOG on oligodendrocytes and activate the complement cascade through the classical pathway leading to olygodendrocyte damage; 4. Local inflammation recruits T cells and monocytes/macrophages; and 5. MOG-IgGs recycling in the blood stream seems to contribute to the persistence of the mechanism of damage. Figure created with Biorender.com. Abbreviations: AQP4, aquaporin-4; AQP4+NMOSD, aquaporin-4-IgG positive neuromyelitis optica spectrum disorder; IL-6, interleukin-6; MOG, myelin oligodendrocyte glycoprotein; MOGAD, myelin oligodendrocyte glycoprotein antibody-associated disease.

AQP4+NMOSD (50%)[31] but also occurs in 20% to 40% of adult and 15% to 20% of pediatric MOGAD.[14] Similar to optic neuritis, attacks are usually moderate or severe at nadir, with a median expanded disability status scale (EDSS) of 7.0 in AQP4+NMOSD and 5.5 in MOGAD.[38] More than 30% of patients are wheelchair dependent at nadir in both diseases,[39] and there is a potential need for admission to the intensive care unit for mechanic ventilation due to respiratory failure, especially in AQP4+NMOSD (2%–7%).[40,41] In the long term, only 6% to 7% of MOGAD compared with 37% to 44% of AQP4+NMOSD will need a gait aid.[38,39] In MOGAD, residual sphincteric dysfunction may persist over time in more than 50% of patients with history of myelitis with many requiring ongoing intermittent urinary catheterization.[38] The presence of an accompanying itch,[42] or the development of painful paroxysmal tonic spasms[43] should prompt AQP4-IgG testing because they are more typical of AQP4+NMOSD. In contrast, the presence of acute flaccid weakness with areflexia may suggest MOGAD and could reflect the involvement of the anterior gray matter. This presentation may mimic the acute flaccid myelitis that has been reported to follow enterovirus infection.[39]

Besides the clinical involvement of the optic nerve and the spinal cord, patients with AQP4+NMOSD and MOGAD can also manifest with symptoms related to infratentorial or cerebral involvement:

- *(Acute) brainstem/cerebellar syndromes*: signs or symptoms referable to infratentorial involvement can be observed in both AQP4+NMOSD and MOGAD. In AQP4+NMOSD, the area postrema syndrome, characterized by intractable vomiting or hiccups for days to several weeks, is the most frequent manifestation of brainstem involvement (16%–60% of patients).[1,44] It is usually associated with a lesion in the area postrema, sometimes representing the extension of a cervical spinal cord lesion.[45] In MOGAD, brainstem or cerebellar symptoms usually occur in the context of polyfocal cerebral involvement or ADEM, and are mainly represented by ataxia (45%) or diplopia (26%).[44] Attacks of isolated facial numbness and diplopia and trigeminal neuralgia are all much more common in MS than AQP4+NMOSD or MOGAD.
- *Cerebral manifestations*: The frequency and manifestations of cerebral involvement are very different between AQP4+NMOSD and MOGAD.

  Approximately 3% of patients with AQP4+NMOSD may present with symptoms of diencephalic involvement (eg, narcolepsy, inappropriate antidiuretic hormone secretion syndrome, hyperphagia, thermic homeostasis dysregulation, and dysfunction of the hypothalamus–hypophysis axis).[46,47] Other cerebral manifestations, including encephalopathy, ADEM, posterior-reversible encephalopathy, and seizures have been reported as well but are rare.[48,49]

  In MOGAD, ADEM represents the most common presenting manifestation in pediatric patients (20%–60%), especially in those aged younger than 12 years.[2,14] It is defined by the concomitant presence of polyfocal CNS symptoms, unexplained encephalopathy, and large poorly demarcated lesions in the gray and white matter at MRI.[50] Severe encephalopathy or status epilepticus can lead to inability to protect the airway and the need for mechanical ventilation.[41] Despite the potential severity of the acute phase, recovery is usually good although deficits in cognition have been reported.[51–53]

  Finally, patients with MOGAD may present with cerebral cortical encephalitis, a recently described phenotype characterized by clinical manifestations (ie, headache [79%], seizures [68%], encephalopathy [63%], and fever [42%])[54] and typical T2-FLAIR cortical hyperintensity with corresponding leptomeningeal or cortical gadolinium enhancement.[54,55] It is observed in almost 7% of all patients but is more common in children (13.5%) than in adults (3.6%).[54] Cerebral cortical encephalitis often precedes other short-term MOGAD attacks. Radiological abnormalities resolve in more than 90% of patients[54] and can occasionally improve without acute immunotherapy.[56]

### *Major MRI Features*

MRI is useful when it comes to differentiating between AQP4+NMOSD and MOGAD. Details are provided below:

- *Optic nerve imaging*: It is essential to order orbital MRI with fat-saturated images to have sufficient sensitivity to confirm optic neuritis but also to be able to adequately identify discriminators because conventional MRI brain is inadequate for the evaluation of the optic nerve. Optic neuritis is frequently bilateral and severe in both AQP4+NMOSD and MOGAD. In both cases long-segments of inflammation (ie, T2-hyperintensity or gadolinium enhancement involving more than half the distance from the orbit to the chiasm) are common.[1,2,57] However, lesions usually involve the anterior portion of the optic nerves in MOGAD (sometimes with optic nerve head swelling visible on MRI)[2] and are commonly posteriorly located involving the chiasm and the optic tracts in AQP4+NMOSD.[1,33] Isolated optic chiasm involvement is more characteristic of AQP4+NMOSD but MOGAD optic nerve enhancement may extend to involve the chiasm relatively frequently with MOGAD optic neuritis.[58] Enhancement of the optic nerve sheath (perioptic enhancement/optic perineuritis) and extension to the orbital fat can also be observed in 50% of MOGAD-related optic neuritis[36] and may help discriminate from MS.[59] In both disorders asymptomatic enhancement may be observed at the site of prior optic neuritis in approximately 20% of patients, possibly representing subclinical blood–brain barrier leakage or residual inflammation.[60,61] Chronic atrophy of the optic nerve or optic disc occurs in 12% to 83% of AQP4+NMOSD,[57,62] and can be clinically observed in MOGAD. Examples of acute and chronic MRI findings are shown in **Fig. 2**, with the corresponding schematic representation in **Fig. 3**.

- *Spinal cord imaging*: During acute myelitis, AQP4+NMOSD and MOGAD involve similar regions of the cord, although conus involvement favors MOGAD.[39,63] Approximately 85% of patients with AQP4+NMOSD and 70% of patients with MOGAD with acute myelitis demonstrate longitudinally extensive spinal cord T2-lesions,[39] which by definition extend over at least 3 vertebral segments on

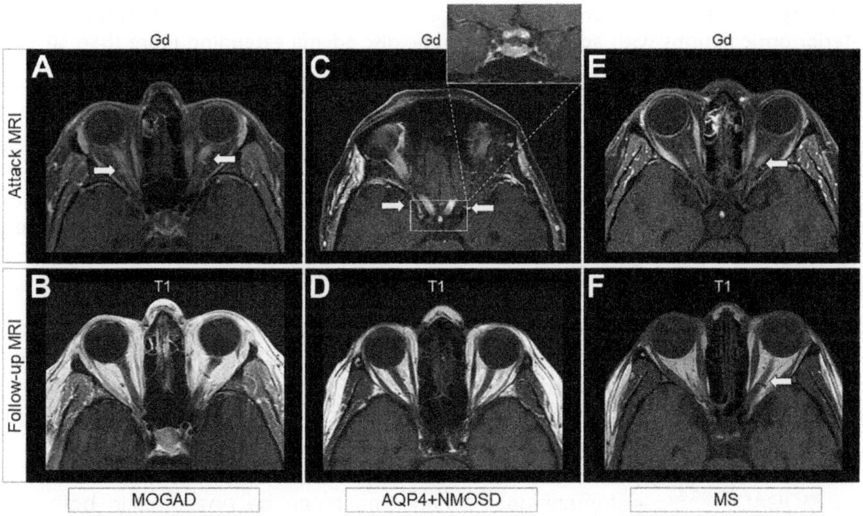


**Fig. 2. MRI examples of optic neuritis in patients with MOGAD, AQP4+NMOSD, and MS.** Top row shows MRI findings during the acute phase (postcontrast T1-weighted images with fat saturation), whereas follow-up imaging is displayed in the bottom row (precontrast T1-weighted images without fat saturation). Unless otherwise specified, images are all shown in axial view. MOGAD: Bilateral anterior optic neuritis (*A, arrows*) extending more than 50% of optic nerve length on the right side (ie, long optic neuritis), and short on the left side, with no or minimal residual optic nerve atrophy (*B*). AQP4+NMOSD: Bilateral optic neuritis (*C, arrows*) involving the chiasm (zoom-in picture, coronal detail) with mild residual atrophy (*D*). MS: Unilateral short left optic neuritis (*E, arrow*) with mild residual focal atrophy (*F*). Abbreviations: AQP4+NMOSD, aquaporin-4-IgG positive neuromyelitis optica spectrum disorder; Gd, postcontrast T1-weighted images; MOGAD, myelin oligodendrocyte glycoprotein antibody-associated disease; MS, multiple sclerosis; T1, precontrast T1-weighted images.

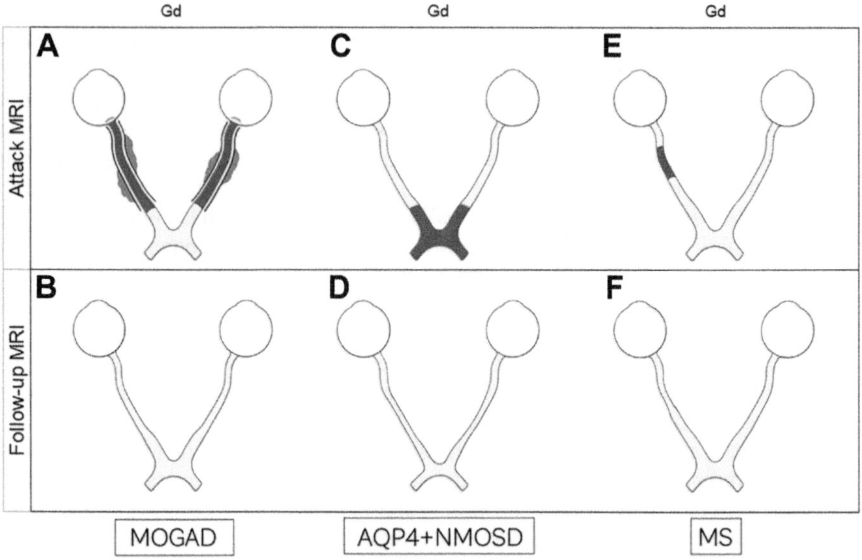


**Fig. 3. Optic neuritis in patients with MOGAD, AQP4+NMOSD, and MS**. Top row shows schematic representation of the optic nerve during the acute phase, while follow-up imaging is displayed in the bottom row. All images are shown in axial view. MOGAD: Bilateral anterior optic neuritis with accompanying optic disc edema extending more than 50% of optic nerve length bilaterally with optic nerve sheaths and perioptic fat involvement (*A*) and minimal residual optic nerve atrophy (*B*). AQP4+NMOSD: Bilateral optic neuritis involving the chiasm (*C*) with residual atrophy (*D*). MS: Unilateral short right optic neuritis (*E*) with residual focal atrophy (*F*). (Used with permission of Mayo Foundation for Medical Education and Research, all rights reserved.) Abbreviations: AQP4+NMOSD, aquaporin-4-IgG positive neuromyelitis optica spectrum disorder; Gd, postcontrast T1-weighted images; MOGAD, myelin oligodendrocyte glycoprotein antibody-associated disease; MS, multiple sclerosis.

sagittal T2-weighted images.[2,46] By contrast, longitudinally-extensive lesions in MS myelitis occur in less than 1%, although occasionally coalescence of multiple short lesions can artifactually appear longitudinally-extensive, and hazy longitudinally-extensive T2-hyperintensity can be sometimes encountered in chronic MS .[64] T2-lesions are more likely to be solitary in AQP4+NMOSD and multiple in MOGAD.[39] Acute gadolinium enhancement (elongated ring-like, patchy) is almost invariably present in AQP4+NMOSD but less frequent and more faint in MOGAD[39,65,66]; leptomeningeal enhancement can be observed in both diseases.[65,67] To note, around 10% of acute myelitis in MOGAD initially have a normal MRI, which will usually reveal spinal cord abnormalities after a median delay of 6 days.[68]

T2-lesions on axial images are usually central and involve the gray and the white matter,[2,69] although T2-hyperintensity restricted to the gray matter in an H-shaped fashion (*H-sign*) is more frequent in MOGAD than AQP4+NMOSD.[39] Marked central canal T2-hyperintensity may occur with AQP4+NMOSD and MOGAD but is rare in MS and this signal change usually resolves in follow-up.[70] It may reflect a potential space from incomplete closure of the central canal that becomes apparent in the setting of central spinal cord inflammation and swelling.[70] Another transient radiological sign helpful in differentiating AQP4+NMOSD from MS and potentially MOGAD is the evidence of spinal cord lesions with areas of T2-hyperintensity at least equal to the cerebrospinal fluid (*brighter spotty lesions*), which tend to be more extensive than just an enlarged central canal and are more common in AQP4+NMOSD.[71–73]

The severity of chronic atrophy is proportional to the number of myelitis in AQP4+NMOSD and MOGAD,[74] is mainly lesional rather than diffuse, and long segments of atrophy can be a clue to AQP4+NMOSD diagnosis.[38,69]

Examples of acute and chronic MRI findings are shown in **Fig. 4**, with the corresponding schematic representation in **Fig. 5**.

• *Brain imaging*: Brain lesions are observed in up to 80% of patients with AQP4+NMOSD.[75] MRI findings have been extensively analyzed and classified in 2015, with the definition of typical and nonspecific lesions.[46] Typical lesions are usually observed at periependymal level,[46] following regions of high AQP4 expression.[76] Among them, periependymal lesions along the lateral ventricles are the most common (12%–40%),[46] especially in the course of cerebral attacks.[77] Corresponding pencil-thin linear ependymal enhancement is typical of AQP4+NMOSD and is neither found in MOGAD nor found in MS.[78]

During the acute phase, lesions may demonstrate typical patterns of heterogeneous appearance (*marbled pattern*) or homogeneous involvement of the splenium (*arch bridge pattern*), which may help diagnosis.[46] Of note, callosal lesions can also be observed in patients with MOGAD at a similar frequency but their size rarely exceeds 2.5 cm (11%) and the extracallosal brain involvement is common (55%).[77] Callosal lesions can resolve in the chronic phase, although with a higher rate in MOGAD than AQP4+NMOSD (56% vs 15%).[77] The shape of callosal lesions may also help differentiate MS, where lesions are usually focal ovoid, with sharp margins, and with the major axis perpendicular to the lateral ventricles.[79]

Other periependymal lesions in AQP4+NMOSD may surround the third ventricle resulting in diencephalic involvement (ie, thalamus, hypothalamus, and anterior border of the midbrain) that may be asymptomatic. Diencephalic lesions favor AQP4+NMOSD over MS, although rarely encountered (6% of patients with AQP4+NMOSD).[75] Finally, periependymal lesions around the cerebral aqueduct and the fourth ventricle are also relatively frequent (7%–46% of patients with AQP4+NMOSD), and those in the dorsal medulla can involve the area postrema causing the hallmark clinical syndrome with intractable nausea, vomiting and hiccups.[46] Other brain lesions considered typical of AQP4+NMOSD are those in the cerebral peduncles and corticospinal tracts and large hemispheric lesions in the white matter (ie, with maximum transverse diameter of >3 cm, often spindle-like or with a radial shape). Similar lesions have also been reported in patients with MOGAD.[80] Tumefactive lesions (≥2 cm) are more frequent in MOGAD than AQP4+NMOSD (22% vs 5%).[81]

Small nonspecific lesions (ie, <3 mm) in the subcortical and deep white matter, similar to those encountered in aging, small vessel disease or migraine, are the most common type of brain lesions in patients with AQP4+NMOSD (35%–84%).[46]

Other than the ependymal enhancement, also cloud-like, nodular, and leptomeningeal enhancement were considered typical of AQP4+NMOSD. However, more recent investigations suggest that cloud-like and nodular enhancement may be encountered with a similar frequency also in MOGAD and MS,[78,81] whereas the leptomeningeal enhancement is much more common in MOGAD (46% of cerebral attacks) and can actually help discriminate from AQP4+NMOSD (7%) and MS (4%).[78] Persistent enhancement over 3 months is rare in all these disorders.[78]

Similar to the variety of cerebral manifestations, the radiological features of brain MRI in MOGAD are heterogeneous. Brain lesions can be found in 42% to 53% of patients with MOGAD,[82] and include lesions in the deep gray matter, cortical lesions, subcortical

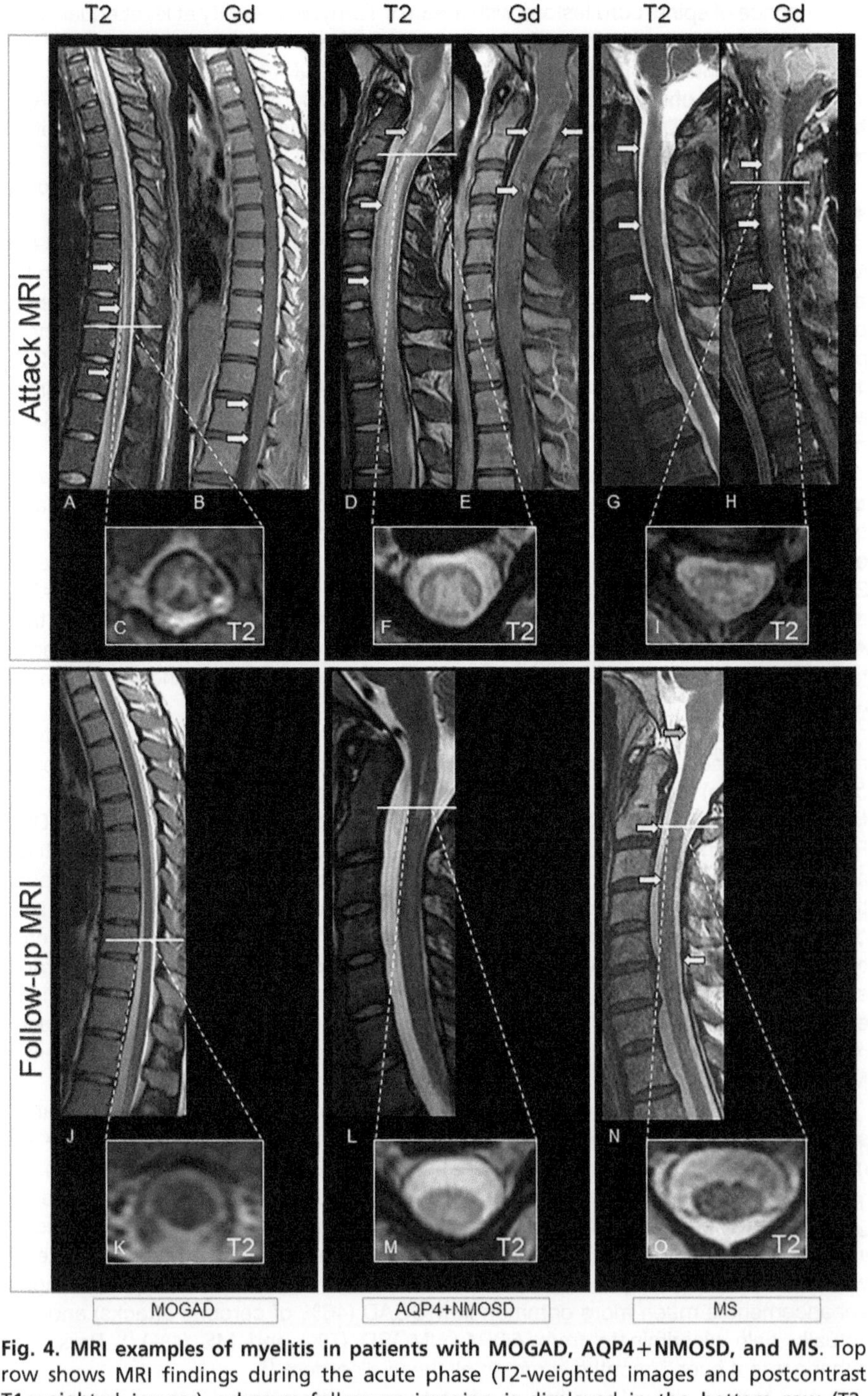


**Fig. 4. MRI examples of myelitis in patients with MOGAD, AQP4+NMOSD, and MS.** Top row shows MRI findings during the acute phase (T2-weighted images and postcontrast T1-weighted images), whereas follow-up imaging is displayed in the bottom row (T2-weighted images). MOGAD: Longitudinally extensive myelitis (ie, T2-lesion extending over at least 3 continuous vertebral segments) with a linear appearance involving the thoracic

or juxtacortical lesions, brainstem and cerebellar lesions, large hemispheric lesions, and, rarely, leukodystrophy-like patterns.[63,82,83] Among all these locations, lesions in the deep gray matter[63,82] and large lesions in the middle cerebellar peduncles[44] are the most characteristic and more common in MOGAD than in AQP4+NMOSD. Diffuse involvement of the pons and/or adjacent to the fourth ventricle (anterior location) may also favor MOGAD over AQP4+NMOSD, although not confirmed in all studies.[44,82]

Brain lesions in this disease are usually poorly demarcated (fluffy),[84] in line with what is observed in patients with ADEM,[50] of which conversely 50% test positive for MOG-IgG.[85] Transient faint T1-hypointensity can occur in the acute phase of MOGAD but chronic T1 hypointensities are rare and are much more suggestive of MS.[81] Cortical lesions in MOGAD usually occur during episodes of cerebral cortical encephalitis, are visible on fluid-attenuated inversion recovery (FLAIR) images and involve large cortical areas.[54,55] This contrasts with MS, where the assessment of cortical lesions may be less visible on conventional sequences and are better identified using advanced sequences such as double inversion recovery, phase sensitive inversion recovery, or magnetization-prepared rapid gradient-echo.[86,87] Furthermore, evidence of cortical lesions also favors MOGAD over AQP4+NMOSD, as in the latter cortical involvement was absent[75,88,89] or rarely[90,91] found.

Examples of acute and chronic MRI findings with the corresponding schematic representation are shown in **Figs. 6** and **7** (MOGAD), **Figs. 8** and **9** (AQP4+NMOSD), and **Figs. 10** and **11** (MS).

## REMISSION MRI

Finally, although not specifically covered by the diagnostic criteria, remission MRI may be relevant for the differentiation of AQP4+NMOSD, MOGAD, and MS given their different behavior in terms of T2-lesion resolution and accumulation of asymptomatic lesions.

After the acute event, brain T2-lesion resolution is very common in MOGAD (60%–79%),[2,81,92–94] can occasionally be observed in AQP4+NMOSD (14%–27%),[44,81,93,95] and is very rare in MS (0%–17%).[44,81,92,93] Similar findings are observed in the spinal

cord down to the conus (A, *arrows*, sagittal view). There is associated H-sign (ie, exclusive involvement of the gray matter; C, axial view). Enhancement is absent, except for a mild leptomeningeal enhancement of the conus (B, *arrows*, sagittal view). The T2-lesion completely resolved on T2-weighted images at follow-up (J, sagittal view and K, axial view), with no evident atrophy. AQP4+NMOSD: Longitudinally extensive myelitis with a T2-lesion starting from the area postrema and involving the cervical cord (D, *arrows*, sagittal view) with associated swelling. Intralesional increased focal T2-hyperintensity similar to the cerebrospinal fluid (CSF; ie, brighter spotty lesion) is also present (D, green *arrow*). The T2-lesion is centrally located in both the gray and the white matter (F). Enhancement is inhomogeneous (E, *arrows*, sagittal view). At follow-up, the T2-lesion reduced in size on T2-weighted images (L, sagittal view and M, axial view) although still present. Residual atrophy of the cord is particularly evident on axial view (M). MS: Multiple focal short spinal cord T2-lesions (G, *arrows*, sagittal view) located in the peripheral white matter (I, axial view). All lesions enhance, with the bottom lesion showing a ring-pattern of enhancement (H, *arrows*, sagittal view). T2-lesions reduce in size and prominence of T2-hyperintensity persists on follow-up T2-weighted images (N, *arrows*, sagittal view and O, axial view). The patient also developed an interval T2-lesion (N, green *arrow*). Abbreviations: AQP4+NMOSD, aquaporin-4-IgG positive neuromyelitis optica spectrum disorder; Gd, postcontrast T1-weighted images; MOGAD, myelin oligodendrocyte glycoprotein antibody-associated disease; MS, multiple sclerosis; T2, T2-weighted images.

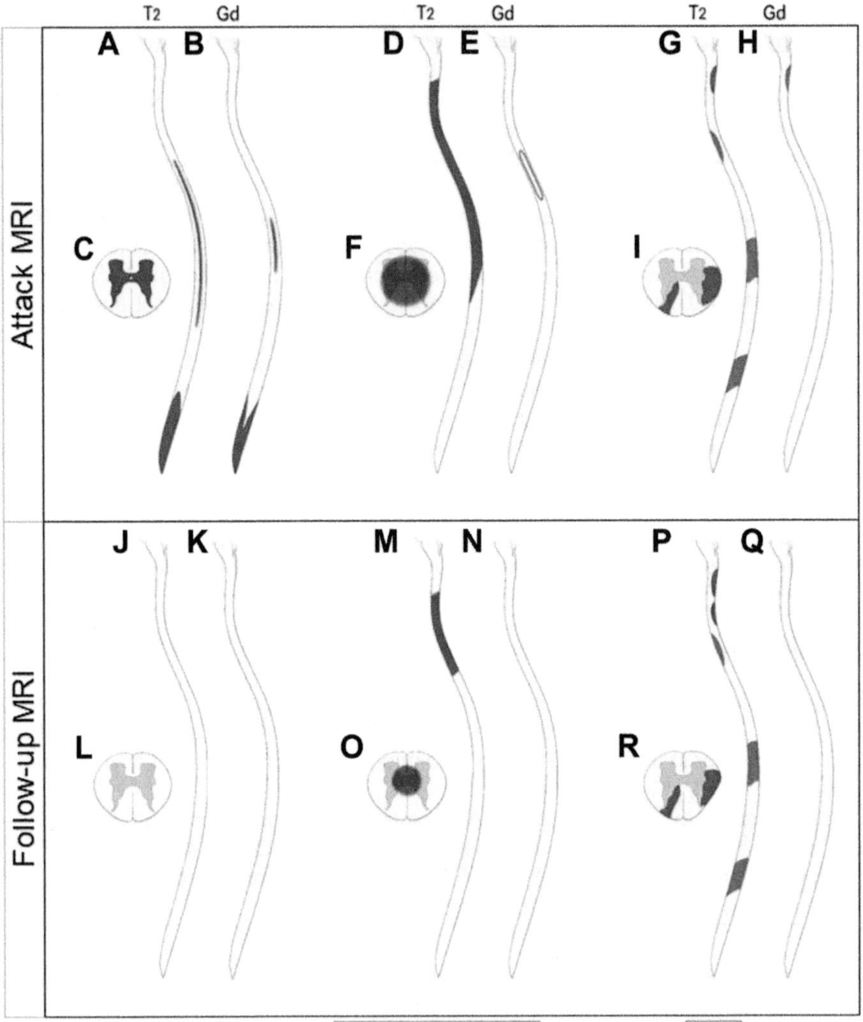


**Fig. 5. Myelitis in patients with MOGAD, AQP4+NMOSD, and MS**. Top row shows spinal cord findings during the acute phase (T2-weighted images and postcontrast T1-weighted images), whereas follow-up imaging is displayed in the bottom row (T2-weighted images). MOGAD: Longitudinally extensive myelitis with a linear T2-lesion appearance involving the lower cervical and upper to middle thoracic cord and another lesion in the conus (A, sagittal view). There is associated H-sign with the T2-lesion restricted to gray matter (C, axial view). Minimum linear enhancement and leptomeningeal enhancement of the conus (B, sagittal view). The T2-lesion completely resolved on T2-weighted images at follow-up (J, sagittal view and L, axial view), with no evident atrophy. Gadolinium enhancement resolved (K). AQP4+NMOSD: Longitudinally extensive myelitis with a T2-lesion involving the cervical and thoracic cord (D, sagittal view) with elongated ring enhancement (E). The T2-lesion is centrally located in both the gray and the white matter (F, axial view). At follow-up, the lesion is smaller on T2-weighted images (M, sagittal and O, axial view) although still present. Gadolinium enhancement resolved (N). MS: Multiple focal short spinal cord T2-lesions (G, sagittal view) located in the peripheral white matter (I, axial view). One lesion shows

cord, where 67% to 79% of lesions will ultimately resolve in MOGAD.[92–94] T2-lesion resolution in MOGAD occurs at approximately 3 months from appearance but can be faster for small lesions.[94] Steroid administration favors resolution of large lesions (ie, $\geq$1 cm) but is not a necessary condition because spontaneous resolution is observed in more than half T2-lesions not undergoing any acute treatment.[94] In contrast, concomitant T1-hypointensity during the acute phase reduces the likelihood of lesions resolving over time.[94] Altogether, these observations (ie, spontaneous resolution, steroid response, effect of T1-hypointensity, and timing of resolution) suggest that this phenomenon is part of the natural history of MOGAD and relies on at least 3 factors: edema reabsorption, mild tissue damage, and postacute healing processes such as, for instance, remyelination.[94]

Large reductions and progressive fragmentation is typical in AQP4+NMOSD, although complete resolution is rare,[92,93,96] and persistence of T2-lesions is the rule in MS.[92,93]

Surveillance MRI outside of attacks is standard of care in MS as new asymptomatic lesions or enlarging T2-lesions are well recognized to occur particularly with low or moderate efficacy medication and their presence may lead to treatment escalation. However, new asymptomatic T2-lesions or enlarging T2-lesions are far less common in MS when high-efficacy treatments are used. The presence of new or enlarging T2-lesions has been commonly used in MS clinical trials as a surrogate end-point.[97] In AQP4+NMOSD and MOGAD, the frequency of new or enlarging asymptomatic T2-lesions is rare and estimated between 3% and 13%[98–101] and between 3% and 14%,[100–102] respectively. This has implications for clinical practice because surveillance MRIs are generally not recommended in AQP4+NMOSD or MOGAD. Moreover, it has implications for upcoming clinical trials in these disorders because this will be a less useful clinical trial endpoint.

**Table 2** summarizes the main radiological features of AQP4+NMOSD, MOGAD, and MS.

### *AQP4-IgG and MOG-IgG Testing*

Some basic knowledge of the antibody testing methodology, the optimal specimen and technique, and potential pitfalls is crucial given their importance in diagnosis of AQP4+NMOSD and MOGAD. The cell-based assay (CBA) technique and analysis in serum is generally recommended for AQP4-IgG and MOG-IgG, with live CBA conferring some advantages over the fixed technique.[2,103]

*AQP4-IgG testing*: Live or fixed CBA with immunofluorescence or flow cytometry/fluorescence-activated cell sorting (FACS)-based detection or quantification are recommended for AQP4-IgG testing because they demonstrated high sensitivity (69.7%–100.0%) and the highest specificity (85.8%–100.0%) in independent cohorts.[95,104,105] Older generation techniques using mouse tissue-based immunofluorescence have lower sensitivity although reasonably high specificity.[106] The enzyme-linked immunosorbent assay has lower sensitivity and a false-positive rate 5-fold higher than CBA,

homogeneous nodular enhancement (H, sagittal view). T2-lesions reduce in size and persist on follow-up T2-weighted images (P, sagittal view and R, axial view) with development of focal left-sided spinal cord atrophy particularly evident on axial images (R). A new interval T2-lesion is also present (P). Gadolinium enhancement resolved (Q). (Used with permission of Mayo Foundation for Medical Education and Research, all rights reserved.) Abbreviations: AQP4+NMOSD, aquaporin-4-IgG positive neuromyelitis optica spectrum disorder; Gd, postcontrast T1-weighted images; MOGAD, myelin oligodendrocyte glycoprotein antibody-associated disease; MS, multiple sclerosis; T2, T2-weighted images.

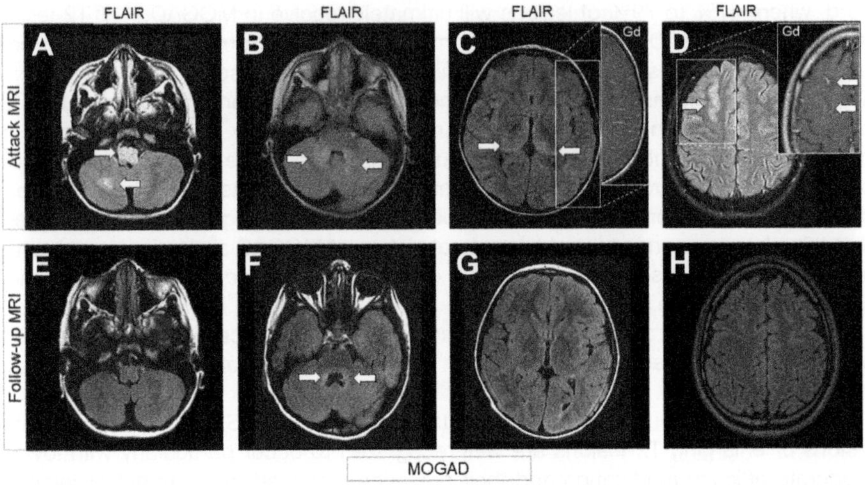


**Fig. 6. MRI examples of brain lesions in patients with MOGAD**. Top row shows MRI findings during the acute phase, whereas follow-up imaging is displayed in the bottom row. Images are in axial view. Poorly defined (ie, fluffy) T2-lesions in the entire medulla and cerebellum (*A, arrows*), completely resolving at follow-up imaging (*E*). Bilateral fluffy T2-lesions in the middle cerebellar peduncles (*B, arrows*) with reduction in size but persistence at follow-up (*F, arrows*) with accompanying fourth ventricle ex vacuo enlargement. Bilateral fluffy T2-lesions of the thalami (*C, arrows*) in a patient with prominent leptomeningeal enhancement (zoom-in picture, postcontrast T1-weighted sequence) undergoing complete resolution at follow-up (*G*). Patient with cerebral cortical encephalitis showing an extensive cortical T2-lesion (*D, arrow*) with focal enhancement (zoom-in picture, postcontrast T1-weighted sequence), completely resolved at follow-up (*H*). Abbreviations: FLAIR, fluid-attenuated inversion recovery; Gd, postcontrast T1-weighted images; MOGAD, myelin oligodendrocyte glycoprotein antibody-associated disease.

particularly with low-positive results.[104,105] False positives are usually low titers and confirmatory testing with one or more different assays is recommended.[1] However, evidence of low-positive results in the context of live CBA assays can be considered reliable because different live CBA assays demonstrated a strong agreement irrespective of antibody titer (100% concordance in high positive and 79% in low-positive patients).[107]

False negatives may be also encountered (especially in patients receiving immunosuppressive treatments or when tested just after plasma exchange)[1] and retesting in these scenarios should be considered,[1] although less than 1% of individuals initially testing negative for AQP4-IgG will subsequently seroconvert to AQP4-IgG-positive.[108]

Finally, although AQP4-IgG can also be found in the CSF,[16,109] antibody testing with modern CBA or FACS on serum are more sensitive.[16] The presence of CSF positivity seems related to high AQP4-IgG titers in serum (higher likelihood of a CSF-positive test in patients with AQP4-IgG titer in serum >1:100) and is more common during clinical attacks.[16] Therefore, serum testing is generally sufficient for AQP4-IgG testing, although in highly suspicious cases CSF AQP4-IgG can be considered but isolated CSF AQP4-IgG positives are exceedingly rare.[16]

*MOG-IgG testing*: In contrast to AQP4-IgG, MOG-IgG testing is more complex and has historically represented a challenge. In fact, initial reports using Western Blot or enzyme-linked immunosorbent assay (ELISA) targeting denatured MOG proteins, yielded the presence of MOG-IgG in serum of many patients with MS and healthy

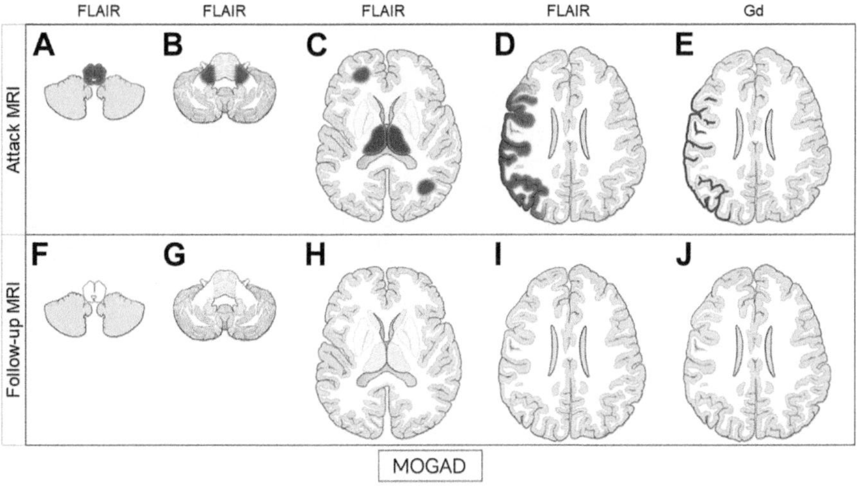


**Fig. 7. Brain lesions in patients with MOGAD**. Top row shows brain findings during the acute phase, while follow-up imaging is displayed in the bottom row. Images are all shown on axial view. T2-lesion involving the entire medulla (*A*), completely resolving at follow-up (*F*). Bilateral fluffy T2-lesions in the middle cerebellar peduncles (*B*) resolved at follow-up (*G*). Bilateral fluffy T2-lesions of the thalami and additional lesions in the white matter (*C*) undergoing complete resolution at follow-up (*H*). Cerebral cortical encephalitis with an extensive cortical T2-lesion (*D*) accompanied by leptomeningeal enhancement (*E*). Both cortical lesion and enhancement completely resolved at follow-up (*I*, *J*). (Used with permission of Mayo Foundation for Medical Education and Research, all rights reserved.) Abbreviations: FLAIR, fluid-attenuated inversion recovery; Gd, postcontrast T1-weighted images; MOGAD, myelin oligodendrocyte glycoprotein antibody-associated disease.

controls,[110–112] leading to the misconception that these antibodies may represent an epiphenomenon of demyelination. The association between MOG-IgG and specific demyelinating phenotypes such as ADEM and optic neuritis (but not MS), was first highlighted by using a laboratory assay expressing MOG in its native tridimensional conformation[4] and was subsequently confirmed by CBAs expressing full-length human MOG.[113,114] ELISA testing demonstrated a poor diagnostic performance and reproducibility and is therefore not recommended or suitable for diagnosing MOGAD.[2,107]

However, in contrast with AQP4-IgG testing,[104,107] an excellent agreement between different CBA assays was only reached with clear positive (82%) and clear negative results (97.5%), with a slight improvement when only live CBA were considered.[107] The agreement on borderline positives was poor (33%).[107] Caution is needed with low-positive CBA results given MOG-IgG can be found at low titer in 1% to 2% of disease controls.[107,115,116] The positive predictive value of MOG-IgG increases when ordered in high probability situations and with higher antibody titers.[115] MOG-IgG is still a very useful test with high specificity (≈98%–99%), and this is exemplified by a recent study that showed no MOG-IgG positive among 703 pediatric healthy controls.[117]

These observations highlight two fundamental principles that should be considered when testing MOG-IgG: (1) CBA methodologies providing quantitative or semiquantitative data can be useful and (2) testing should be reserved to patients with a high a priori probability of having MOGAD. Universal testing of all patients with MS is not recommend given the potential for 1% to 2% to have low-positive results that may

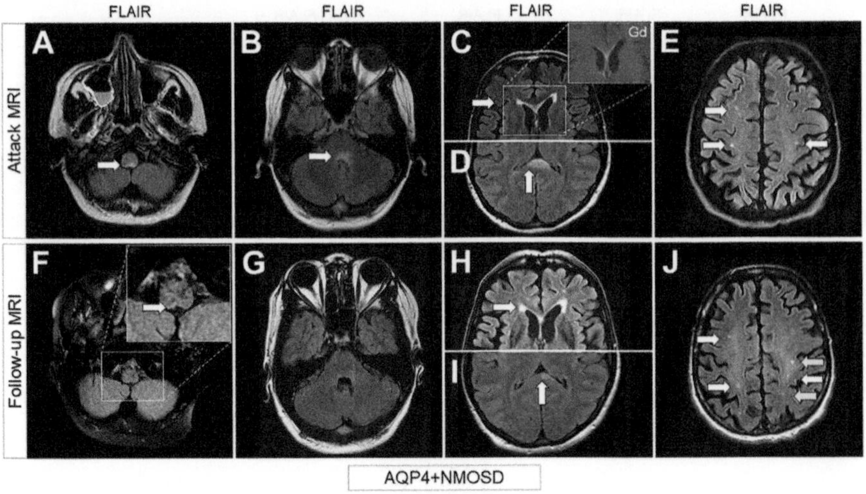


**Fig. 8. MRI examples of brain lesions in patients with AQP4+NMOSD.** Top row shows MRI findings during the acute phase, whereas follow-up imaging is displayed in the bottom row. Images are shown in axial view.T2-lesion in the area postrema (*A, arrow*) almost invisible but still present at follow-up (*F,* zoom-in picture, *arrow*). T2-lesion involving the dorsal pons abutting to the fourth ventricle (*B, arrow*) with complete resolution at follow-up (*G*). Periependymal T2-lesion (*C, arrow*) with corresponding linear ependymal enhancement (zoom-in picture, postcontrast T1-weighted sequence), persisting at follow-up (*H, arrow*). T2-lesion involving the splenium of the corpus callosum in another patient (*D, arrow*), significantly reduced in size but still visible at follow-up (*I, arrow*). Multiple small nonspecific T2-lesions in the subcortical white matter (*E, arrows*), persisting unchanged at follow-up (*J, arrows*). Additional interval T2-lesions are observed as well (*J, green arrows*). Abbreviations: AQP4+NMOSD, aquaporin-4-IgG positive neuromyelitis optica spectrum disorder; FLAIR, fluid-attenuated inversion recovery; Gd, postcontrast T1-weighted images.

lead to confusion about the diagnosis. It is preferred to select those with features that are suggestive of MOGAD and avoid testing in patients with classic features of MS.

Finally, recent investigations have highlighted a role for CSF testing in MOGAD. In fact, although serum is overall more sensitive to MOG-IgG detection, concomitant detection of MOG-IgG in serum and CSF occurs in 41% to 87% of patients.[17–20,118–120] CSF positivity can be observed in isolation in 3% to 29%,[17–20,118–120] and in suspicious cases negative for MOG-IgG in serum, CSF MOG-IgG testing should be undertaken. Patients with evidence of intrathecal synthesis of MOG-IgG or CSF MOG-IgG positivity seem to have a worse clinical prognosis.[19,20] Because false-positive MOG-IgG in CSF can be rarely encountered in MS and other diseases,[19,20] the result should always be put into clinical context.

*Additional CSF analysis and other laboratory features in MOGAD and AQP4+NMOSD*: Other than disease-specific antibody testing, additional laboratory analysis can be helpful in the differential diagnosis process, although not included in the diagnostic criteria. CSF usually reveals pleocytosis in more than 50% of patients with MOGAD (median 31–40 cells/μL)[121,122] and AQP4+NMOSD (median 19 cells/μL)[123] but rarely in MS. Cells are usually predominantly lymphocytes[121–123] although also monocytes (MOGAD),[121,122] neutrophils (both AQP4+NMOSD and MOGAD),[121–123] or eosinophils (AQP4+NMOSD)[123] can be found. In MOGAD, CSF abnormalities may vary by phenotype and are more common in patients with brain and/or spinal

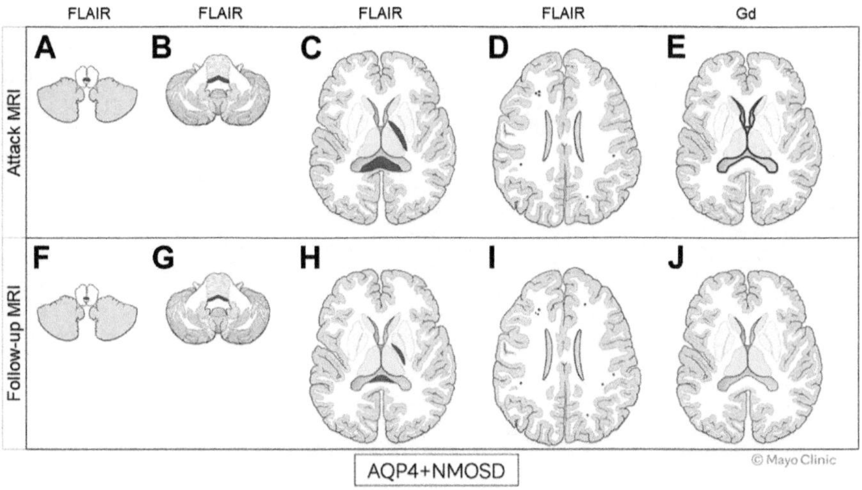


**Fig. 9. Brain lesions in patients with AQP4+NMOSD**. Top row shows brain findings during the acute phase, whereas follow-up imaging is displayed in the bottom row. Images are all shown on axial view. T2-lesion in the area postrema (*A*) smaller but still present at follow-up (*F*). Posterior T2-lesion abutting to the fourth ventricle (*B*) smaller but still present at follow-up (*G*). T2-lesion in the corticospinal tract and splenium of the corpus callosum (*C*) smaller but still present at follow-up (*H*). Multiple small nonspecific T2-lesions in the subcortical white matter (*D*), persisting unchanged at follow-up (*I*). Additional interval T2-lesions are observed as well (*I*). The presence of linear ependymal enhancement (*E*), resolving at follow-up (*J*) is typical of AQP4+NMOSD. (Used with permission of Mayo Foundation for Medical Education and Research, all rights reserved.) Abbreviations: AQP4+NMOSD, aquaporin-4-IgG positive neuromyelitis optica spectrum disorder; FLAIR, fluid-attenuated inversion recovery; Gd, postcontrast T1-weighted images.

cord lesions.[124] CSF oligoclonal bands are rarely encountered in patients with MOGAD and AQP4+NMOSD (approximately 10%–20%)[121–124] compared with 88% of patients with MS.[125]

Approximately 2% to 3% of patients with AQP4+NMOSD can have coexistent myasthenia gravis.[126,127] Although AQP4+NMOSD diagnosis usually follows that of myasthenia,[128] antiacetylcholine receptor antibody in serum should be checked in case of compatible clinical manifestations. Rarely MOG-IgG was also found coexisting with AQP4-IgG and in most cases is likely related to its background rate being found in 1% to 2% of disease controls. Most patients with dual AQP4-IgG and MOG-IgG positivity had high-titer AQP4-IgG and low-titer MOG-IgG and a phenotype more suggestive of AQP4+NMOSD.[129]

The laboratory features and antibody testing of AQP4+NMOSD and MOGAD are summarized in **Table 3**.

### *Diagnostic Criteria*

The latest diagnostic criteria for AQP4+NMOSD and MOGAD are dated 2015 and 2023, respectively, and are summarized in **Table 4**.

In both cases, the diagnostic algorithm starts from the evidence of core clinical features, and then dichotomizes based on antibody-serostatus. Clear evidence of the pathogenetic antibody in a patient with typical clinical manifestations allows the achievement of the diagnosis; alternatively, additional clinical or MRI requirements

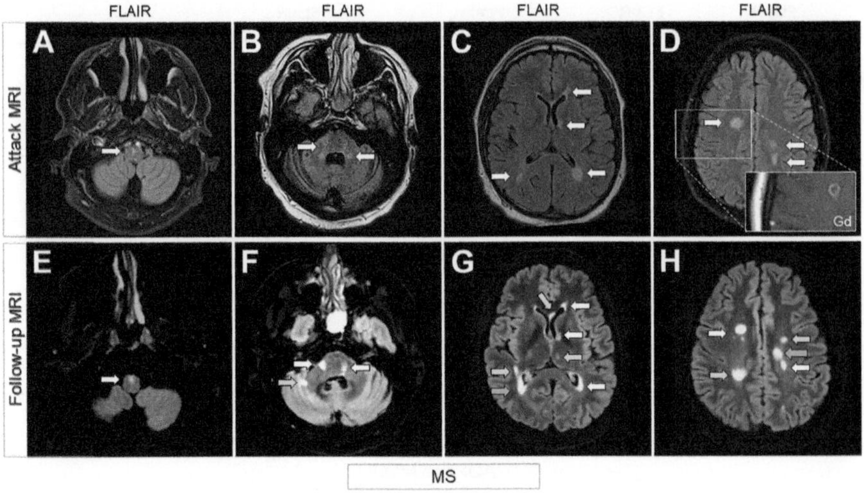


**Fig. 10. MRI examples of brain lesions in patients with MS**. Top row shows MRI findings during the acute phase, whereas follow-up imaging is displayed in the bottom row. Unless otherwise specified, images are all shown on FLAIR sequences, axial view. Small T2-lesion in the anterior medulla (*A, arrow*), unchanged at follow-up (*E, arrow*). Multiple T2-lesions in the peripheral pons and abutting on the fourth ventricles (*B, arrows*), still visible at follow-up (*F, arrows*) with additional interval T2-lesions (*F*, green *arrow*). Multiple ovoid periventricular T2-lesions abutting on the lateral ventricles (*C, arrows*). T2-lesions persisted at follow-up (*G, arrows*), at times increasing in size (*G*, blue *arrow*). Additional interval T2-lesions (*G*, green *arrows*) are shown as well. White matter T2-lesions (*D, arrows*), one showing ring enhancement (zoom-in picture, postcontrast T1-weighted sequence). T2-lesions persisted at follow-up (*H, arrows*), at times increasing in size (*H*, blue *arrow*). Additional interval T2-lesions (*H*, green *arrows*) are shown as well. Abbreviations: FLAIR, fluid-attenuated inversion recovery; Gd, postcontrast T1-weighted images; MS, multiple sclerosis.

are needed. The comparison of AQP4+NMOSD and MOGAD diagnostic criteria highlights several differences. First, for AQP4+NMOSD diagnosis, but not MOGAD, there is a seronegative or unknown antibody status category.[1] Because MOG-IgG is found in up to 30% of seronegative patients with NMOSD,[130,131] future iterations of AQP4-IgG seronegative NMOSD will likely require a negative MOG-IgG test. The reason for this is that MOG-IgG positive patients with a compatible syndrome should be diagnosed with MOGAD rather than AQP4-IgG seronegative NMOSD. MOGAD diagnostic criteria, but not AQP4+NMOSD, have additional requirements for low-positive or CSF MOG-IgG positive tests given the challenges with low-positive results and limited data on CSF MOG-IgG, respectively.

## AQP4+NMOSD AND MOGAD TREATMENT

Treatment in autoimmune disorders has two main goals: (1) promote recovery after an acute attack and (2) prevent subsequent relapses. In this section, we will describe the main treatment strategies in AQP4+NMOSD and MOGAD.

### *Acute Treatment of Attacks*

Acute treatment in both AQP4+NMOSD and MOGAD is similar to MS. It mainly includes intravenous steroids and plasma exchange although occasionally, intravenous

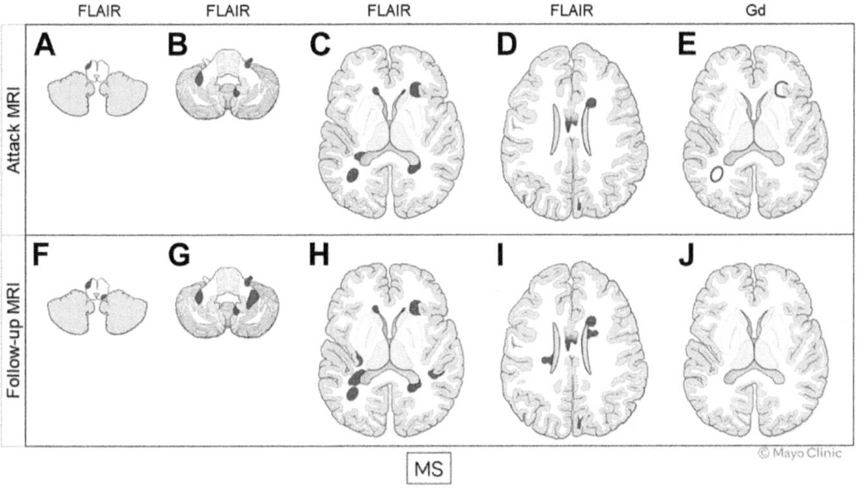


**Fig. 11. Brain lesions in patients with MS**. Top row shows brain findings during the acute phase, whereas follow-up imaging is displayed in the bottom row. Images are all shown on axial view. Small peripheral T2-lesion in the anterior medulla (*A*), substantially unchanged at follow-up with additional interval T2-lesion (*F*). Multiple T2-lesions in the peripheral pons, trigeminal nerve, and abutting on the fourth ventricles (*B*), substantially unchanged at follow-up with additional interval lesion (*G*). Multiple ovoid periventricular, juxtacortical, and deep white matter T2-lesions (*C*). T2-lesions persisted at follow-up (*H*), at times increasing in size. Additional juxtacortical interval T2-lesions are also visible (*H*). White matter T2-lesions and one cortical T2-lesion (*D*) persisting at follow-up with additional interval lesions development (*I*). Two of the lesions shown in C demonstrate open or closed ring enhancement, which is typically observed in MS (*E*) and resolves at follow-up (*J*). (Used with permission of Mayo Foundation for Medical Education and Research, all rights reserved.) Abbreviations: FLAIR, fluid-attenuated inversion recovery; Gd, postcontrast T1-weighted images; MS, multiple sclerosis.

immunoglobulin (IVIg) is also used. The details are summarized in **Table 5**. There is evidence that early treatment (ie, <7 day-delay from symptoms onset) reduces the likelihood of residual deficits in both AQP4+NMOSD and MOGAD.[132] Moreover, the use of both steroids and plasma exchange may be more common in these conditions, given the greater severity of symptoms at nadir and the high efficacy of early plasma exchange or apheresis by immunoadsorption in patients with AQP4+NMOSD.[133–135] In AQP4+NMOSD, transitional corticosteroids for a few weeks are often used while awaiting attack-prevention treatments to work, and the duration varies depending on the type of immunosuppressant used.[103,136] In MOGAD, longer steroid tapers for many months have sometimes been used to prevent early relapses but the majority of patients will not have an early relapse and prolonged steroids has a large side effect burden, particularly in growing children.[10,137,138] Therefore, using such an approach in all patients is problematic and further studies are needed to determine the role of a more prolonged corticosteroid taper.

### *Chronic Attack-Preventive Treatment*

Because AQP4-IgG positive patients with AQP4+NMOSD at first clinical attack are at high risk of relapses in the first year (70%) and disability worsening is strongly associated with acute attacks, all newly diagnosed patients should undergo a chronic treatment aimed to prevent attacks.[103] In contrast with AQP4+NMOSD, approximately

**Table 2**
**Imaging findings in AQP4+NMOSD, MOGAD, and MS**

| | AQP4+NMOSD | MOGAD | MS |
|---|---|---|---|
| Optic nerve | | | |
| Bilateral involvement | ++ | ++ | - |
| Longitudinally extensive lesions (>50% length of optic nerve) | ++ | ++ | - |
| Location | Posterior with chiasm | Anterior | Anterior/middle |
| Optic nerve enhancement | +++ | +++ | +++ |
| Optic nerve sheath enhancement | - | ++ | - |
| Perioptic fat enhancement | - | ++ | - |
| Spinal cord | | | |
| Multiple lesions | - | ++ | +++ |
| Longitudinally extensive lesions | +++ | +++ | - |
| Location (axial) | Central | Central | Peripheral |
| Gray matter involved | +++ | +++ | + |
| White matter involved | ++ | + | +++ |
| Location (sagittal) | Cervico-thoracic | Cervico-thoracic | Cervico-thoracic |
| Conus involved | + | ++ | + |
| Parenchymal enhancement | Lens-shape, heterogeneous | Faint, ill-defined | Ring, nodular |
| Leptomeningeal enhancement | + | ++ | - |
| Brain | | | |
| Shape | Along white matter tracts | Poorly demarcated | Ovoid |
| Cortical lesions | - | + | ++ |
| Juxtacortical lesions | - | ++ | +++ |
| Subcortical lesions | ++ | + | - |
| Periventricular lesions | Peri-3rd/4th ventricle and peri-ependymal lateral ventricles | - | Dawson's fingers |

| | | | |
|---|---|---|---|
| Corpus callosum lesions | ++ | ++ | +++ |
| Deep gray matter lesions | + | ++ | - |
| Diffuse pons/middle cerebellar peduncle lesions | + | +++ | - |
| T1-hypointense lesions | + | + | +++ |
| Ring enhancement | - | - | ++ |
| Ependymal enhancement | ++ | - | - |
| Leptomeningeal enhancement | - | ++ | -[a] |
| T2-lesion resolution | + | +++ | - |
| Interattack asymptomatic accumulation of new T2-lesions | - | - | ++[b] |

Note that: "-" indicates rare findings (<5%), "+" infrequent findings (5%–30%), "++" common findings (30%–69%), "+++" very common findings (>=70%).

*Abbreviations:* AQP4+NMOSD, aquaporin-4-IgG positive neuromyelitis optica spectrum disorder; MOGAD, myelin-oligodendrocyte glycoprotein antibody-associated disease; MS, multiple sclerosis.

[a] May be seen with more sophisticated MRI techniques (eg, postcontrast fluid-attenuated inversion recovery or at 7.0 T field strength).

[b] Dependent on treatment and is common with low or moderate efficacy MS disease modifying treatments but rare with high-efficacy treatments.

**Table 3**
**Recommendations and laboratory features of AQP4+NMOSD and MOGAD**

| | AQP4+NMOSD | MOGAD |
|---|---|---|
| Antibody | AQP4-IgG1 | MOG-IgG1 |
| Sample | | |
| Serum | Yes (preferred) | Yes (preferred) |
| CSF | No (isolated CSF AQP4-IgG extremely rare) | Yes (≈10% isolated CSF MOG-IgG) |
| Test assay | | |
| Live CBA | Yes (gold standard) | Yes (gold standard) |
| Fixed CBA | Yes | Yes |
| Murine tissue-based assays | Intermediate sensitivity but very good specificity | May have white matter staining when CSF tested but very insensitive[24] |
| ELISA | Good performance but reduced sensitivity and risk of false positives at low titer vs CBAs | Not recommended due to inconsistent results |
| Quantitative results important | No | Yes (risk of false positives at low titer) |
| Seroconversion important | No | Yes (relapse-risk) |
| CSF findings | | |
| Pleocytosis | ++ | ++ |
| High protein | ++ | ++ |
| Oligoclonal bands | + (<20%) | + (<20%) |

Note that: "-" indicates rare findings (<5%), "+" infrequent findings (5%–30%), "++" common findings (30%–69%), "+++" very common findings (>=70%).

*Abbreviations:* AQP4, aquaporin-4; AQP4+NMOSD, aquaporin-4-IgG positive neuromyelitis optica spectrum disorder; CBA, cell-based assay; CSF, cerebrospinal fluid; ELISA, enzyme-linked immunosorbent assay; MOG, myelin oligodendrocyte glycoprotein; MOGAD, myelin-oligodendrocyte glycoprotein antibody-associated disease.

**Table 4**
**Diagnostic criteria of AQP4+NMOSD and MOGAD**

| | | AQP4+NMOSD | MOGAD |
|---|---|---|---|
| Antibody test (CBA) positive (AQP4+NMOSD) or clear positive (MOGAD) | Core clinical features | Optic neuritis | Optic neuritis |
| | | Myelitis | Myelitis |
| | | Area postrema syndrome | Brainstem or cerebellar deficits |
| | | Acute brainstem syndrome | |
| | | Symptomatic cerebral syndrome with AQP4+NMOSD-typical brain MRI lesions | ADEM |
| | | Symptomatic narcolepsy or acute diencephalic clinical syndrome with AQP4+NMOSD-typical diencephalic MRI lesions | Cerebral monofocal or polyfocal deficits |
| | | | Cerebral cortical encephalitis often with seizures |
| Antibody test (CBA) negative/ unknown (AQP4+NMOSD) or low positive/positive without titer in serum or negative in serum but CSF positive (MOGAD) | Supporting features | | |
| | Optic neuritis | Normal findings or only nonspecific white matter lesions in the brain | Bilateral simultaneous clinical involvement |
| | | Longitudinal optic nerve involvement (>50% length of the optic nerve on T2 or postgadolinium T1) | Longitudinal optic nerve involvement (>50% length of the optic nerve) |
| | | Optic chiasm | Perineural optic sheath enhancement |
| | | | Optic disc edema |
| | Myelitis | Longitudinally extensive myelitis | Longitudinally extensive myelitis |
| | | Longitudinally extensive focal spinal cord atrophy in patients | Central cord lesion or H-sign |

(*continued on next page*)

**Table 4**
***(continued)***

| | | AQP4+NMOSD | MOGAD |
|---|---|---|---|
| | | with history compatible with acute myelitis | |
| | | | Conus lesion |
| | Area postrema syndrome | Dorsal medulla/area postrema lesions | - |
| | Brain, brainstem, or cerebral syndromes | Periependymal brainstem lesions | Multiple ill-defined T2 hyperintense lesions in supratentorial and often infratentorial white matter<br>Deep gray matter involvement<br>Ill-defined T2-hyperintensity involving pons, middle cerebellar peduncle, or medulla<br>Cortical lesion with or without lesional and overlying meningeal enhancement |
| | Exclusion of better diagnoses including MS | Yes | Yes |

*Abbreviations:* AQP4+NMOSD, aquaporin-4-IgG positive neuromyelitis optica spectrum disorder; CBA, cell-based assay; CSF, cerebrospinal fluid; MOGAD, myelin oligodendrocyte glycoprotein antibody-associated disease.

**Table 5**
**Main treatment protocols in AQP4+NMOSD and MOGAD**

| | Protocol | AQP4+NMOSD | MOGAD |
|---|---|---|---|
| Acute treatment of attacks | | | |
| Importance | - | Residual disability | Residual disability |
| Steroids | Intravenous methylprednisolone 1000 mg/d for 5 d[a] | +++ | +++ |
| Plasma exchange[b] | Every other day for 5–7 cycles | +++ | ++ |
| Steroid tapering | Oral steroids 20–40 mg followed by a taper | Weeks[c] | Weeks–months |
| Chronic attack-preventive treatment[d] | | | |
| Importance | - | Affects long-term prognosis | Unknown |
| Start at first clinical attack | - | +++ | + |
| Complement inhibitors | | | |
| Eculizumab | 900 mg intravenous every week for the first 4 wk, then 1200 mg every 2 wk | +++ | Not tried in trials |
| Ravulizumab | Body-weight-based intravenous loading dose (2400–3000 mg) plus a body-weight-based maintenance dose (3000–3600 mg) on day 15, then once every 8 wk | +++ | Not tried in trials |
| B cells depleters | | | |
| Rituximab | 375 mg/m$^2$ intravenous every week for the first 4 wk, or 1000 mg × 2 doses 2 wk apart and then 1000 mg 2 wk apart every 6 mo | +++ | Trial ongoing |
| Inebilizumab | 300 mg intravenous every 15 d × 2 doses, and then every 6 mo | +++ | Limited data |
| IL-6 receptors inhibitors | | | |
| Satralizumab | 120 mg subcutaneously every 4 wk | +++ | Trial ongoing |

Note that: "-" indicates rare (<5%), "+" infrequent (5%–30%), "++" common (30%–69%), "+++" very common/very high efficacy (>=70%).

[a] Alternatively, oral steroids bioequivalent (ie, prednisone 1250 mg) may be considered given its similar efficacy in patients with optic neuritis.[163]

[b] IVIg may be sometimes administered instead of expanded Disability Status Scale (EDSS).

[c] Duration may vary depending on steroid-sparing treatment making effect.

[d] We focused here on level 1 evidence of efficacy, although biosimilars of rituximab, tocilizumab, mycophenolate, and azathioprine may be used and a trial on rozanolixizumab is ongoing in MOGAD.

50% of patients with MOGAD will ultimately have a relapsing disease course.[12] Therefore, treatment is usually recommended only after the second clinical event in patients with MOGAD, although exceptions may be made in those with a severe first attack with residual disability.

AQP4+NMOSD represents one of the few neurological disorders with tailored proven treatments available, where drugs target key elements of disease pathophysiology, namely (1) IL-6 (satralizumab), (2) B cells and their subsets (inebilizumab and rituximab), and (3) complement (eculizumab, ravulizumab). The very high efficacy of these biologic drugs was demonstrated in phase 3 clinical trials (level 1 evidence of efficacy), although only in AQP4+NMOSD. Biosimilars of rituximab are potential alternatives to reduce costs. In resource-limited settings, azathioprine and mycophenolate mofetil have been used but their efficacy appears to be less,[139] and they have drawbacks including the need for at least 6 months of concomitant corticosteroids with its high side effect burden and risk of secondary lymphoproliferative disorders with long-term use.[140,141] Tocilizumab is another off-label IL-6 blocking medications with some data supporting its use.[142] In this review, we will focus on treatments that have class 1 evidence. A summary of treatment efficacy and the main side effects during the trials and in the open label phase (if available) are provided below and in **Table 5**.

## *Complement Inhibitors*

### *Eculizumab*

This humanized monoclonal antibody inhibits C5 preventing the membrane attack complex formation. The phase-3 trial included only adult patients with AQP4+NMOSD and the treatment showed a 94% relapse-risk reduction compared with the placebo arm,[143] and similar results during the open-label extension.[144] Although eculizumab was administered as add-on therapy in most patients, efficacy was confirmed in the subgroup of patients receiving eculizumab monotherapy[145] and was not influenced by the main demographic/clinical variables, including age, sex, race, disease duration, annualized relapse rate, EDSS, prior treatment with rituximab, and additional autoimmune conditions.[146]

All patients received *Neisseria meningitidis* vaccination before eculizumab administration to reduce the risk of capsulated bacterial infection, with no evidence of meningitis during the trial and its extension so far,[144] although one case occurred in the initial phase 2 open label trial of this medication.[147] Adverse effects were generally mild or moderate. Headache, upper respiratory tract infections, nasopharyngitis, and urinary tract infections were the most common.[143,144] A single death from pulmonary empyema was registered.[143,144]

### *Ravulizumab*

Ravulizumab is a humanized monoclonal antibody similar to eculizumab that also targets C5. The main difference with eculizumab is that the complementary binding region and the neonatal fragment crystallizable region were modified in ravulizumab to lengthen its half-life. It was administered to AQP4-IgG seropositive patients with AQP4+NMOSD in a phase-3 open label trial using the placebo arm of the PREVENT trial as the control group.[148] No patients relapsed during the trial, leading to a 98.6% reduction in relapse-risk. In addition, investigators found a significant improvement of the ambulation index at study end.[148] Similar to eculizumab, adverse events were generally mild to moderate and included coronavirus disease 2019 infection, headache, back pain, arthralgia, and urinary tract infections.[148] However, despite prior vaccination, two patients developed meningococcal meningitis but recovered with treatment.[148]

### *B Cell Depletion*

#### *Rituximab*

Rituximab is a chimeric monoclonal antibody targeting the surface CD20 biomarker expressed on B cells. Its efficacy was proven in patients with AQP4+NMOSD in a randomized placebo-controlled clinical trial. In this study, no treated patients relapsed although the total number of patients (19 in each study arm) was smaller than some of the other clinical trials. In addition, an improvement in the quantification of nerve and spinal cord impairment scale was observed. No deaths occurred. Infusion reactions, headache, nasopharyngitis, and upper respiratory tract infections were the most common adverse effects, confirming rituximab's good safety profile.[149]

#### *Inebilizumab*

This humanized monoclonal antibody targets surface CD19, which is a B-cell lineage biomarker with a wider expression than CD20 because it is also present on plasmablasts and, to a lesser extent, on plasma cells. It was administered in monotherapy to both patients with AQP4+NMOSD and AQP4-IgG seronegative patients with NMOSD (18 patients), showing an overall relapse-risk reduction of 77% when in patients with AQP4+NMOSD.[150] Secondary endpoints such as the risk of EDSS worsening, radiological activity, and hospitalization were also met.[150,151] No significant benefit of treatment were observed among AQP4-IgG seronegative patients,[150] although a post hoc analysis suggested that treated patients had a lower annualized-relapse rate at study end than preenrollment.[152]

Post hoc analyses also provided interesting insights into treatment response showing that patients with early and persisting B cell depletion ($\leq$4 cells/$\mu$L at 6 months) were clinically stable for more than 2 years.[153]

Adverse events mainly included urinary tract infections, arthralgias, and infusion-related reactions. In the open-label phase, a decrease of immunoglobulins over time was observed, and further long-term analysis will be needed to determine its frequency and impact on risk of infections.[154] Two deaths due to respiratory failure within a relapse and an indeterminate neurological condition occurred.[150]

### *IL-6 Receptor Inhibitors*

#### *Satralizumab*

Satralizumab is a humanized monoclonal antibody inhibiting the IL-6 receptor. It was administered monotherapy or add-on in patients with AQP4+NMOSD and AQP4-IgG seronegative patients with NMOSD, demonstrating an overall relapse-risk reduction of 74% to 79% in patients with AQP4+NMOSD.[155,156] In contrast to the other medications, satralizumab administration is a subcutaneous injection, so it can be given at home. The adverse effects included upper respiratory or urinary infections and injection-related reactions. Efficacy and safety results were confirmed in the open label extension of the trial, and no deaths were reported.[157] Seronegative patients did not show a benefit but larger cohort studies are needed.[155,156]

So far, no level 1 evidence of treatment efficacy is available in patients with MOGAD, and empiric treatment decisions are based on retrospective analyses and expert opinion.[158,159] Treatment currently administered in clinical practice includes old immunosuppressants (azathioprine, mycophenolate mofetil), B cell depleting therapies (rituximab), IL-6 receptor inhibitors (tocilizumab), and IVIg.[160] Among them, multicenter retrospective studies demonstrated that rituximab and IVIg[161] are effective maintenance treatments. However, rituximab seems less effective in MOGAD than AQP4-IgG positive AQP4+NMOSD, despite B cell depletion.[162] Thus, IVIg or tocilizumab are often favored in clinical practice. Clinical trials evaluating the efficacy of rituximab

(NCT05545384), satralizumab (NCT05271409), and rozanolixizumab (an inhibitor of the neonatal Fc receptor, NCT05063162) versus placebo are currently ongoing.

## SUMMARY

The recent identification of AQP4+NMOSD and MOGAD as separate disorders has prompted the development of separate diagnostic criteria for MOGAD diagnosis. The stratification of patients based on the presence/absence of AQP4-IgG in NMOSD and stratification by antibody-titer in MOGAD represents the main differences between the two criteria. Using CBA in serum, AQP4-IgG and MOG-IgG are sensitive and highly specific but caution is needed with low-positive MOG-IgG, which is found in 1% to 2% of disease controls. In addition, specific MRI features of the diseases are described and included as supportive criteria in uncertain cases. NMOSD negative for AQP4-IgG and MOG-IgG likely represents a heterogenous group of disorders that should be a focus of research to potentially discover new antibodies that associate with demyelination. A number of highly effective attack-prevention treatments are now available for AQP4+NMOSD and should be started promptly at diagnosis. Empiric attack-prevention treatments in MOGAD are generally reserved for those with 2 or more attacks. However, level 1 evidence is lacking in MOGAD. The approach to developing treatments in AQP4+NMOSD will be a useful template for MOGAD and randomized clinical trials are now underway with the hope for a proven attack-prevention treatment in the near future.

## CLINICS CARE POINTS

- AQP4+NMOSD and MOGAD are separate antibody-mediated CNS disorders with different antigenic targets.
- Bilateral optic neuritis and extensive myelitis are common features of both AQP4+NMOSD and MOGAD; cerebral involvement can be encountered with both diseases, although ADEM favors MOGAD.
- It is important to recognize the MRI features of MOGAD and AQP4+NMOSD because it helps to select those that should be tested for MOG-IgG and AQP4-IgG.
- Caution is needed with low-positive MOG-IgG because it can occur in 1% to 2% of other diseases.
- Long-term attack-prevention treatment is required after the first attack in AQP4+NMOSD but not MOGAD, where it is typically reserved for those with 2 or more attacks.
- In AQP4+NMOSD, level 1 evidence of efficacy is available for complement inhibitors (eculizumab, ravulizumab), B cell depleting agents (rituximab, inebilizumab), and IL-6 receptor inhibitors (satralizumab).
- High-level evidence of treatment efficacy is not available for MOGAD yet but clinical trials are now underway.

## DISCLOSURE

L. Cacciaguerra received speaker and consultant honoraria from ACCMED, Roche, BMS Celgene, Sanofi and travel support for conferences by Merck Serono. E.P. Flanagan was a site primary investigator in a randomized clinical trial on Inebilizumab in neuromyelitis optica spectrum disorder run by Medimmune/Viela-Bio/Horizon Therapeutics, has received funding from the NIH, United States (R01NS113828), and is a member of the medical advisory board of the MOG project. Dr E.P. Flanagan is an editorial board member of the Journal of the Neurological Sciences and Neuroimmunology Reports, and a patent has been submitted on DACH1-IgG as a biomarker of paraneoplastic autoimmunity.

## REFERENCES


1. Wingerchuk DM, Banwell B, Bennett JL, et al. International consensus diagnostic criteria for neuromyelitis optica spectrum disorders. Neurology 2015; 85(2):177–89.
2. Banwell B, Bennett JL, Marignier R, et al. Diagnosis of myelin oligodendrocyte glycoprotein antibody-associated disease: International MOGAD Panel proposed criteria. Lancet Neurol 2023;22(3):268–82.
3. Lennon VA, Kryzer TJ, Pittock SJ, et al. IgG marker of optic-spinal multiple sclerosis binds to the aquaporin-4 water channel. J Exp Med 2005;202(4):473–7.
4. O'Connor KC, McLaughlin KA, De Jager PL, et al. Self-antigen tetramers discriminate between myelin autoantibodies to native or denatured protein. Nat Med 2007;13(2):211–7.
5. Kunchok A, Chen JJ, Saadeh RS, et al. Application of 2015 Seronegative Neuromyelitis Optica Spectrum Disorder Diagnostic Criteria for Patients With Myelin Oligodendrocyte Glycoprotein IgG-Associated Disorders. JAMA Neurol 2020; 77(12):1572–5.
6. Flanagan EP, Cabre P, Weinshenker BG, et al. Epidemiology of aquaporin-4 autoimmunity and neuromyelitis optica spectrum. Ann Neurol 2016;79(5): 775–83.
7. Papp V, Magyari M, Aktas O, et al. Worldwide Incidence and Prevalence of Neuromyelitis Optica: A Systematic Review. Neurology 2021;96(2):59–77.
8. O'Connell K, Hamilton-Shield A, Woodhall M, et al. Prevalence and incidence of neuromyelitis optica spectrum disorder, aquaporin-4 antibody-positive NMOSD and MOG antibody-positive disease in Oxfordshire, UK. J Neurol Neurosurg Psychiatry 2020;91(10):1126–8.
9. de Mol CL, Wong Y, van Pelt ED, et al. The clinical spectrum and incidence of anti-MOG-associated acquired demyelinating syndromes in children and adults. Mult Scler 2020;26(7):806–14.
10. Jurynczyk M, Messina S, Woodhall MR, et al. Clinical presentation and prognosis in MOG-antibody disease: a UK study. Brain 2017;140(12):3128–38.
11. Ramanathan S, Mohammad S, Tantsis E, et al. Clinical course, therapeutic responses and outcomes in relapsing MOG antibody-associated demyelination. J Neurol Neurosurg Psychiatry 2018;89(2):127–37.
12. Cobo-Calvo A, Ruiz A, Rollot F, et al. Clinical Features and Risk of Relapse in Children and Adults with Myelin Oligodendrocyte Glycoprotein Antibody-Associated Disease. Ann Neurol 2021;89(1):30–41.
13. Papadopoulos MC, Verkman AS. Aquaporin 4 and neuromyelitis optica. Lancet Neurol 2012;11(6):535–44.
14. Marignier R, Hacohen Y, Cobo-Calvo A, et al. Myelin-oligodendrocyte glycoprotein antibody-associated disease. Lancet Neurol 2021;20(9):762–72.
15. Fujihara K, Bennett JL, de Seze J, et al. Interleukin-6 in neuromyelitis optica spectrum disorder pathophysiology. Neurol Neuroimmunol Neuroinflamm 2020;7(5).
16. Majed M, Fryer JP, McKeon A, et al. Clinical utility of testing AQP4-IgG in CSF: Guidance for physicians. Neurol Neuroimmunol Neuroinflamm 2016;3(3):e231.

17. Mariotto S, Gajofatto A, Batzu L, et al. Relevance of antibodies to myelin oligodendrocyte glycoprotein in CSF of seronegative cases. Neurology 2019;93(20): e1867–72.
18. Pace S, Orrell M, Woodhall M, et al. Frequency of MOG-IgG in cerebrospinal fluid versus serum. J Neurol Neurosurg Psychiatry 2022;93(3):334–5.
19. Kwon YN, Kim B, Kim JS, et al. Myelin Oligodendrocyte Glycoprotein-Immunoglobulin G in the CSF: Clinical Implication of Testing and Association With Disability. Neurol Neuroimmunol Neuroinflamm 2022;9(1).
20. Carta S, Cobo Calvo A, Armangue T, et al. Significance of Myelin Oligodendrocyte Glycoprotein Antibodies in CSF: A Retrospective Multicenter Study. Neurology 2023;100(11):e1095–108.
21. Lucchinetti CF, Mandler RN, McGavern D, et al. A role for humoral mechanisms in the pathogenesis of Devic's neuromyelitis optica. Brain 2002;125(Pt 7):1450–61.
22. Hoftberger R, Guo Y, Flanagan EP, et al. The pathology of central nervous system inflammatory demyelinating disease accompanying myelin oligodendrocyte glycoprotein autoantibody. Acta Neuropathol 2020;139(5):875–92.
23. Takai Y, Misu T, Kaneko K, et al. Myelin oligodendrocyte glycoprotein antibody-associated disease: an immunopathological study. Brain 2020;143(5):1431–46.
24. Spadaro M, Winklmeier S, Beltran E, et al. Pathogenicity of human antibodies against myelin oligodendrocyte glycoprotein. Ann Neurol 2018;84(2):315–28.
25. Kohyama K, Nishida H, Kaneko K, et al. Complement-dependent cytotoxicity of human autoantibodies against myelin oligodendrocyte glycoprotein. Front Neurosci 2023;17:1014071.
26. Yandamuri SS, Filipek B, Obaid AH, et al. MOGAD patient autoantibodies induce complement, phagocytosis, and cellular cytotoxicity. JCI Insight 2023.
27. Keller CW, Lopez JA, Wendel EM, et al. Complement Activation Is a Prominent Feature of MOGAD. Ann Neurol 2021;90(6):976–82.
28. Macrini C, Gerhards R, Winklmeier S, et al. Features of MOG required for recognition by patients with MOG antibody-associated disorders. Brain 2021;144(8): 2375–89.
29. Mader S, Ho S, Wong HK, et al. Dissection of complement and Fc-receptor-mediated pathomechanisms of autoantibodies to myelin oligodendrocyte glycoprotein. Proc Natl Acad Sci U S A 2023;120(13). e2300648120.
30. Kaneko K, Sato DK, Nakashima I, et al. CSF cytokine profile in MOG-IgG+ neurological disease is similar to AQP4-IgG+ NMOSD but distinct from MS: a cross-sectional study and potential therapeutic implications. J Neurol Neurosurg Psychiatry 2018;89(9):927–36.
31. Mealy MA, Wingerchuk DM, Greenberg BM, et al. Epidemiology of neuromyelitis optica in the United States: a multicenter analysis. Arch Neurol 2012;69(9):1176–80.
32. Wingerchuk DM, Hogancamp WF, O'Brien PC, et al. The clinical course of neuromyelitis optica (Devic's syndrome). Neurology 1999;53(5):1107–14.
33. Ramanathan S, Prelog K, Barnes EH, et al. Radiological differentiation of optic neuritis with myelin oligodendrocyte glycoprotein antibodies, aquaporin-4 antibodies, and multiple sclerosis. Mult Scler 2016;22(4):470–82.
34. Chen JJ, Bhatti MT. Clinical phenotype, radiological features, and treatment of myelin oligodendrocyte glycoprotein-immunoglobulin G (MOG-IgG) optic neuritis. Curr Opin Neurol 2020;33(1):47–54.
35. Jitprapaikulsan J, Chen JJ, Flanagan EP, et al. Aquaporin-4 and Myelin Oligodendrocyte Glycoprotein Autoantibody Status Predict Outcome of Recurrent Optic Neuritis. Ophthalmology 2018;125(10):1628–37.

36. Chen JJ, Flanagan EP, Jitprapaikulsan J, et al. Myelin Oligodendrocyte Glycoprotein Antibody-Positive Optic Neuritis: Clinical Characteristics, Radiologic Clues, and Outcome. Am J Ophthalmol 2018;195:8–15.
37. Wilejto M, Shroff M, Buncic JR, et al. The clinical features, MRI findings, and outcome of optic neuritis in children. Neurology 2006;67(2):258–62.
38. Mariano R, Messina S, Kumar K, et al. Comparison of Clinical Outcomes of Transverse Myelitis Among Adults With Myelin Oligodendrocyte Glycoprotein Antibody vs Aquaporin-4 Antibody Disease. JAMA Netw Open 2019;2(10): e1912732.
39. Dubey D, Pittock SJ, Krecke KN, et al. Clinical, Radiologic, and Prognostic Features of Myelitis Associated With Myelin Oligodendrocyte Glycoprotein Autoantibody. JAMA Neurol 2019;76(3):301–9.
40. Elsone L, Goh YY, Trafford R, et al. How often does respiratory failure occur in neuromyelitis optica? J Neurol Neurosurg Psychiatry 2013;84(11):e2.
41. Zhao-Fleming HH, Valencia Sanchez C, Sechi E, et al. CNS Demyelinating Attacks Requiring Ventilatory Support With Myelin Oligodendrocyte Glycoprotein or Aquaporin-4 Antibodies. Neurology 2021;97(13):e1351–8.
42. Elsone L, Townsend T, Mutch K, et al. Neuropathic pruritus (itch) in neuromyelitis optica. Mult Scler 2013;19(4):475–9.
43. Usmani N, Bedi G, Lam BL, et al. Association between paroxysmal tonic spasms and neuromyelitis optica. Arch Neurol 2012;69(1):121–4.
44. Banks SA, Morris PP, Chen JJ, et al. Brainstem and cerebellar involvement in MOG-IgG-associated disorder versus aquaporin-4-IgG and MS. J Neurol Neurosurg Psychiatry 2020.
45. Dubey D, Pittock SJ, Krecke KN, et al. Association of Extension of Cervical Cord Lesion and Area Postrema Syndrome With Neuromyelitis Optica Spectrum Disorder. JAMA Neurol 2017;74(3):359–61.
46. Kim HJ, Paul F, Lana-Peixoto MA, et al. MRI characteristics of neuromyelitis optica spectrum disorder: an international update. Neurology 2015;84(11):1165–73.
47. Etemadifar M, Nouri H, Khorvash R, et al. Frequency of diencephalic syndrome in NMOSD. Acta Neurol Belg 2022;122(4):961–7.
48. Magana SM, Matiello M, Pittock SJ, et al. Posterior reversible encephalopathy syndrome in neuromyelitis optica spectrum disorders. Neurology 2009;72(8): 712–7.
49. McKeon A, Lennon VA, Lotze T, et al. CNS aquaporin-4 autoimmunity in children. Neurology 2008;71(2):93–100.
50. Krupp LB, Tardieu M, Amato MP, et al. International Pediatric Multiple Sclerosis Study Group criteria for pediatric multiple sclerosis and immune-mediated central nervous system demyelinating disorders: revisions to the 2007 definitions. Mult Scler 2013;19(10):1261–7.
51. Bartels F, Baumgartner B, Aigner A, et al. Impaired Brain Growth in Myelin Oligodendrocyte Glycoprotein Antibody-Associated Acute Disseminated Encephalomyelitis. Neurol Neuroimmunol Neuroinflamm 2023;10(2).
52. Hahn CD, Miles BS, MacGregor DL, et al. Neurocognitive outcome after acute disseminated encephalomyelitis. Pediatr Neurol 2003;29(2):117–23.
53. Kuni BJ, Banwell BL, Till C. Cognitive and behavioral outcomes in individuals with a history of acute disseminated encephalomyelitis (ADEM). Dev Neuropsychol 2012;37(8):682–96.
54. Valencia-Sanchez C, Guo Y, Krecke KN, et al. Cerebral Cortical Encephalitis in Myelin Oligodendrocyte Glycoprotein Antibody-Associated Disease. Ann Neurol 2023;93(2):297–302.

55. Ogawa R, Nakashima I, Takahashi T, et al. MOG antibody-positive, benign, unilateral, cerebral cortical encephalitis with epilepsy. Neurol Neuroimmunol Neuroinflamm 2017;4(2):e322.
56. Budhram A, Sechi E, Nguyen A, et al. FLAIR-hyperintense Lesions in Anti-MOG-associated Encephalitis With Seizures (FLAMES): Is immunotherapy always needed to put out the fire? Mult Scler Relat Disord 2020;44. 102283.
57. Tatekawa H, Sakamoto S, Hori M, et al. Imaging Differences between Neuromyelitis Optica Spectrum Disorders and Multiple Sclerosis: A Multi-Institutional Study in Japan. AJNR Am J Neuroradiol 2018;39(7):1239–47.
58. Tajfirouz D, Padungkiatsagul T, Beres S, et al. Optic chiasm involvement in AQP-4 antibody-positive NMO and MOG antibody-associated disorder. Mult Scler 2022;28(1):149–53.
59. Jarius S, Paul F, Aktas O, et al. MOG encephalomyelitis: international recommendations on diagnosis and antibody testing. J Neuroinflammation 2018;15(1):134.
60. Shah SS, Morris P, Buciuc M, et al. Frequency of Asymptomatic Optic Nerve Enhancement in a Large Retrospective Cohort of Patients With Aquaporin-4+ NMOSD. Neurology 2022;99(8):e851–7.
61. Pacheco JM, Tajfirouz D, Madhavan A, et al. Asymptomatic Optic Nerve Enhancement in Myelin Oligodendrocyte Glycoprotein Associated Disease. Invest Ophthalmol Vis Sci 2022;63(7):1215.
62. Srikajon J, Siritho S, Ngamsombat C, et al. Differences in clinical features between optic neuritis in neuromyelitis optica spectrum disorders and in multiple sclerosis. Mult Scler J Exp Transl Clin 2018;4(3). 2055217318791196.
63. Kitley J, Waters P, Woodhall M, et al. Neuromyelitis optica spectrum disorders with aquaporin-4 and myelin-oligodendrocyte glycoprotein antibodies: a comparative study. JAMA Neurol 2014;71(3):276–83.
64. Asnafi S, Morris PP, Sechi E, et al. The frequency of longitudinally extensive transverse myelitis in MS: A population-based study. Mult Scler Relat Disord 2020;37:101487.
65. Fadda G, Alves CA, O'Mahony J, et al. Comparison of Spinal Cord Magnetic Resonance Imaging Features Among Children With Acquired Demyelinating Syndromes. JAMA Netw Open 2021;4(10):e2128871.
66. Cacciaguerra L, Sechi E, Rocca MA, et al. Neuroimaging features in inflammatory myelopathies: A review. Front Neurol 2022;13:993645.
67. Asgari N, Flanagan EP, Fujihara K, et al. Disruption of the leptomeningeal blood barrier in neuromyelitis optica spectrum disorder. Neurol Neuroimmunol Neuroinflamm 2017;4(4):e343.
68. Sechi E, Krecke KN, Pittock SJ, et al. Frequency and characteristics of MRI-negative myelitis associated with MOG autoantibodies. Mult Scler 2021;27(2):303–8.
69. Cacciaguerra L, Valsasina P, Mesaros S, et al. Spinal Cord Atrophy in Neuromyelitis Optica Spectrum Disorders Is Spatially Related to Cord Lesions and Disability. Radiology 2020;297(1):154–63.
70. Webb LM, Cacciaguerra L, Krecke KN, et al. Marked central canal T2-hyperintensity in MOGAD myelitis and comparison to NMOSD and MS. J Neurol Sci 2023;450:120687.
71. Hyun JW, Lee HL, Park J, et al. Brighter spotty lesions on spinal MRI help differentiate AQP4 antibody-positive NMOSD from MOGAD. Mult Scler 2022;28(6):989–92.

72. Hyun JW, Kim SH, Jeong IH, et al. Bright spotty lesions on the spinal cord: an additional MRI indicator of neuromyelitis optica spectrum disorder? J Neurol Neurosurg Psychiatry 2015;86(11):1280–2.
73. Yonezu T, Ito S, Mori M, et al. "Bright spotty lesions" on spinal magnetic resonance imaging differentiate neuromyelitis optica from multiple sclerosis. Mult Scler 2014;20(3):331–7.
74. Chien C, Scheel M, Schmitz-Hubsch T, et al. Spinal cord lesions and atrophy in NMOSD with AQP4-IgG and MOG-IgG associated autoimmunity. Mult Scler 2019;25(14):1926–36.
75. Cacciaguerra L, Meani A, Mesaros S, et al. Brain and cord imaging features in neuromyelitis optica spectrum disorders. Ann Neurol 2019;85(3):371–84.
76. Pittock SJ, Weinshenker BG, Lucchinetti CF, et al. Neuromyelitis optica brain lesions localized at sites of high aquaporin 4 expression. Arch Neurol 2006;63(7):964–8.
77. Chia NH, Redenbaugh V, Chen JJ, et al. Corpus callosum involvement in MOG antibody-associated disease in comparison to AQP4-IgG-seropositive neuromyelitis optica spectrum disorder and multiple sclerosis. Mult Scler 2023;29(6):748–52.
78. Elsbernd P, Cacciaguerra L, Krecke KN, et al. Cerebral enhancement in MOG antibody-associated disease. J Neurol Neurosurg Psychiatry 2023.
79. Cai MT, Zhang YX, Zheng Y, et al. Callosal lesions on magnetic resonance imaging with multiple sclerosis, neuromyelitis optica spectrum disorder and acute disseminated encephalomyelitis. Mult Scler Relat Disord 2019;32:41–5.
80. Mastrangelo V, Asioli GM, Foschi M, et al. Bilateral extensive corticospinal tract lesions in MOG antibody-associated disease. Neurology 2020;95(14):648–9.
81. Cacciaguerra L, Morris P, Tobin WO, et al. Tumefactive Demyelination in MOG Ab-Associated Disease, Multiple Sclerosis, and AQP-4-IgG-Positive Neuromyelitis Optica Spectrum Disorder. Neurology 2023;100(13):e1418–32.
82. Cobo-Calvo A, Ruiz A, Maillart E, et al. Clinical spectrum and prognostic value of CNS MOG autoimmunity in adults: The MOGADOR study. Neurology 2018;90(21):e1858–69.
83. Chen C, Liu C, Fang L, et al. Different magnetic resonance imaging features between MOG antibody- and AQP4 antibody-mediated disease: A Chinese cohort study. J Neurol Sci 2019;405:116430.
84. Jurynczyk M, Geraldes R, Probert F, et al. Distinct brain imaging characteristics of autoantibody-mediated CNS conditions and multiple sclerosis. Brain 2017;140(3):617–27.
85. Lopez-Chiriboga AS, Majed M, Fryer J, et al. Association of MOG-IgG Serostatus With Relapse After Acute Disseminated Encephalomyelitis and Proposed Diagnostic Criteria for MOG-IgG-Associated Disorders. JAMA Neurol 2018;75(11):1355–63.
86. Wattjes MP, Ciccarelli O, Reich DS, et al. 2021 MAGNIMS-CMSC-NAIMS consensus recommendations on the use of MRI in patients with multiple sclerosis. Lancet Neurol 2021;20(8):653–70.
87. Nelson F, Poonawalla A, Hou P, et al. 3D MPRAGE improves classification of cortical lesions in multiple sclerosis. Mult Scler 2008;14(9):1214–9.
88. Calabrese M, Oh MS, Favaretto A, et al. No MRI evidence of cortical lesions in neuromyelitis optica. Neurology 2012;79(16):1671–6.
89. Sinnecker T, Dorr J, Pfueller CF, et al. Distinct lesion morphology at 7-T MRI differentiates neuromyelitis optica from multiple sclerosis. Neurology 2012;79(7):708–14.

90. Tahara M, Ito R, Tanaka K, et al. Cortical and leptomeningeal involvement in three cases of neuromyelitis optica. Eur J Neurol 2012;19(5):e47–8.
91. Kim W, Lee JE, Kim SH, et al. Cerebral Cortex Involvement in Neuromyelitis Optica Spectrum Disorder. J Clin Neurol 2016;12(2):188–93.
92. Redenbaugh V, Chia NH, Cacciaguerra L, et al. Comparison of MRI T2-lesion evolution in pediatric MOGAD, NMOSD, and MS. Mult Scler 2023. 13524585231166834.
93. Sechi E, Krecke KN, Messina SA, et al. Comparison of MRI Lesion Evolution in Different Central Nervous System Demyelinating Disorders. Neurology 2021;97(11):e1097–109.
94. Cacciaguerra L, Redenbaugh V, Chen JJ, et al. Timing and Predictors of T2-Lesion Resolution in Patients With Myelin-Oligodendrocyte-Glycoprotein-Antibody-Associated Disease. Neurology 2023.
95. Redenbaugh V, Montalvo M, Sechi E, et al. Diagnostic value of aquaporin-4-IgG live cell based assay in neuromyelitis optica spectrum disorders. Mult Scler J Exp Transl Clin 2021;7(4). 20552173211052656.
96. Tackley G, Kuker W, Palace J. Magnetic resonance imaging in neuromyelitis optica. Mult Scler 2014;20(9):1153–64.
97. Sormani MP, Bruzzi P. MRI lesions as a surrogate for relapses in multiple sclerosis: a meta-analysis of randomised trials. Lancet Neurol 2013;12(7):669–76.
98. Paolilo RB, Rimkus CM, da Paz JA, et al. Asymptomatic MRI lesions in pediatric-onset AQP4-IgG positive NMOSD. Mult Scler Relat Disord 2022;68:104215.
99. Lee MY, Yong KP, Hyun JW, et al. Incidence of interattack asymptomatic brain lesions in NMO spectrum disorder. Neurology 2020;95(23):e3124–8.
100. Camera V, Holm-Mercer L, Ali AAH, et al. Frequency of New Silent MRI Lesions in Myelin Oligodendrocyte Glycoprotein Antibody Disease and Aquaporin-4 Antibody Neuromyelitis Optica Spectrum Disorder. JAMA Netw Open 2021;4(12):e2137833.
101. S BSM, Chen JJ, Morris P, et al. Frequency of New or Enlarging Lesions on MRI Outside of Clinical Attacks in Patients With MOG-Antibody-Associated Disease. Neurology 2022;99(18):795–9.
102. Fadda G, Banwell B, Waters P, et al. Silent New Brain MRI Lesions in Children with MOG-Antibody Associated Disease. Ann Neurol 2021;89(2):408–13.
103. Wingerchuk DM, Lucchinetti CF. Neuromyelitis Optica Spectrum Disorder. N Engl J Med 2022;387(7):631–9.
104. Waters P, Reindl M, Saiz A, et al. Multicentre comparison of a diagnostic assay: aquaporin-4 antibodies in neuromyelitis optica. J Neurol Neurosurg Psychiatry 2016;87(9):1005–15.
105. Prain K, Woodhall M, Vincent A, et al. AQP4 Antibody Assay Sensitivity Comparison in the Era of the 2015 Diagnostic Criteria for NMOSD. Front Neurol 2019;10:1028.
106. Waters PJ, McKeon A, Leite MI, et al. Serologic diagnosis of NMO: a multicenter comparison of aquaporin-4-IgG assays. Neurology 2012;78(9):665–71, discussion 669.
107. Reindl M, Schanda K, Woodhall M, et al. International multicenter examination of MOG antibody assays. Neurol Neuroimmunol Neuroinflamm 2020;7(2).
108. Majed M, Sanchez CV, Bennett JL, et al. Alterations in aquaporin-4-IgG serostatus in 986 patients: a laboratory-based longitudinal analysis. Ann Neurol 2023.
109. McKeon A, Pittock SJ, Lennon VA. CSF complements serum for evaluating paraneoplastic antibodies and NMO-IgG. Neurology 2011;76(12):1108–10.

110. Berger T, Rubner P, Schautzer F, et al. Antimyelin antibodies as a predictor of clinically definite multiple sclerosis after a first demyelinating event. N Engl J Med 2003;349(2):139–45.
111. Kuhle J, Pohl C, Mehling M, et al. Lack of association between antimyelin antibodies and progression to multiple sclerosis. N Engl J Med 2007;356(4):371–8.
112. Lampasona V, Franciotta D, Furlan R, et al. Similar low frequency of anti-MOG IgG and IgM in MS patients and healthy subjects. Neurology 2004;62(11): 2092–4.
113. Chan A, Decard BF, Franke C, et al. Serum antibodies to conformational and linear epitopes of myelin oligodendrocyte glycoprotein are not elevated in the preclinical phase of multiple sclerosis. Mult Scler 2010;16(10):1189–92.
114. Ketelslegers IA, Van Pelt DE, Bryde S, et al. Anti-MOG antibodies plead against MS diagnosis in an Acquired Demyelinating Syndromes cohort. Mult Scler 2015; 21(12):1513–20.
115. Sechi E, Buciuc M, Pittock SJ, et al. Positive Predictive Value of Myelin Oligodendrocyte Glycoprotein Autoantibody Testing. JAMA Neurol 2021;78(6):741–6.
116. Held F, Kalluri SR, Berthele A, et al. Frequency of myelin oligodendrocyte glycoprotein antibodies in a large cohort of neurological patients. Mult Scler J Exp Transl Clin 2021;7(2). 20552173211022767.
117. Gaudioso CM, Mar S, Casper TC, et al. MOG and AQP4 Antibodies among Children with Multiple Sclerosis and Controls. Ann Neurol 2023;93(2):271–84.
118. Akaishi T, Takahashi T, Misu T, et al. Difference in the Source of Anti-AQP4-IgG and Anti-MOG-IgG Antibodies in CSF in Patients With Neuromyelitis Optica Spectrum Disorder. Neurology 2021;97(1):e1–12.
119. Matsumoto Y, Kaneko K, Takahashi T, et al. Diagnostic implications of MOG-IgG detection in sera and cerebrospinal fluids. Brain 2023.
120. Jarius S, Ruprecht K, Kleiter I, et al. MOG-IgG in NMO and related disorders: a multicenter study of 50 patients. Part 1: Frequency, syndrome specificity, influence of disease activity, long-term course, association with AQP4-IgG, and origin. J Neuroinflammation 2016;13(1):279.
121. Jarius S, Lechner C, Wendel EM, et al. Cerebrospinal fluid findings in patients with myelin oligodendrocyte glycoprotein (MOG) antibodies. Part 2: Results from 108 lumbar punctures in 80 pediatric patients. J Neuroinflammation 2020;17(1):262.
122. Jarius S, Pellkofer H, Siebert N, et al. Cerebrospinal fluid findings in patients with myelin oligodendrocyte glycoprotein (MOG) antibodies. Part 1: Results from 163 lumbar punctures in 100 adult patients. J Neuroinflammation 2020;17(1):261.
123. Jarius S, Paul F, Franciotta D, et al. Cerebrospinal fluid findings in aquaporin-4 antibody positive neuromyelitis optica: results from 211 lumbar punctures. J Neurol Sci 2011;306(1–2):82–90.
124. Sechi E, Buciuc M, Flanagan EP, et al. Variability of cerebrospinal fluid findings by attack phenotype in myelin oligodendrocyte glycoprotein-IgG-associated disorder. Mult Scler Relat Disord 2021;47:102638.
125. Dobson R, Ramagopalan S, Davis A, et al. Cerebrospinal fluid oligoclonal bands in multiple sclerosis and clinically isolated syndromes: a meta-analysis of prevalence, prognosis and effect of latitude. J Neurol Neurosurg Psychiatry 2013; 84(8):909–14.
126. McKeon A, Lennon VA, Jacob A, et al. Coexistence of myasthenia gravis and serological markers of neurological autoimmunity in neuromyelitis optica. Muscle Nerve 2009;39(1):87–90.

127. Kunchok A, Flanagan EP, Snyder M, et al. Coexisting systemic and organ-specific autoimmunity in MOG-IgG1-associated disorders versus AQP4-IgG+ NMOSD. Mult Scler 2021;27(4):630–5.
128. Leite MI, Coutinho E, Lana-Peixoto M, et al. Myasthenia gravis and neuromyelitis optica spectrum disorder: a multicenter study of 16 patients. Neurology 2012; 78(20):1601–7.
129. Kunchok A, Chen JJ, McKeon A, et al. Coexistence of Myelin Oligodendrocyte Glycoprotein and Aquaporin-4 Antibodies in Adult and Pediatric Patients. JAMA Neurol 2020;77(2):257–9.
130. Sato DK, Callegaro D, Lana-Peixoto MA, et al. Distinction between MOG antibody-positive and AQP4 antibody-positive NMO spectrum disorders. Neurology 2014;82(6):474–81.
131. Carnero Contentti E, Lopez PA, Pettinicchi JP, et al. What percentage of AQP4-ab-negative NMOSD patients are MOG-ab positive? A study from the Argentinean multiple sclerosis registry (RelevarEM). Mult Scler Relat Disord 2021;49: 102742.
132. Stiebel-Kalish H, Hellmann MA, Mimouni M, et al. Does time equal vision in the acute treatment of a cohort of AQP4 and MOG optic neuritis? Neurol Neuroimmunol Neuroinflamm 2019;6(4):e572.
133. Kleiter I, Gahlen A, Borisow N, et al. Neuromyelitis optica: Evaluation of 871 attacks and 1,153 treatment courses. Ann Neurol 2016;79(2):206–16.
134. Bonnan M, Valentino R, Debeugny S, et al. Short delay to initiate plasma exchange is the strongest predictor of outcome in severe attacks of NMO spectrum disorders. J Neurol Neurosurg Psychiatry 2018;89(4):346–51.
135. Kleiter I, Gahlen A, Borisow N, et al. Apheresis therapies for NMOSD attacks: A retrospective study of 207 therapeutic interventions. Neurol Neuroimmunol Neuroinflamm 2018;5(6):e504.
136. Costello F. Neuromyelitis Optica Spectrum Disorders. Continuum (Minneap Minn) 2022;28(4):1131–70.
137. Nosadini M, Eyre M, Giacomini T, et al. Early Immunotherapy and Longer Corticosteroid Treatment Are Associated With Lower Risk of Relapsing Disease Course in Pediatric MOGAD. Neurol Neuroimmunol Neuroinflamm 2023;10(1).
138. Huda S, Whittam D, Jackson R, et al. Predictors of relapse in MOG antibody associated disease: a cohort study. BMJ Open 2021;11(11):e055392.
139. Huang W, Wang L, Xia J, et al. Efficacy and safety of azathioprine, mycophenolate mofetil, and reduced dose of rituximab in neuromyelitis optica spectrum disorder. Eur J Neurol 2022;29(8):2343–54.
140. O'Neill BP, Vernino S, Dogan A, et al. EBV-associated lymphoproliferative disorder of CNS associated with the use of mycophenolate mofetil. Neuro Oncol 2007;9(3):364–9.
141. Kandiel A, Fraser AG, Korelitz BI, et al. Increased risk of lymphoma among inflammatory bowel disease patients treated with azathioprine and 6-mercaptopurine. Gut 2005;54(8):1121–5.
142. Zhang C, Zhang M, Qiu W, et al. Safety and efficacy of tocilizumab versus azathioprine in highly relapsing neuromyelitis optica spectrum disorder (TANGO): an open-label, multicentre, randomised, phase 2 trial. Lancet Neurol 2020;19(5):391–401.
143. Pittock SJ, Berthele A, Fujihara K, et al. Eculizumab in Aquaporin-4-Positive Neuromyelitis Optica Spectrum Disorder. N Engl J Med 2019;381(7):614–25.
144. Wingerchuk DM, Fujihara K, Palace J, et al. Long-Term Safety and Efficacy of Eculizumab in Aquaporin-4 IgG-Positive NMOSD. Ann Neurol 2021;89(6):1088–98.

145. Pittock SJ, Fujihara K, Palace J, et al. Eculizumab monotherapy for NMOSD: Data from PREVENT and its open-label extension. Mult Scler 2022;28(3):480–6.
146. Palace J, Wingerchuk DM, Fujihara K, et al. Benefits of eculizumab in AQP4+ neuromyelitis optica spectrum disorder: Subgroup analyses of the randomized controlled phase 3 PREVENT trial. Mult Scler Relat Disord 2021;47:102641.
147. Pittock SJ, Lennon VA, McKeon A, et al. Eculizumab in AQP4-IgG-positive relapsing neuromyelitis optica spectrum disorders: an open-label pilot study. Lancet Neurol 2013;12(6):554–62.
148. Pittock SJ, Barnett M, Bennett JL, et al. Ravulizumab in Aquaporin-4-Positive Neuromyelitis Optica Spectrum Disorder. Ann Neurol 2023.
149. Tahara M, Oeda T, Okada K, et al. Safety and efficacy of rituximab in neuromyelitis optica spectrum disorders (RIN-1 study): a multicentre, randomised, double-blind, placebo-controlled trial. Lancet Neurol 2020;19(4):298–306.
150. Cree BAC, Bennett JL, Kim HJ, et al. Inebilizumab for the treatment of neuromyelitis optica spectrum disorder (N-MOmentum): a double-blind, randomised placebo-controlled phase 2/3 trial. Lancet 2019;394(10206):1352–63.
151. Marignier R, Bennett JL, Kim HJ, et al. Disability Outcomes in the N-MOmentum Trial of Inebilizumab in Neuromyelitis Optica Spectrum Disorder. Neurol Neuroimmunol Neuroinflamm 2021;8(3).
152. Marignier R, Pittock SJ, Paul F, et al. AQP4-IgG-seronegative patient outcomes in the N-MOmentum trial of inebilizumab in neuromyelitis optica spectrum disorder. Mult Scler Relat Disord 2022;57:103356.
153. Bennett JL, Aktas O, Rees WA, et al. Association between B-cell depletion and attack risk in neuromyelitis optica spectrum disorder: An exploratory analysis from N-MOmentum, a double-blind, randomised, placebo-controlled, multicentre phase 2/3 trial. EBioMedicine 2022;86:104321.
154. Rensel M, Zabeti A, Mealy MA, et al. Long-term efficacy and safety of inebilizumab in neuromyelitis optica spectrum disorder: Analysis of aquaporin-4-immunoglobulin G-seropositive participants taking inebilizumab for ≱4 years in the N-MOmentum trial. Mult Scler 2022;28(6):925–32.
155. Yamamura T, Kleiter I, Fujihara K, et al. Trial of Satralizumab in Neuromyelitis Optica Spectrum Disorder. N Engl J Med 2019;381(22):2114–24.
156. Traboulsee A, Greenberg BM, Bennett JL, et al. Safety and efficacy of satralizumab monotherapy in neuromyelitis optica spectrum disorder: a randomised, double-blind, multicentre, placebo-controlled phase 3 trial. Lancet Neurol 2020;19(5):402–12.
157. Yamamura T, Weinshenker B, Yeaman MR, et al. Long-term safety of satralizumab in neuromyelitis optica spectrum disorder (NMOSD) from SAkuraSky and SAkuraStar. Mult Scler Relat Disord 2022;66:104025.
158. Thakolwiboon S, Zhao-Fleming H, Karukote A, et al. Meta-analysis of effectiveness of steroid-sparing attack prevention in MOG-IgG-associated disorder. Mult Scler Relat Disord 2021;56:103310.
159. Spagni G, Sun B, Monte G, et al. Efficacy and safety of rituximab in myelin oligodendrocyte glycoprotein antibody-associated disorders compared with neuromyelitis optica spectrum disorder: a systematic review and meta-analysis. J Neurol Neurosurg Psychiatry 2023;94(1):62–9.
160. Sechi E, Cacciaguerra L, Chen JJ, et al. Myelin Oligodendrocyte Glycoprotein Antibody-Associated Disease (MOGAD): A Review of Clinical and MRI Features, Diagnosis, and Management. Front Neurol 2022;13:885218.

161. Chen JJ, Huda S, Hacohen Y, et al. Association of Maintenance Intravenous Immunoglobulin With Prevention of Relapse in Adult Myelin Oligodendrocyte Glycoprotein Antibody-Associated Disease. JAMA Neurol 2022;79(5):518–25.
162. Durozard P, Rico A, Boutiere C, et al. Comparison of the Response to Rituximab between Myelin Oligodendrocyte Glycoprotein and Aquaporin-4 Antibody Diseases. Ann Neurol 2020;87(2):256–66.
163. Morrow SA, Fraser JA, Day C, et al. Effect of Treating Acute Optic Neuritis With Bioequivalent Oral vs Intravenous Corticosteroids: A Randomized Clinical Trial. JAMA Neurol 2018;75(6):690–6.

# Advances in Multiple Sclerosis Neurotherapeutics, Neuroprotection, and Risk Mitigation Strategies

Ahmad Abdelrahman, MD, MPh[a], Enrique Alvarez, MD, PhD[b,*]

**KEYWORDS**

• Relapsing multiple sclerosis • Treatment • Disease modifying therapies • Efficacy • Safety • De-escalation • Remyelination • Neurorepair

**KEY POINTS**

- The treatment landscape has improved dramatically over the past few years for patients with multiple sclerosis (MS).
- New treatments for MS can significantly reduce the inflammatory process of relapsing MS.
- Treatments that induce neurorepair are much more limited, and neuroprotection involves preventing or at least limiting the inflammatory component of relapsing MS and encouraging a healthy lifestyle.
- Risk management strategies can help balance the risk of these newer disease-modifying therapies.
- Stopping or de-escalating treatment is an emerging risk management strategy.

## INTRODUCTION

We live in an exciting time for the treatment of patients with multiple sclerosis (MS). We now possess a vast armamentarium of effective therapies, which offer neuroprotection by mitigating neural damage and disability from the inflammatory processes involved in relapsing MS.[1] This is particularly important to do early in the disease course given our limited ability to induce neurorepair. Developing risk management strategies for these disease-modifying therapies (DMTs) can improve their safety and is important to achieve given that they will often need to be used for many years and can induce a variable amount of immunosuppression. This article will focus on recent advances in neurotherapeutics for relapsing MS and risk mitigation strategies.

[a] Department of Neurology, Rocky Mountain MS Center at the University of Colorado Anschutz Medical Center, Aurora, CO, USA; [b] Department of Neurology, Rocky Mountain MS Center at the University of Colorado Anschutz Medical Center, University of Colorado, Aurora, CO, USA
* Corresponding author. 12469 East 17th Place, Room 224, Aurora, CO 80045.
*E-mail address:* enrique.alvarez@cuanschutz.edu

Neurol Clin 42 (2024) 115–135
https://doi.org/10.1016/j.ncl.2023.08.002 **neurologic.theclinics.com**

## TREATMENT OF MULTIPLE SCLEROSIS ACUTE EXACERBATIONS

Early treatment of acute exacerbations may improve early functional recovery, helping to reduce deconditioning, and provide some neuroprotection.[2,3] The gold standard initial therapy consists of high-dose, short-term glucocorticoids: prednisone (oral 1000–1250 mg daily) or methylprednisolone (intravenous [IV] or oral 1000 mg daily) for 3 to 5 days. Adrenocorticotropic hormone (ACTH) has been postulated to have additional therapeutic advantages over glucocorticoids, but this remains to be shown clinically.[4] For severe relapses or those that do not respond to glucocorticoids, plasmapheresis should be considered.[5]

## TREATMENT OF RELAPSING MULTIPLE SCLEROSIS

When a patient is diagnosed with relapsing MS, one of the most reassuring discussions is the number of available DMT options (**Fig. 1**). Initial strategies on how to use these medications and how to leverage real-world evidence of comparative DMT performance are discussed in other articles in this MS issue. Additionally, further information on B-cell depletion and their role in progressive MS including risk mitigation and the promising therapies of Bruton tyrosine kinase inhibitors (BTKi) and autologous hematopoietic stem cell therapy are also discussed in other articles in this MS issue. Here, we will focus on newer neurotherapeutics and developments in their use.

Because of the number of DMTs that are now available for treating relapsing MS, they are sometimes discussed initially by route of administration (infusion, oral, or injection), efficacy (low, moderate, or high), or mechanism of action, as we will discuss here. See **Table 1** for a summary of DMTs used in patients with MS.

## B-CELL–DEPLETING THERAPIES

It was initially thought that MS was driven by T-cells, based on MS animal models showing the ability to transfer the disease to healthy animals with T-cells from affected animals.[6] However, targeted B-cell therapy was suggested by the presence of B-cells in cerebrospinal fluid and in inflammatory MS lesions, along with the presence of intrathecal antibody production including oligoclonal bands of roughly 95% of patients with MS.[7,8] The use of monoclonal antibodies directed against CD-20 that result in B-cell depletion has highlighted the importance of this cell in driving the pathophysiology of MS given their reduction in clinical and radiological measures of MS. The pathology is likely linked to altered interactions between T-cells, B-cells, and other immune cell populations since the main gene associated with MS is the major histocompatibility II factor by which B-cells (and other antigen-presenting cells) communicate with T-cells.[9]

There are currently 3 approved anti-CD20 monoclonal antibodies by the Food and Drug Administration (FDA) in the United States— ocrelizumab, ofatumumab, and ublituximab. Additionally, rituximab is often used off-label in the treatment of patients with MS. This drug class now accounts for over 50% of new prescriptions written for patients with MS. Ocrelizumab is a humanized anti-CD20 monoclonal antibody, which was approved in 2017 for relapsing MS and remains the only medication also approved for primary progressive MS. Ofatumumab is unique in its dosing as it is a subcutaneous injection monthly. Ublituximab is the most recent addition as it was approved in December 2022 and can be infused over 1 hour. Although rituximab is not approved for MS, it has the longest experience as it was approved initially in 1996 for non-Hodgkin lymphoma and tried in relapsing MS initially in the Heart failure

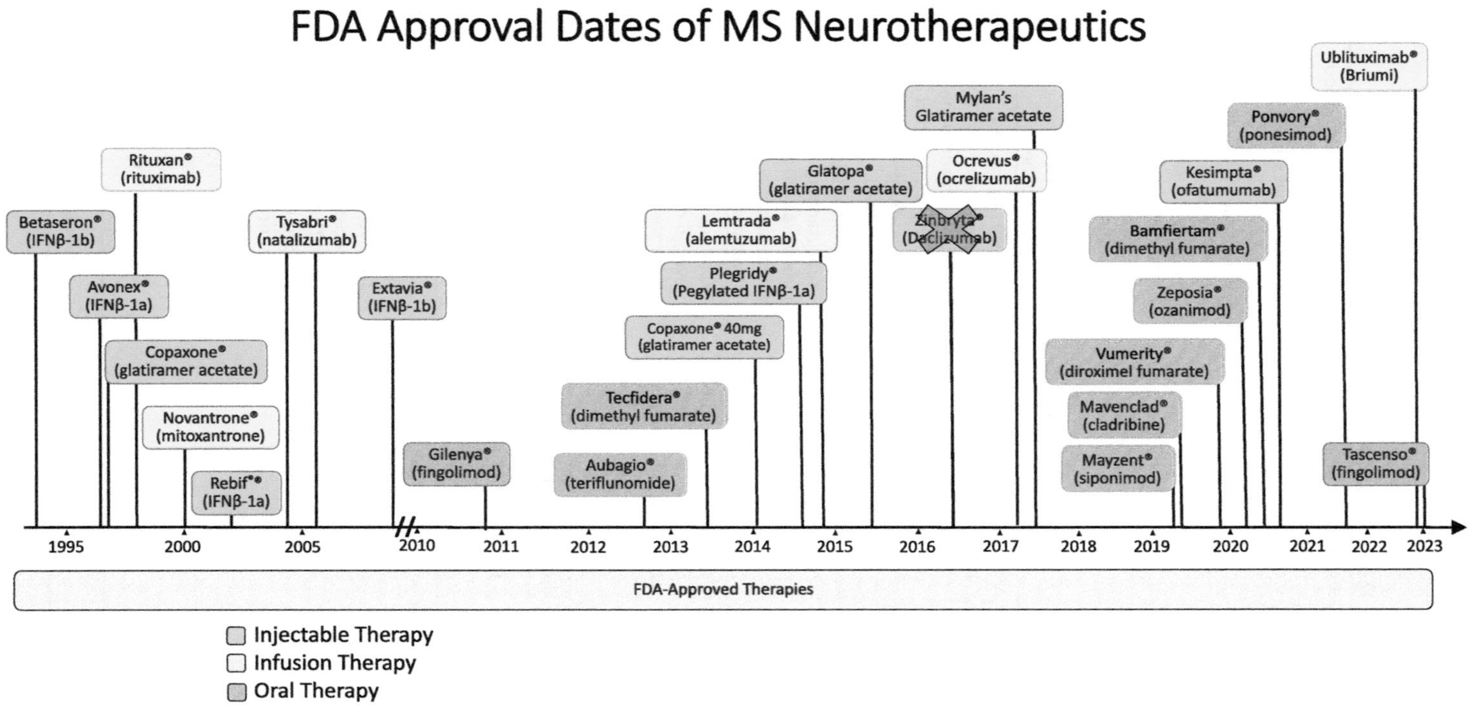


**Fig. 1.** Dates of approval of multiple sclerosis (MS) disease-modifying therapies by the Food and Drug Administration (FDA). Natalizumab was withdrawn in 2015 due to 3 cases of progressive multifocal leukoencephalopathy and reapproved in 2016. Daclizumab was withdrawn in 2018 due to safety concerns. mg, milligrams.

**Table 1**
**Disease-modifying therapies used for the treatment of patients with multiple sclerosis**

| Drug Name | Mechanisms of Action | Dosage and Route of Administration |
| --- | --- | --- |
| Ocrelizumab | Anti-CD20 humanized monoclonal antibody; B-cell depletion | 600 mg infused intravenously every 6 mo;<br>1st dose is split with 300 mg on day 1 and 15<br>Premedications can include (administered 30–60 min prior to infusion)<br>1. 100–125 mg IV methylprednisolone<br>2. Antihistamine (eg, diphenhydramine, cetirizine)<br>3. Acetaminophen |
| Rituximab | Anti-CD20 chimeric monoclonal antibody; B-cell depletion | 500–1000 mg infused intravenously every 6 mo;<br>Sometimes an additional 1000 mg is infused at 2 wk.<br>Premedications–same as ocrelizumab. |
| Ofatumumab | Anti-CD20 fully humanized monoclonal antibody; B-cell depletion | 20 mg administered via subcutaneous injection<br>Initial titration–at week 0, 1, 2<br>Maintenance dosing—every 4 wk starting on week 4 |
| Ublituximab | Glycoengineered anti-CD20 chimeric monoclonal antibody; B-cell depletion | 450 mg infused intravenously every 6 mo starting 2 wk after the initial dose of 150 mg<br>Premedications—same as ocrelizumab |
| Natalizumab | Humanized monoclonal antibody to alpha-4 integrin; blocks transmigration of activated lymphocytes into the CNS | 300 mg infused intravenously every 4–6 wk |
| Alemtuzumab | Anti-CD52 humanized monoclonal antibody; depletion of T-cells and B-cells predominantly with some effect on natural killer cells and monocytes | 12 mg infused intravenously for 5 consecutive days, followed by 12 mg daily for 3 consecutive days 12 months later. This can be repeated as needed every 12 mo. Monitor blood pressure.<br>Premedication—1000 mg methylprednisolone or equivalent and herpes prophylaxis for 2 mo or CD4+ cells are $\leq$ 200 cells/microliter. |

(*continued on next page*)

**Table 1**
**(*continued*)**

| Drug Name | Mechanisms of Action | Dosage and Route of Administration |
|---|---|---|
| Dimethyl Fumarate | Nuclear factor erythroid-derived 2-related factor (Nrf2)–dependent and independent pathways | 240 mg orally twice daily<br>Initial titration—120 mg orally twice daily for 7 d |
| Diroximel Fumarate | Nuclear factor erythroid-derived 2-related factor (Nrf2)–dependent and independent pathways | 462 mg orally twice daily<br>Initial titration—231 mg orally twice daily for 7 d |
| Monomethyl Fumarate | Nuclear factor erythroid-derived 2-related factor (Nrf2)–dependent and independent pathways | 190 mg orally twice daily<br>Initial titration—95 mg orally twice daily for 7 d |
| Teriflunomide | Inhibits dihydro-orotate dehydrogenase, involved in the de novo pyrimidine synthesis pathway | 7 or 14 mg orally once daily |
| Fingolimod | Sphingosine 1-phosphate receptor (S1PR) modulator | 0.5 mg orally once daily<br>Requires a first dose observation which must be repeated if there is a 2-wk interruption |
| Siponimod | Sphingosine 1-phosphate receptor (S1PR) modulator | 1 mg orally once daily (no CYP2C9*3 allele)<br>2 mg orally once daily (if CYP2C9*1/*3 or *2/*3) and contraindicated if CYP2C9*3/*3<br>Initial titration—start 0.25 mg daily and increase to these doses; repeat if there is a 4-d interruption |
| Ozanimod | Sphingosine 1-phosphate receptor (S1PR) modulator | 0.92 mg orally once daily<br>Initial titration—0.23 mg daily on day 1–4 followed by 0.46 mg daily on days 5–7, which must be repeated if there is a 2-wk interruption |
| Ponesimod | Sphingosine 1-phosphate receptor (S1PR) modulator | 20 mg orally once daily<br>Initial titration—start 2 mg orally daily and increase over 15 d; repeat if there is a 4-d interruption |
| Cladribine | Deoxyadenosine analog that is activated only in selected cell types, resulting in a reduction of B and T-cells | 3.5 mg/kg of body weight orally divided into 2 yearly treatment courses. Each course is separated into 2 treatment cycles of 4 to 5 days separated by roughly 4 weeks |

(*continued on next page*)

Table 1
*(continued)*

| Drug Name | Mechanisms of Action | Dosage and Route of Administration |
|---|---|---|
| Interferon beta-1b | Increases anti-inflammatory signals while downregulating proinflammatory cytokines | 0.25 mg (1 mL) subcutaneous injection every other day<br>Initial titration—0.25 mL every other day for weeks 1–2, followed by 0.50 mL every other day for weeks 3–4, and then 0.75 mL every other day for weeks 5–6 |
| Interferon beta-1a | Increases anti-inflammatory signals while downregulating proinflammatory cytokines | 30 mcg weekly intramuscular injection<br>Initial titration—7.5 mcg increasing by 7.5 mcg weekly until reach 30 μg. |
| Interferon beta-1a | Increases anti-inflammatory signals while downregulating proinflammatory cytokines | 22 or 44 mcg subcutaneous injection 3 times per week<br>Initial titration—For 22 mcg dose, 4.4 mcg 3 times per week for 2 wk, then 11 mcg 3 times per week for 2 wk.<br>For 44 mcg dose, 8.8 mcg 3 times per week for 2 wk, then 22 mcg 3 times per week for 2 wk. |
| Pegylated Interferon beta-1a | Increases anti-inflammatory signals while downregulating proinflammatory cytokines | 125 mcg subcutaneous or intramuscular injection every 2 wk.<br>Initial titration—63 mcg on day 194 mcg on day 15, and 125 mcg on day 29 and thereafter. |
| Glatiramer acetate | Binds major histocompatibility complex and inhibits inflammatory responses. Induces anti-inflammatory cytokines. | 20 mg daily or 40 mg 3 times per week subcutaneously |

*Abbreviations:* CNS, central nervous system; IV, intravenous; mcg, micrograms; mg, milligrams; ml, milliliter.

Events reduction with Remote Monitoring and eHealth Support trial.[10] Here, the proportion of patients with clinical relapses was statistically significantly reduced by 58% at 24 weeks ($P = .02$) and 49% at 48 weeks ($P = .04$) compared to patients receiving placebo. These medications have achieved relapse rate reductions in the range of 50% to 60% against active comparators including interferon beta-1a and teriflunomide.[11–13] They also showed reductions of 94% or greater in the number of contrast-enhancing lesions.

Treatment with B-cell–depleting therapies is commonly associated with infusion-related reactions (IRRs). These reactions are common (20%–48%) but are seldom life-threatening.[11–13] Although often thought to be a reaction to the drug themselves, they are more likely related to the release of cytokines upon B-cell apoptosis, creating a cytokine storm type reaction. These reactions are more common in patients who still have B-cells present during an infusion.[14] Ofatumumab has been associated with fewer treatment reactions likely because the subcutaneous route of administration causes a more gradual destruction of B-cells. Premedication with steroids is helpful in reducing IRRs.[15] Acetaminophen is also likely to be helpful as IRRs were more common with ublituximab, which omitted acetaminophen in the phase 3 trials.[13] In subsequent infusions, premedication may be simplified, as intravenous diphenhydramine can often cause sedation. Additionally, infusions can be done at a slower rate if IRRs in a patient are common.

Due to the immunosuppression associated with B-cell depletion, infections need to be monitored in patients receiving these medications. Upper respiratory tract, lower urinary tract, and skin infections are the most common infections.[11] Other infections and immune-mediated conditions reported in the post-marketing setting include herpes simplex virus and varicella zoster virus infections, hepatitis B reactivation, progressive multifocal leukoencephalopathy (PML), and colitis.[16–18] In the event of an active infection, treatment should be delayed until the infection has resolved. Patients are encouraged to receive all necessary live or live-attenuated vaccines at least 4 weeks prior to starting ocrelizumab infusions. They are also not recommended until B-cells have been repleted after discontinuing treatment. All non-live vaccines may be taken up to 2 weeks prior to starting infusions.

## NATALIZUMAB

Natalizumab disrupts the leukocyte-endothelial interaction and prevents the transmigration of activated leukocytes from the circulating bloodstream into the central nervous system by blocking the alpha-4 subunit on integrin.[19–21] In the phase III study versus placebo, natalizumab decreased sustained progression of disability by 42%, annualized relapse rate by 68%, new and enlarging T2 lesions by 83%, and the mean number of contrast-enhancing lesion by 92% over placebo.[20] Natalizumab was initially approved by the FDA in November 2004 but was withdrawn in February 2005 after 3 deaths from PML. After development of the risk-minimization and monitoring TOUCH program, natalizumab was reapproved in June 2006. The main safety concern is the development of PML that has been associated with longer natalizumab exposure, older age, and higher titers of the John Cunningham virus serology.[22,23] Infusions can be extended to every 6 weeks, which appears to reduce the rates of PML.[24] IRRs can occur but are much less common than with B-cell–depleting treatments and have been associated with anti-natalizumab antibodies. These antibodies should be checked when IRRs occur, as well as when breakthrough disease is suspected, as they have been associated with reduced efficacy of natalizumab.[25]

## ALEMTUZUMAB

Alemtuzumab is a monoclonal antibody directed against CD52-expressing T-cells, B-cells, natural killer cells, and monocytes.[26] The reduction in relapse rates versus interferon beta-1a ranges from 49.4% to 55%.[27,28] The main concern with the use of alemtuzumab is the type of adverse events, which include IRRs, infections, and autoimmune disorders (thyroid disorders, hemophagocytic lymphohistiocytosis, acquired hemophilia A), malignancy (thyroid cancer, melanoma, lymphoproliferative disorders), and vascular events (ischemic stroke, hemorrhagic stroke, arterial dissection, and myocardial infarction occurring shortly after initiation of alemtuzumab treatment).[27–33] Because of these concerns, alemtuzumab is recommended in the following settings: (1) for highly active relapsing-remitting multiple sclerosis (RRMS) that has been unresponsive to at least 2 or more DMTs by the FDA and (2) for highly active RRMS unresponsive to at least 1 DMT or in patients with rapidly worsening disease according to the European Medicines Agency.

## FUMARATES

The fumarate class of DMTs includes dimethyl fumarate, diroximel fumarate, and monomethyl fumarate.[33–35] Dimethyl and diroximel fumarate are both metabolized to monomethyl fumarate, which is believed to be the active component of these medications. In the CONFIRM and DEFINE phase 3 trial of dimethyl fumarate versus placebo, reductions of 44% and 53% were seen for relapses and 74% and 90% were observed for contrast-enhancing lesions.[34,35] Diroximel fumarate had similar efficacy to diroximel fumarate. However, it was better tolerated with fewer gastrointestinal-related side effects and missed days of work.[36,37] This is likely due to less methanol (<10%) produced with diroximel fumarate.[37] These effects can be ameliorated by taking the medication with food and improve after the first month of being on treatment. Although dimethyl fumarate is associated with more discontinuations due to gastrointestinal side effects, its efficacy is similar to that of fingolimod in several real-world studies.[38–41] Aspirin can help with flushing if this side effect becomes clinically significant.

## TERIFLUNOMIDE

Teriflunomide, the active metabolite of leflunomide, inhibits pyrimidine biosynthesis and disrupts the interaction between antigen-presenting cells, such as B-cells and T-cells.[36] Teriflunomide has become the comparator DMT in most of the newer clinical trials for higher efficacy therapies. However, teriflunomide demonstrated annualized relapse rate (ARR) reductions of 31.5% and 36.3% versus placebo and 80% reduction in contrast-enhancing lesions.[42,43] Although side effects associated with teriflunomide are common (**Table 2**), they can often be easily mitigated, especially given the long-term experience with leflunomide in rheumatological conditions (see **Table 1**).

## SPHINGOSINE 1-PHOSPHATE RECEPTOR MODULATORS

The sphingosine 1-phosphate receptor (S1PR) modulators include fingolimod, siponimod, ozanimod, and ponesimod. The efficacy of these medications appears to be similar, although comparative studies are currently difficult as the number of patients on siponimod, ozanimod, and ponesimod remains limited.[44] Fingolimod demonstrated an ARR reduction of 54% and had an 82% reduction in contrast-enhancing lesions versus placebo.[45] The efficacy of fingolimod appears to be similar to that of dimethyl fumarate although with better tolerability.[38,39,42]

The newer S1PR modulators gradually became more selective with the hope of minimizing their side effect profiles.[44] However, their side effect profile has remained similar and described in **Table 2**. Due to these similarities, complete blood count including lymphocyte counts, electrocardiogram, liver functions tests, and ophthalmic evaluation are recommended prior to starting S1PR modulators. The dosing for siponimod is variable and dependent on the *CYP2C9* genotype due to metabolism of this drug. Otherwise, all S1PR modulators can prolong the QT interval, resulting in the first dose observation required for fingolimod. This has been resolved with the newer generation

**Table 2**
**Most common risk mitigations associated with disease-modifying therapies used in patients with multiple sclerosis**

| Disease Modifying Therapy | Risk Factor | Risk Mitigation |
| --- | --- | --- |
| Anti-CD20 therapies (ocrelizumab, rituximab, ofatumumab, ublituximab) | Infusion Reactions | Infuse slower. Consider additional premedication or eliminating part of premedication if the reaction is to current premedication. If B-cells have reconstituted, then consider infusing more frequently or a higher dose |
| | Infections | Baseline and surveillance CBC with differential. Baseline hepatitis B core antibody, consider getting surface antibody if will vaccinate and surface antigen; monitor lymphocyte and immunoglobulin levels. Reconsideration of risk-benefit as disability and/or age increases |
| | Elevated Liver Enzymes | Baseline and surveillance LFTs throughout treatment |
| Natalizumab | PML | JCV serology testing every 6 mo. Repeat monitoring MRI every 6–12 mo. Infuse at extended interval – 6 wk. Reconsideration of risk-benefit though REMS program (TOUCH®) |
| | Infusion Reaction | Consider pretreatment medication. Check for natalizumab neutralizing antibodies |
| | Lymphopenia | Baseline and surveillance CBC with differential auto diff throughout treatment |
| | Elevated Liver Enzymes | Baseline and surveillance LFTs throughout treatment |

(*continued on next page*)

**Table 2**
***(continued)***

| Disease Modifying Therapy | Risk Factor | Risk Mitigation |
|---|---|---|
| Alemtuzumab | Infusion Reaction | Pretreatment with corticosteroids, antipyretics, and antihistamines. Control blood pressure |
| | Infection | Monitor for UTI, URI. REMS: baseline VZV IgG (consider vaccination if negative), TB testing |
| | Humoral Autoimmunity (thyroid, ITP, Goodpasture) | REMS: baseline and monthly for 48 mo after last dose—CBC with differential, serum creatinine, urinalysis with urine cell counts, LFTs, and TSH (every 3 mo) |
| | Malignancy | Monitor for thyroid cancer, melanoma, lymphoproliferative disorders, and lymphoma |
| Fumarates (dimethyl fumarate, diroximel fumarate, monomethyl fumarate) | Gastrointestinal Symptoms | Symptomatic treatment. Administer with food |
| | Flushing | Aspirin |
| | Pruritis | Antihistamine |
| | Lymphopenia | Baseline and surveillance CBC with differential throughout treatment. Absolute lymphocyte count of >500 cells/microliter recommended to reduce PML risk |
| | Elevated Liver Enzymes | Baseline and surveillance LFTs throughout treatment |
| Teriflunomide | Teratogenic | Baseline pregnancy test. Reliable method of contraception. Immediate washout with cholestyramine if become or planning on becoming pregnant |
| | Liver Toxicity | Baseline and surveillance LFTs, monthly for the first 6 mo and then periodically |
| | Lymphopenia | Baseline and surveillance CBC with differential throughout treatment |
| | Reactivation of Latent TB | Baseline TB screening with purified protein derivative or QuantiFERON |
| | Hair Thinning | Biotin supplementation |

| | | |
|---|---|---|
| Sphingosine 1-phosphate receptor (S1PR) modulator (fingolimod, siponimod, ozanimod, ponesimod) | Cardiac Anomalies (bradycardia, AV block, cardiac arrest, arrhythmias) | Baseline ECG and 6-h observation during the first dose (fingolimod). Avoid in patients with QT prolongation or medications that can increase the QT interval |
| | Zoster Infections (Herpes, Varicella) | Zoster virus serology screening and vaccinations. Early and/or chronic preventative treatment |
| | Macular Edema | Ophthalmologic monitoring or OCT at baseline and 3 mo after starting treatment |
| | Lymphopenia | Baseline and surveillance CBC with differential |
| | Elevated Liver Enzymes | Baseline and surveillance LFTs |
| Cladribine | Teratogenic | Baseline pregnancy test. Reliable method of contraception |
| | Lymphopenia | Baseline and surveillance CBC with differential. ALC reconstitution to within normal limits necessary for starting Year 2 of treatment |
| | Elevated Liver Enzymes | Baseline and surveillance LFTs |
| | Infection | Exclude HIV infection, TB, and active hepatitis at baseline. Monitor for zoster infections and consider vaccination |
| | Malignancy | Avoid if there is a current malignancy and monitor |
| Interferon (interferon beta-1a, interferon beta-1b, pegylated interferon beta-1a) | Flu-like Symptoms | NSAIDs, hydration |
| | Leukopenia | Baseline and surveillance CBC with differential |
| | Elevated Liver Enzymes | Baseline and surveillance LFTs |
| | Depression/Suicidal | Screening and monitoring for depression and suicidal ideation. Consider antidepressant medications and/or referral to therapy. |
| Glatiramer acetate | Acute post-injection systemic reaction | Reassurance that reaction is self-limiting. |

*Abbreviations:* CBC, complete blood count; ECG, electrocardiogram, HIV, human immunodeficiency virus; ITP, immune thrombocytopenic purpura; JCV, john cunningham virus; LFT, liver function tests; NSAIDS, nonsteroidal anti-inflammatory drugs; OCT, optical coherence tomography; PML, progressive multifocal leucoencephalitis; REMS, risk evaluation and mitigation strategy; TB, tuberculosis; TSH, thyroid-stimulating hormone; URI, upper respiratory infection; UTI, urinary tract infection; VZV, varicella zoster virus.

S1PR modulators by using a dose titration to gradually start medication. It is too early to compare infections between these medications, but the newer generation S1PR modulators also appear to have better vaccine responses than fingolimod.[46] These differences may provide an advantage of the newer S1PR modulators over fingolimod.

## CLADRIBINE

Cladribine works by suppressing purine synthesis and targets specific lymphocyte subtypes by controlling activation of this medication. Over 96 weeks, the ARR was reduced by 57.6% over placebo and contrast-enhancing lesions by 85.7%.[47] The percentage of patients who had a relapse gradually increased over the following 2 years to 25%.[48] The concern for malignancies delayed the approval of this medication, and it is usually reserved as a second-line therapy. It is contraindicated in patients with active chronic infections, malignancy, pregnancy, breastfeeding, and patients of reproductive potential not willing to use effective contraception for at least 6 months after treatment.[49] Due to these contraindications and adverse events, patients should be screened for pregnancy, malignancies, and active infections prior to initiating cladribine therapy.

## INTERFERON BETA-1

Interferons (IFN) are cytokines that regulate the responsiveness of the immune system via multiple mechanisms. Four medications are included in this group: recombinant human interferon beta (IFN-b)1b, intramuscular IFN-b1a, subcutaneous IFN-b1a, and pegylated IFN-b1a. The first approved medication for patients with MS was IFN-b1b in 1993 by the FDA. IFN-b1a is produced in mammalian hosts and is glycosylated, while IFN-b1b is produced in bacterial hosts and is not glycosylated. These DMTs have lower efficacy, reducing relapses by about a third with the lower dose once weekly intramuscular IFN-b1a being at the lower end of the group.[50–52] Adverse events are similar and include injection site reactions (eg, abscess, cellulitis, or necrosis), flu-like symptoms, liver abnormalities, thyroid dysfunction, leukopenia, and decreased mood. The low efficacy and difficulty with tolerability have led to decreased use of these DMTs over the past few years.

## GLATIRAMER ACETATE

Glatiramer is composed of random polymers of the 4 amino acids most commonly found in myelin basic protein. Glatiramer affects the immune system by binding to major histocompatibility complex molecules and competes with various myelin antigens in presenting to T-cells. Glatiramer is also a potent inducer of specific T helper 2 type suppressor cells that migrate to the brain, resulting in bystander suppression and anti-inflammatory cytokine production.[50] Glatiramer acetate has a similar level of efficacy as subcutaneous INF-b1a and INF-b1b.[53,54] Glatiramer is not associated with an increased risk of infection but can be associated with local injection site reactions and, less commonly, transient systemic post-injection reactions (eg, chest pain, flushing, dyspnea, palpitations, and/or anxiety). The safety of glatiramer acetate has led to the development of a monthly depot formulation with an ongoing phase 3 clinical trial being conducted (NCT04121221).

## NOVEL TREATMENTS UNDER DEVELOPMENT

New therapies for relapsing MS include BTKi and stem cell transplantation, which are discussed more in other sections. Phase 3 studies are currently underway for multiple

BTKi in treating relapsing and progressive MS including evobrutinib, tolebrutinib, fenebrutinib, remibrutinib, and BIIB091, with results for evobrutinib expected at the end of 2023. Phase 3 studies are also underway for IMU-838 (vidofludimus calcium),a more selective inhibitor of dihydroorotate dehydrogenase than teriflunomide, which is being compared to placebo. Additionally, biosimilars are being developed for natalizumab, which may acquire FDA approval by the end of 2023. Xacrel, a biosimilar to ocrelizumab, is currently being studied in Iran. Frexalimab (SAR441344) is a monoclonal antibody that binds CD40 L and will soon be entering phase 3 studies after reporting an 89% reduction in contrast-enhancing lesions in patients with relapsing MS (NCT04879628). Many other compounds have completed phase 1 and 2 trials, suggesting that we will continue to see drugs with new mechanisms of action for the treatment MS.

## REMYELINATION

A pathway to consider in neurorepair is neuronal remyelination. Remyelination is mediated by the recruitment and differentiation of surrounding oligodendroglial precursor cells to restore conduction through axons.[55] Because of the increasing loss of neurons, it may prove difficult to achieve this goal later in the disease. However, since dalfampridine is theorized to work on demyelinated neurons, remyelination should be achievable in at least some patients. Current drugs being explored in clinical trials for possible remyelinating potential include clemastine, GSK239512, opicinumab, GNbAC1, simvastatin, biotin, and domperidone (**Table 3**).[55] Despite the extraordinary strides being made in identifying remyelinating therapies, there has yet to be an effective treatment.

## MULTIPLE SCLEROSIS RISK MITIGATION

Risk mitigation strategies refer to the identification of therapy risks based on the individual patient's characteristics.[56] As with any medication, DMTs are associated with different risks and adverse events. Therefore, it is vital to not only know what those risks/adverse events are but also how to minimize and address them if they are precipitated. **Table 2** summarizes the most common risk mitigation strategies associated with each of the MS DMTs.

One of the most important aspects in risk mitigation is determining whether a patient still needs to be on a DMT. Much like there can be therapeutic inertia, which can slow down therapy escalation when breakthrough disease occurs, there can be therapeutic inertia that keeps patients on treatment that they may not need. In the past, this was less common as patients often tired of using the frequent injectable platform medications, and they would self-discontinue treatment. There was also a recognition that patients tended to have less inflammatory activity as they aged and remained stable for several years. This led to the first randomized trial evaluating DMT discontinuation. The Discontinue Disease Modifying Therapies in MS (DISCOMS) study randomized patients over the age of 55 years who were clinically stable for 5 years and radiologically stable for 3 years to continue or stop treatment. In this patient population, DMT discontinuation was not non-inferior to continuing therapy (ie, 12.2% of patients who discontinued DMT had a relapse or a new/expanding brain MRI lesion vs 4.7% who continued therapy).[57] It therefore appears to be safe to discontinue medication in this patient population, although most of these patients were on platform medications.

There was a shift toward the approval of more highly efficacious and tolerable DMTs following the approval of natalizumab and fingolimod. With patients increasingly likely to be on higher efficacy therapies, another risk mitigation approach to be considered is de-escalation when appropriate (eg, increased safety concerns, aging patient

Table 3
Remyelinating treatments tried in patients with MS

| Medication | Mechanism of Action | Study Information |
| --- | --- | --- |
| Clemastine | First-generation histamine H1 receptor blocker | Remyelinating potential identified in a high-throughput in vitro screening.[62]<br>The ReBUILD clinical study involved 50 RRMS patients and investigated the remyelinating potential of clemastine in chronic demyelinating optic neuropathy. Remyelination was assessed using the shortening of the P100 latency delay in VEP, which was reduced by 3.2 ms/eye if the results were analyzed as a "delayed treatment trial," or 1.7 ms/eye when analyzed as a "crossover trial."[63] |
| GSK239512 | CNS-penetrant antihistamine that targets $H_3$ receptors | Phase II, randomized, parallel-group, placebo-controlled, double-blind, multicenter study of adults with relapsing MS (NCT01772199). While the study failed to meet its primary and secondary endpoints, post hoc analysis using MTR to assess in vivo myelin content showed small mean improvements in lesional MTR relative to placebo.[64] |
| Opicinumab | Antibody against LINGO-1 (leucine-rich repeat and immunoglobulin-like domain–containing nogo receptor–interacting protein 1).[65,66]<br>Loss of LINGO-1 enhances myelin sheath formation and myelination.[65,66] | The Phase 2 RENEW showed non statistically significant improvement in the recovery of optic nerve conduction latency by measuring VEP in patients with ON. The phase 2b SYNERGY trial also did not meet its primary endpoint, but post hoc analyses showed an increased clinical effect in a subgroup of patients with earlier disease and certain baseline MRI characteristics. Based on these results a third phase 2 trial, AFFINITY, was done which was not successful. |
| GNbAC1 | Antibody against the envelope protein (ENV) of multiple sclerosis–associated retrovirus.<br>ENV protein can be silenced via epigenetic control and certain environmental factors such as viruses (eg, EBV and HHV8) result in its re-expression. ENV can limit OPC differentiation via toll-like receptor 4.[67,68] | In the CHANGE-MS trial, 270 patients were enrolled and showed significant benefit of GNbAC1 on cortical and thalamic atrophy, with relative volume loss reductions of 31% and 72%. Furthermore, there was a 63% reduction in the number of T1 hypointense lesions when compared to the control group. Finally, a benefit in magnetization transfer ratio in both normal appearing white matter and cerebral cortex, suggests an effect on remyelination. |

| | | |
|---|---|---|
| Simvastatin | β-Hydroxy β-methylglutaryl-CoA (HMG-CoA) reductase inhibitor | Previous trials showed that statins stimulated OPC differentiation. The phase 4 SIMCOMBIN trial assessed whether simvastatin could be efficacious as an add-on therapy to interferon beta-1a in relapsing MS.[69] No difference in the annualized relapse rate was seen. However, a second trial (MS-STAT) which enrolled 140 secondary progressive MS patients showed that simvastatin led to a 43% reduction in mean annualized brain atrophy rate. A larger 3-y MS-STAT2 study is now planned to enroll 1180 patients.[70] |
| Biotin | Vitamin B Coenzyme<br>May increase myelin production by increasing adenosine triphosphate and stimulating fatty acid synthesis.[71] | The MS-SPI trial enrolled 154 patients and increased the proportion of patients with disability reversal by 12.6% vs placebo. However, the phase 3 SPI2 with 642 subjects failed to show a significant improvement in disability.[72] |
| Domperidone | A D2/D3 dopamine receptor antagonist<br>May increase production of prolactin.[73] | Prolactin can stimulate remyelination in animal models which prompted the initiation of a phase 2 clinical trial in secondary progressive MS (NCT02308137).[74] |
| Elezanumab | Fully human monoclonal antibody directed against repulsive guidance molecule A (RGMa)<br>RGMa is a modulator of axonal growth, myelination, and downstream immunoregulatory molecules that inhibiting oligodendroglial regeneration[75] | Phase 2 trials involving 123 patients in progressive MS (RADIUS-P) and 208 patients in relapsing MS (RADIUS-R) vs placebo in addition to their standard of care disease modifying therapy were completed in 2021. However, elezanumab did not outperform placebo.[76] |

*Abbreviations:* ENV, envelope protein; MS, multiple sclerosis; ms, millisecond; MTR, magnetization transfer ratio; ON, optic neuritis; OPC, oligodendrocyte precursor cells; VEP, visual evoked potentials.

population with associated immunosenescence that may incur additional risks).[58] Although advancing age remains an important factor in considering when a patient may no longer need a DMT to treat their MS, another factor to consider is increasing disability due to its association with serious infections.[59] For example, patients with MS on rituximab were 8.56 times more likely to have a serious infection than if they did not require a walking device.[60] In this multivariable model using stepwise selection, age became non-significant. Additionally, during the coronavirus disease 2019 pandemic, mortality was much more associated with being non-ambulatory (OR = 25.4) than age (OR = 1.77 for every 10-year increase) or treatment, which was not significant.[61] However, B-cell–depleting therapies were associated with higher rates of hospitalizations.

In summary, risk management of being on a DMT should include monitoring when a patient should discontinue or de-escalate their treatment.

## SUMMARY

There have been great advances in the treatment of relapsing MS. Since the introduction of the first FDA approved DMT for relapsing MS in 1993, new therapies have continued to be developed with higher efficacy and better safety profiles and tolerability. The inflammation associated with relapses results in neuronal damage that disproportionally affects patients when they are younger. The risks of infections associated with higher efficacy DMTs escalate with increasing disability. This proves another reason to maximize neuroprotection early in the disease course as part of the risk mitigation strategy. By controlling relapses, the contribution of progressive MS has become clearer and highlights the continued need to pursue therapies to stop progression and offer neurorepair.

## CLINICS CARE POINTS

- Once a diagnosis of relapsing MS is secured, treatment options should be discussed with the patient to minimize the risk of future disabling relapses and maximize neuroprotection.
- A risk mitigation strategy should be developed early to maximize the benefit-risk potential of the disease-modifying therapy.
- More investigation is needed in the treatment of progressive disease and inducing neurorepair.

## DISCLOSURES/ FUNDING

AA has nothing to disclose. EA has received compensation for activities such as advisory boards, lectures and consultancy with the following companies and organizations: Alexion, Biogen, Celgene/BMS, EMD Serono/Merck, Genentech/Roche, Horizon, Motric Bio, Novartis, Sanofi, and TG Therapeutics and research support from: Biogen, Genentech/Roche, Novartis, TG Therapeutics, Patient-Centered Outcomes Research Initiative, National Multiple Sclerosis Society, National Institutes of Health, and Rocky Mountain MS Center. This review was non-funded.

## REFERENCES

1. Amin M, Hersh CM. Updates and advances in multiple sclerosis neurotherapeutics. Neurodegener Dis Manag 2023;13(1):47–70.

2. Brusaferri F, Candelise L. Steroids for multiple sclerosis and optic neuritis: a meta-analysis of randomized controlled clinical trials. J Neurol 2000;247(6): 435–42.
3. Lublin FD, Baier M, Cutter G. Effect of relapses on development of residual deficit in multiple sclerosis. Neurology 2003;61(11):1528–32.
4. Filippini G, Brusaferri F, Sibley WA, et al. Corticosteroids or ACTH for acute exacerbations in multiple sclerosis. Cochrane Database Syst Rev 2000;4: CD001331.
5. Cortese I, Chaudhry V, So YT, et al. Evidence-based guideline update: Plasmapheresis in neurologic disorders: report of the Therapeutics and Technology Assessment Subcommittee of the American Academy of Neurology. Neurology 2011;76(3):294–300.
6. Sospedra M, Martin R. Immunology of multiple sclerosis. Annu Rev Immunol 2005;23:683–747.
7. Dobson R, Ramagopalan S, Davis A, et al. Cerebrospinal fluid oligoclonal bands in multiple sclerosis and clinically isolated syndromes: a meta-analysis of prevalence, prognosis and effect of latitude. J Neurol Neurosurg Psychiatry 2013;84(8): 909–14.
8. Esiri MM. Multiple sclerosis: a quantitative and qualitative study of immunoglobulin-containing cells in the central nervous system. Neuropathol Appl Neurobiol 1980;6(1):9–21.
9. International Multiple Sclerosis Genetics Consortium, Wellcome Trust Case Control Consortium 2, Sawcer S, Hellenthal G, et al. Genetic risk and a primary role for cell-mediated immune mechanisms in multiple sclerosis. Nature 2011; 476(7359):214–9.
10. Hauser SL, Waubant E, Arnold DL, et al, HERMES Trial Group. B-cell depletion with rituximab in relapsing-remitting multiple sclerosis. N Engl J Med 2008; 358(7):676–88.
11. Hauser SL, Bar-Or A, Comi G, et al. OPERA I and OPERA II Clinical Investigators. Ocrelizumab versus Interferon Beta-1a in Relapsing Multiple Sclerosis. N Engl J Med 2017;376(3):221–34.
12. Hauser SL, Bar-Or A, Cohen JA, et al. ASCLEPIOS I and ASCLEPIOS II Trial Groups. Ofatumumab versus Teriflunomide in Multiple Sclerosis. N Engl J Med 2020;383(6):546–57.
13. Steinman L, Fox E, Hartung HP, et al. ULTIMATE I and ULTIMATE II Investigators. Ublituximab versus Teriflunomide in Relapsing Multiple Sclerosis. N Engl J Med 2022;387(8):704–14.
14. Alvarez E, Nair KV, Sillau S, et al. Tolerability and Safety of Switching from Rituximab to Ocrelizumab: Evaluating Factors Associated with Infusion Related Reactions. Mult Scler J Exp Transl Clin 2022;8(1). 20552173211069359.
15. Tachi T, Yasuda M, Usui K, et al. Risk factors for developing infusion reaction after rituximab administration in patients with B-cell non-Hodgkin's lymphoma. Pharmazie 2015;70(10):674–7.
16. Ocrevus (ocrelizumab) prescribing information. Available at: https://www.accessdata.fda.gov/drugsatfda_docs/label/2022/761053s029s030lbl.pdf Accessed August 05, 2022. No abstract available.
17. Patel A, Sul J, Gordon ML, et al. Progressive Multifocal Leukoencephalopathy in a Patient With Progressive Multiple Sclerosis Treated With Ocrelizumab Monotherapy. JAMA Neurol 2021;78(6):736–40.

18. Ciardi MR, Iannetta M, Zingaropoli MA, et al. Reactivation of Hepatitis B Virus With Immune-Escape Mutations After Ocrelizumab Treatment for Multiple Sclerosis. Open Forum Infect Dis 2018;6(1):ofy356.
19. Niino M, Bodner C, Simard ML, et al. Natalizumab effects on immune cell responses in multiple sclerosis. Ann Neurol 2006;59(5):748–54. Erratum in: Ann Neurol. 2006 Jun;59(6):990. PMID: 16634035.
20. Stüve O, Marra CM, Jerome KR, et al. Immune surveillance in multiple sclerosis patients treated with natalizumab. Ann Neurol 2006;59(5):743–7.
21. Polman CH, O'Connor PW, Havrdova E, et al. A randomized, placebo-controlled trial of natalizumab for relapsing multiple sclerosis. N Engl J Med 2006;354(9): 899–910.
22. Kappos L, Bates D, Hartung HP, et al. Natalizumab treatment for multiple sclerosis: recommendations for patient selection and monitoring. Lancet Neurol 2007;6(5):431–41.
23. Ransohoff RM. Natalizumab for multiple sclerosis. N Engl J Med 2007;356(25): 2622–9.
24. Foley JF, Defer G, Ryerson LZ, et al. NOVA study investigators. Comparison of switching to 6-week dosing of natalizumab versus continuing with 4-week dosing in patients with relapsing-remitting multiple sclerosis (NOVA): a randomised, controlled, open-label, phase 3b trial. Lancet Neurol 2022;21(7): 608–19.
25. Vollmer BL, Nair K, Sillau S, et al. Rituximab versus natalizumab, fingolimod, and dimethyl fumarate in multiple sclerosis treatment. Ann Clin Transl Neurol 2020; 7(9):1466–76.
26. Ruck T, Bittner S, Wiendl H, et al. Alemtuzumab in Multiple Sclerosis: Mechanism of Action and Beyond. Int J Mol Sci 2015;16(7):16414–39.
27. Cohen JA, Coles AJ, Arnold DL, et al. Alemtuzumab versus interferon beta 1a as first-line treatment for patients with relapsing-remitting multiple sclerosis: a randomised controlled phase 3 trial. Lancet 2012;380(9856): 1819–28.
28. Coles AJ, Twyman CL, Arnold DL, et al, CARE-MS II investigators. Alemtuzumab for patients with relapsing multiple sclerosis after disease-modifying therapy: a randomised controlled phase 3 trial. Lancet 2012;380(9856): 1829–39.
29. Coles AJ, Fox E, Vladic A, et al. Alemtuzumab more effective than interferon β-1a at 5-year follow-up of CAMMS223 clinical trial. Neurology 2012;78(14):1069–78.
30. Lemtrada (alemtuzumab) prescribing information. Available at: https://www.accessdata.fda.gov/drugsatfda_docs/label/2022/103948s5185lbl.pdf (Accessed on June 17, 2022).
31. European Medicines Agency. Measures to minimise risk of serious side effects of multiple sclerosis medicine Lemtrada. https://www.ema.europa.eu/en/documents/referral/lemtrada-article-20-procedure-measures-minimise-risk-serious-side-effects-multiple-sclerosis_en-0.pdf Accessed on May 05, 2020.
32. FDA warns about rare but serious risks of stroke and blood vessel wall tears with multiple sclerosis drug Lemtrada (alemtuzumab). https://www.fda.gov/Drugs/DrugSafety/ucm624247.htm Accessed on November 29, 2018.
33. Azevedo CJ, Kutz C, Dix A, et al. Intracerebral haemorrhage during alemtuzumab administration. Lancet Neurol 2019;18(4):329–31. Erratum in: Lancet Neurol. 2019 Feb 22;: Erratum in: Lancet Neurol. 2019 Sep;18(9):e8. PMID: 30777657.
34. Gold R, Kappos L, Arnold DL, et al, DEFINE Study Investigators. Placebo-controlled phase 3 study of oral BG-12 for relapsing multiple sclerosis. N Engl

J Med 2012;367(12):1098–107. Erratum in: N Engl J Med. 2012 Dec 13;367(24): 2362. PMID: 22992073.
35. Fox RJ, Miller DH, Phillips JT, et al, CONFIRM Study Investigators. Placebo-controlled phase 3 study of oral BG-12 or glatiramer in multiple sclerosis. N Engl J Med 2012;367(12):1087–97. Erratum in: N Engl J Med. 2012 Oct 25;367(17):1673. PMID: 22992072.
36. Wundes A, Wray S, Gold R, et al. Improved gastrointestinal profile with diroximel fumarate is associated with a positive impact on quality of life compared with dimethyl fumarate: results from the randomized, double-blind, phase III EVOLVE-MS-2 study. Ther Adv Neurol Disord 2021;14. 1756286421993999.
37. Wray S, Then Bergh F, Wundes A, et al. Efficacy and Safety Outcomes with Diroximel Fumarate After Switching from Prior Therapies or Continuing on DRF: Results from the Phase 3 EVOLVE-MS-1 Study. Adv Ther 2022;39(4): 1810–31.
38. Vollmer B, Ontaneda D, Harris H, et al. Comparative discontinuation, effectiveness, and switching practices of dimethyl fumarate and fingolimod at 36-month follow-up. J Neurol Sci 2019;407:116498.
39. Zhu C, Kalincik T, Horakova D, et al, MSBase Study Group. Comparison Between Dimethyl Fumarate, Fingolimod, and Ocrelizumab After Natalizumab Cessation. JAMA Neurol 2023;80(7):739–48.
40. Hersh CM, Altincatal A, Belviso N, et al. Real-world effectiveness of dimethyl fumarate versus fingolimod in a cohort of patients with multiple sclerosis using standardized, quantitative outcome metrics. Mult Scler J Exp Transl Clin 2022; 8(1). 20552173211069852.
41. Zeyda M, Poglitsch M, Geyeregger R, et al. Disruption of the interaction of T cells with antigen-presenting cells by the active leflunomide metabolite teriflunomide: involvement of impaired integrin activation and immunologic synapse formation. Arthritis Rheum 2005;52(9):2730–9.
42. O'Connor P, Wolinsky JS, Confavreux C, et al, TEMSO Trial Group. Randomized trial of oral teriflunomide for relapsing multiple sclerosis. N Engl J Med 2011; 365(14):1293–303.
43. Confavreux C, O'Connor P, Comi G, et al, TOWER Trial Group. Oral teriflunomide for patients with relapsing multiple sclerosis (TOWER): a randomised, double-blind, placebo-controlled, phase 3 trial. Lancet Neurol 2014;13(3): 247–56.
44. McGinley MP, Cohen JA. Sphingosine 1-phosphate receptor modulators in multiple sclerosis and other conditions. Lancet 2021;398(10306):1184–94. Erratum in: Lancet. 2021 Sep 25;398(10306):1132. PMID: 34175020.
45. Kappos L, Radue EW, O'Connor P, et al, FREEDOMS Study Group. A placebo-controlled trial of oral fingolimod in relapsing multiple sclerosis. N Engl J Med 2010;362(5):387–401.
46. Baker D, Forte E, Pryce G, et al. The impact of sphingosine-1-phosphate receptor modulators on COVID-19 and SARS-CoV-2 vaccination. Mult Scler Relat Disord 2023;69:104425.
47. Giovannoni G, Comi G, Cook S, et al, CLARITY Study Group. A placebo-controlled trial of oral cladribine for relapsing multiple sclerosis. N Engl J Med 2010;362(5):416–26.
48. Giovannoni G, Soelberg Sorensen P, Cook S, et al. Safety and efficacy of cladribine tablets in patients with relapsing-remitting multiple sclerosis: Results from

the randomized extension trial of the CLARITY study. Mult Scler 2018;24(12): 1594–604.
49. Prescribing information Mavenclad (cladribine) tablets. https://www.accessdata.fda.gov/drugsatfda_docs/label/2022/022561s006lbl.pdf Accessed on October 20, 2022.
50. Rudick RA, Goelz SE. Beta-interferon for multiple sclerosis. Exp Cell Res 2011; 317(9):1301–11.
51. Durelli L, Verdun E, Barbero P, et al. Independent Comparison of Interferon (INCOMIN) Trial Study Group. Every-other-day interferon beta-1b versus once-weekly interferon beta-1a for multiple sclerosis: results of a 2-year prospective randomised multicentre study (INCOMIN). Lancet 2002;359(9316): 1453–60.
52. Arnon R, Aharoni R. Mechanism of action of glatiramer acetate in multiple sclerosis and its potential for the development of new applications. Proc Natl Acad Sci U S A 2004;101(Suppl 2):14593–8.
53. Mikol DD, Barkhof F, Chang P, et al. REGARD study group. Comparison of subcutaneous interferon beta-1a with glatiramer acetate in patients with relapsing multiple sclerosis (the REbif vs Glatiramer Acetate in Relapsing MS Disease [REGARD] study): a multicentre, randomised, parallel, open-label trial. Lancet Neurol 2008;7(10):903–14.
54. Cadavid D, Wolansky LJ, Skurnick J, et al. Efficacy of treatment of MS with IFNbeta-1b or glatiramer acetate by monthly brain MRI in the BECOME study. Neurology 2009;72(23):1976–83.
55. Kremer D, Akkermann R, Küry P, et al. Current advancements in promoting remyelination in multiple sclerosis. Mult Scler 2019;25(1):7–14.
56. Ontaneda D, Cohn S, Fox R. Risk stratification and mitigation multiple sclerosis. Mult Scler Relat Disord 2014;3(5):639–49.
57. Corboy JR, Fox RJ, Kister I, et al. DISCOMS investigators. Risk of new disease activity in patients with multiple sclerosis who continue or discontinue disease-modifying therapies (DISCOMS): a multicentre, randomised, single-blind, phase 4, non-inferiority trial. Lancet Neurol 2023;22(7):568–77.
58. Vollmer BL, Wolf AB, Sillau S, et al. Evolution of Disease Modifying Therapy Benefits and Risks: An Argument for De-escalation as a Treatment Paradigm for Patients With Multiple Sclerosis. Front Neurol 2022;12:799138.
59. Luna G, Alping P, Burman J, et al. Infection Risks Among Patients With Multiple Sclerosis Treated With Fingolimod, Natalizumab, Rituximab, and Injectable Therapies. JAMA Neurol 2020;77(2):184–91. Erratum in: JAMA Neurol. 2021 Sep 7;: null. PMID: 31589278; PMCID: PMC6784753.
60. Vollmer BL, Wallach AI, Corboy JR, et al. Serious safety events in rituximab-treated multiple sclerosis and related disorders. Ann Clin Transl Neurol 2020; 7(9):1477–87.
61. Salter A, Fox RJ, Newsome SD, et al. Outcomes and Risk Factors Associated With SARS-CoV-2 Infection in a North American Registry of Patients With Multiple Sclerosis. JAMA Neurol 2021;78(6):699–708. Erratum in: JAMA Neurol. 2021 Jun 1;78(6):765. PMID: 33739362; PMCID: PMC7980147.
62. Mei F, Fancy SPJ, Shen YA, et al. Micropillar arrays as a high-throughput screening platform for therapeutics in multiple sclerosis. Nat Med 2014;20(8): 954–60.
63. Green AJ, Gelfand JM, Cree BA, et al. Clemastine fumarate as a remyelinating therapy for multiple sclerosis (ReBUILD): a randomised, controlled, double-blind, crossover trial. Lancet 2017;390(10111):2481–9.

64. Schwartzbach CJ, Grove RA, Brown R, et al. Lesion remyelinating activity of GSK239512 versus placebo in patients with relapsing-remitting multiple sclerosis: a randomised, single-blind, phase II study. J Neurol 2017;264(2):304–15.
65. Mi S, Miller RH, Lee X, et al. LINGO-1 negatively regulates myelination by oligodendrocytes. Nat Neurosci 2005;8(6):745–51.
66. Mi S, Pepinsky RB, Cadavid D. Blocking LINGO-1 as a therapy to promote CNS repair: from concept to the clinic. CNS Drugs 2013;27(7):493–503.
67. Perron H, Lang A. The human endogenous retrovirus link between genes and environment in multiple sclerosis and in multifactorial diseases associating neuroinflammation. Clin Rev Allergy Immunol 2010;39(1):51–61.
68. Kremer D, Schichel T, Förster M, et al. Human endogenous retrovirus type W envelope protein inhibits oligodendroglial precursor cell differentiation. Ann Neurol 2013;74(5):721–32.
69. Sorensen PS, Lycke J, Erälinna JP, et al. SIMCOMBIN study investigators. Simvastatin as add-on therapy to interferon β-1a for relapsing-remitting multiple sclerosis (SIMCOMBIN study): a placebo-controlled randomised phase 4 trial. Lancet Neurol 2011;10(8):691–701.
70. Chataway J, Schuerer N, Alsanousi A, et al. Effect of high-dose simvastatin on brain atrophy and disability in secondary progressive multiple sclerosis (MS-STAT): a randomised, placebo-controlled, phase 2 trial. Lancet 2014;383(9936):2213–21.
71. Sedel F, Bernard D, Mock DM, et al. Targeting demyelination and virtual hypoxia with high-dose biotin as a treatment for progressive multiple sclerosis. Neuropharmacology 2016;110(Pt B):644–53.
72. Tourbah A, Lebrun-Frenay C, Edan G, et al, MS-SPI study group. MD1003 (high-dose biotin) for the treatment of progressive multiple sclerosis: A randomised, double-blind, placebo-controlled study. Mult Scler 2016;22(13):1719–31.
73. Fujino T, Kato H, Yamashita S, et al. Effects of domperidone on serum prolactin levels in human beings. Endocrinol Jpn 1980;27(4):521–5.
74. Gregg C, Shikar V, Larsen P, et al. White matter plasticity and enhanced remyelination in the maternal CNS. J Neurosci 2007;27(8):1812–23.
75. Kalluri HV, Rosebraugh MR, Misko TP, et al. Phase 1 Evaluation of Elezanumab (Anti-Repulsive Guidance Molecule A Monoclonal Antibody) in Healthy and Multiple Sclerosis Participants. Ann Neurol 2023;93(2):285–96.
76. Cree BA, Ziemann A, Pfleeger K, Schwefel B, Wundes A, Freedman MS. Safety and Efficacy of Elezanumab in Relapsing and Progressive Forms of Multiple Sclerosis: Results From Two Phase 2 Studies, RADIUS-R and RADIUS-P. OP149, ECTRIMS 2021 Virtual Congress, 13–15 October.

# Role of B Cells in Relapsing-Remitting and Progressive Multiple Sclerosis and Long-Term Effects of B Cell Depletion

Afsaneh Shirani, MD, MSCI[a], Olaf Stuve, MD, PhD[b],
Anne H. Cross, MD[c,*]

**KEYWORDS**

- Multiple sclerosis • Relapsing multiple sclerosis • Progressive multiple sclerosis
- Treatment • Anti-CD20 monoclonal antibody • Mechanisms of action • Safety
- Efficacy

**KEY POINTS**

- Anti-CD20 monoclonal antibodies (mAbs) are highly efficacious treatments to reduce clinical and magnetic resonance disease activity in relapsing MS. These agents deplete circulating B lymphocytes but their mechanisms of action are broader than initially thought and are still being investigated.
- The efficacy of anti-CD20 mAbs in patients with progressive, nonrelapsing multiple sclerosis has not been rigorously tested and is currently unknown. Perceived lower efficacy than in relapsing forms of MS is likely due to both their lack of access across the blood–brain barrier as well as mechanisms of progressive MS that do not involve B cells.
- Anti-CD20 mAbs have a relatively favorable safety profile; however, long-term postmarketing surveillance is critical both to detect less common safety signals and to compare the safety profiles of different anti-CD20 mAbs.

## INTRODUCTION

This article focuses on B cell depletion with anti-CD20 monoclonal antibodies (mAbs) and the beneficial effects, limitations and safety in relapsing multiple sclerosis (RMS) and nonrelapsing progressive MS. As of 2023, approved treatments that reduce clinical and MRI activity in RMS comprise at least 9 different groups based on mechanisms

[a] Division of Multiple Sclerosis, Department of Neurological Sciences, University of Nebraska Medical Center, 988440 Nebraska Medical Center, Omaha, NE 68198-8440, USA; [b] Department of Neurology, University of Texas Southwestern Medical Center, 6000 Harry Hines Boulevard, Dallas, TX 75390-8813, USA; [c] Department of Neurology, Washington University School of Medicine in St. Louis, 660 South Euclid Avenue, CB 8111, St Louis, MO 63110, USA
* Corresponding author.
*E-mail address:* crossa@wustl.edu

Neurol Clin 42 (2024) 137–153
https://doi.org/10.1016/j.ncl.2023.06.001
neurologic.theclinics.com

of action, including anti-CD20 mAbs that eliminate circulating B cells. In contrast, only one agent is approved for slowing disability progression in patients with primary progressive MS (PPMS), the anti-CD20 mAb ocrelizumab.

## PART 1. ANTI-CD20 MONOCLONAL ANTIBODIES IN RELAPSING MULTIPLE SCLEROSIS—EFFICACY AND MECHANISMS OF ACTION

CD20 is expressed on almost all B cells in the blood, including immature B cell, mature naïve B cell, and memory B cell stages (**Fig. 1**). Some plasmablasts and a small proportion of CD3+ T cells express CD20, as well. Three anti-CD20 mAbs are approved for relapsing MS by the United States Food and Drug Administration (US FDA), ocrelizumab (in 2017), ofatumumab (in 2020), and ublituximab (in 2022) (**Table 1**). Ocrelizumab is approved for PPMS but the beneficial effects are less dramatic, as we will discuss later in this article.

The beneficial results in patients with RMS using these anti-CD20 agents have been remarkable. Some differences exist in the 3 approved anti-CD20 mAbs in terms of the epitope of CD20 being recognized and degree of complement-dependent versus cell-dependent lytic mechanisms used. All 3 have rapid onset of benefits within 12 weeks of drug initiation in RMS. In all of the phase 3 studies in RMS, the anti-CD20 mAbs were compared with an active comparator. Ocrelizumab was compared with beta-interferon 1a at 44 μg thrice weekly in the relapsing MS trials and reduced annualized relapse rate (ARR) by 46% and 47% ($P$<.0001 each) in the 2 pivotal phase 3 trials.[1] Ocrelizumab reduced gadolinium-enhanced MRI activity in RMS by 94% and 95% ($P$<.0001 each) and reduced 12-week confirmed disability progression (CDP) by 40% ($P$ = .0006, 2 phase 3 studies combined).

Ofatumumab reduced ARR by 51% and 59% (both $P$ < .001) in patients with RMS in 2 large randomized controlled trials in comparison to oral teriflunomide 14 mg/d.[2] Ofatumumab reduced 3-month CDP by 34.4% ($P$ = .002, 2 studies combined) and gadolinium-enhanced lesions by 98% and 94% (both $P$ < .001) versus teriflunomide.[2]

Ublituximab reduced ARR by 59% and 49% ($P$<.001 and $P$ = .002, respectively) in patients with RMS after 96 weeks in 2 phase 3 trials in comparison to oral teriflunomide 14 mg/d.[3] Gadolinium-enhanced lesions were reduced by ublituximab by 97% and

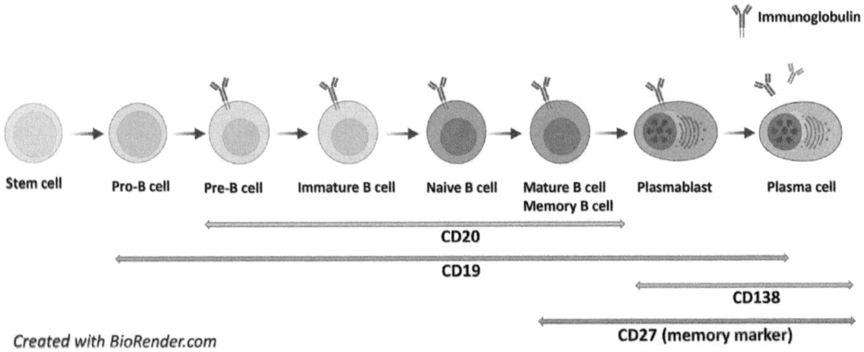


**Fig. 1.** The markers expressed by developing human B cells. CD19 is first expressed at the pro-B cell stage and continues to be expressed into the plasmablast stage and by some plasma cells. CD20 is expressed only on pre-B cells, immature, naïve, and memory B cells and is not expressed by terminally differentiated plasmablasts and plasma cells. CD138 is relatively specific to plasmablasts and plasma cells.

**Table 1**
**Approved anti-CD20 monoclonal antibodies in multiple sclerosis**

| Name | Structure | Dose | Approval by the FDA | Indication | Brand Name |
|---|---|---|---|---|---|
| Ocrelizumab | Humanized | 300 mg i.v. at weeks 0 and 2, then 600 mg i.v. every 6 mo | March 28, 2017 | Relapsing or primary progressive forms of multiple sclerosis | Ocrevus |
| Ofatumumab | Human | 20 mg s.c. at day 1, 7, and 14, then 20 mg every 4 wk | August 20, 2020 | Clinically isolated syndrome, relapsing-remitting multiple sclerosis, and active secondary progressive multiple sclerosis | Kesimpta |
| Ublituximab | Chimeric | 150 mg i.v. at weeks 0, 450 mg at week 2, then 450 mg every 6 mo | December 29, 2022 | Relapsing forms of multiple sclerosis | Briumvi |

96% (both $P<.001$) but 12-week CDP was not significantly different between ublituximab and teriflunomide treatment groups.

Ocrelizumab, a humanized mAb against CD20, was studied versus placebo in people with PPMS, and reduced expanded disability status scale (EDSS) progression by mean 24% ($P = .03$) and worsening of the timed 25-foot walk by mean 25%.[4] However, there are some caveats to the study in PPMS patients, which will be discussed later in this article.

Due to the marked reduction in MS relapse activity seen in patients with RMS with these treatments, a better understanding of the mechanism(s) of action has been sought. Clearly, the anti-CD20 mAbs eliminate circulating CD20+ cells, which includes almost all B cells and the small percentage of T cells that express surface CD20. Yet, the full mechanisms of action of these anti-CD20 lytic mAbs are not understood. All 3 mAbs seem to indiscriminately eliminate circulating cells expressing CD20, although by slightly different lytic mechanisms. In doing so, these agents presumably eliminate pathogenic B cells but also homeostatic and nonpathogenic B cells. We will discuss several studies that examined how removal of B cells and CD20+ T cells might reduce MS activity.

For relapsing MS, the mechanism by which B cell elimination benefits those with the disease likely relates to the important roles B lymphocytes play in T cell activation and in the production of proinflammatory cytokines and chemokines. It was initially thought that perhaps eliminating B cells would be beneficial in MS by reducing (presumed) autoantibodies. However, plasma cells are the source of most antibody production, and they lack surface CD20 expression (see **Fig. 1**). B cells can produce antibodies and are the precursors of plasma cells but antibody (immunoglobulin G) levels in blood and cerebrospinal fluid (CSF) are not affected at early time-points when these anti-CD20 mAbs already dramatically reduce disease activity.[5,6] Thus, reduction in antibody production is not likely to play a major role in the early benefits seen in patients with relapsing MS taking anti-CD20 mAbs.

One means by which the removal of B cells might have a rapid impact on MS activity is through the loss of B cell-derived soluble factors, such as cytokines and chemokines. B cells from MS patients have enhanced expression of proinflammatory cytokines that may contribute to disease pathogenesis.[7] B cells not only can produce antibodies and cytokines themselves but they can induce other cells to produce proinflammatory and anti-inflammatory cytokines and soluble chemotactic factors (chemokines) that can influence MS activity. In an early study in active patients with RMS treated open-label with rituximab, a chimeric anti-CD20 mAb that binds the same CD20 epitope as ocrelizumab, CSF was examined before and 6 months following treatment with the mAb. CSF C-X-C motif chemokine ligand 13 (CXCL13) and C-C motif chemokine ligand 19 (CCL19) levels decreased ($P = .002$ and $P = .03$, respectively) after rituximab treatment compared with pretreatment. However, the CSF IgG index, IgG concentration, and oligoclonal band number were unchanged following the 6 months of treatment.[6]

That same open-label study of rituximab in active patients with RMS found a small reduction (mean 12%) in circulating T cells, and both B cells and T cells were reduced in the CSF.[5,6] CSF B cell levels were decreased or undetectable in all subjects, and CSF T cell levels were reduced in 21 of 26 (81%) of subjects. The mean reduction in CSF cellularity was 95% for B cells and 50% for T cells. Subsequently, similar research has been done in a multicenter open-label study of ocrelizumab ("OBOE," ClinicalTrials.gov Identifier: NCT02688985), with highly similar results of reductions in blood and CSF of both B and T cells. In OBOE, T cells were reduced in CSF by about 50% to 60% and in blood by about 5%. (Cross AH, et al. Presented at ECTRIMS 2022 (Poster P449).

About 3% to 5% of human blood T cells express cell surface CD20.[8] These T cells have generally proinflammatory characteristics, are found in higher proportion in MS patients than controls, and can be either CD4+ or CD8+.[9] Data indicate that ocrelizumab effectively eliminates circulating CD20+ T cells.[10,11] Thus, the rapid reduction in MS activity following anti-CD20 mAb therapy may be partly related to elimination of potentially pathogenic proinflammatory CD20+ T cells.

With regard to effects on T cells of anti-CD20 mAbs, during a phase II clinical trial with ublituximab, blood lymphocyte profiles were examined longitudinally by flow cytometry during 24 weeks. In 48 patients with RMS initiating ublituximab, proportions of naïve CD4+ and CD8+ T cells increased, whereas proportions of both effector and central memory T cells decreased. Moreover, a significant increase in CD4+ regulatory T cells was observed, which was hypothesized to a play a role in the beneficial effects of ublituximab.[12]

Multiple subsets of B cells exist including regulatory B cells, as well as B cells secreting proinflammatory cytokines. From several directions, results point to memory B cells as having a pathogenic role in MS relapses. It has been observed that memory B cells from MS patients have a higher capacity to present myelin antigen to T cells compared with naïve B cells.[13] Anti-CD20 mAb treatment may lyse all circulating CD20+ cells indiscriminately but the reconstitution of B cells after anti-CD20 mAb therapy seems to occur differentially. In particular, naïve CD27-negative B cells rather than memory (CD27+) B cells were noted to be the majority of those repopulating the blood after rituximab.[14] This may be one reason that "rebound" of MS activity has not been reported on stopping anti-CD20 mAb therapies in MS.[15]

Failed trials of blockers of B cell activation and maturation factors in MS have also shed light on the specific subset of B cells that may be pathogenic in MS activity. Atacicept binds to the soluble factors B cell-activating factor (BAFF) and a proliferation-inducing ligand (APRIL), which are involved in B cell differentiation, maturation, and survival. A clinical trial in patients with RMS of the fusion protein atacicept, which binds to and blocks function of both BAFF and APRIL, was terminated early after the data and safety monitoring board detected increased ARR with atacicept.[16] After adjusting for the imbalance in gadolinium-enhancing brain lesions at baseline, an increase in the mean number of gadolinium-enhancing lesions was noted with atacicept treatment compared with placebo. Notably, atacicept preferentially affects naïve B cells while sparing memory B cells. Naïve B cells harbor relatively more regulatory B cells expressing IL-10. Thus, the sparing of memory B cells associated with loss of naïve B cells is thought to be a key factor related to the worsening of MS activity observed with atacicept.

B lymphocytes are also important to the development of ectopic lymphoid follicles (ELFs), which have been noted in the meninges of many but not all MS autopsies and are associated with worse MS course and cortical damage.[17,18] The development of lymphoid structures requires the chemokine CXCL13,[19] and the chemokines CXCL13 and CCL19 have each been implicated in the development of ELFs.[20] CXCL13 is increased in CSF of patients with MS versus controls[21] and, notably, is reduced in CSF and blood by B cell depletion with rituximab[6] and ocrelizumab (Cross, AH et al. unpublished data, 2023). ELFs, as well as less organized cell aggregates within the meninges that include B cells and T cells, have been noted in all clinical subtypes of MS but are more frequently seen in secondary progressive MS. However, lymphocyte aggregates are noted in the meninges of PPMS where they also associate with worse prognosis and younger age of death.[22] Whether and how much the anti-CD20 mAbs affect these meningeal aggregates is questionable. Using MRI, meningeal inflammatory cell collections, including ELFs, are thought to be indicated by leptomeningeal enhancement postgadolinium contrast seen on fluid-attenuated inversion recovery (FLAIR) imaging.[23] A longitudinal study using postcontrast FLAIR 3T brain MRI found no evidence for reduction in enhancing leptomeningeal structures up to 2 years after the initiation of ocrelizumab.[24]

## PART 2. B CELL DEPLETION USING ANTI-CD20 MONOCLONAL ANTIBODIES IN PROGRESSIVE MULTIPLE SCLEROSIS

In contrast to RMS, clinical trials in PPMS have thus far not substantially advanced our knowledge of biological disease mechanisms responsible for progressive MS. Ocrelizumab was the first agent to be approved for patients with PPMS based on the results of the ORATORIO phase 3 randomized placebo-controlled multicenter trial.[4] Approval was granted after ocrelizumab was found to have a significant benefit over placebo control in reducing CDP at 12 weeks, an accepted clinical outcome in progressive MS studies.[4] Although the results of this clinical trial were widely heralded as a milestone in the treatment of PPMS, their true impact is difficult to assess. The assessment of anti-CD20 mAb in patients with PPMS seemed plausible based on the observation that meningeal ELFs had been identified in some patients with secondary-progressive MS[20,22] and B and T lymphocyte aggregates that lacked structural characteristics of secondary lymphoid tissue had also been found in patients with PPMS.[22,25] In each case, the presence of these collections has been associated with worse pathology and worse prognosis.

The definition of MS subtypes is currently restricted to clinical phenotypes of the disease, which is considered by many MS neurologists and neuroimmunologists to be imprecise and ultimately inadequate. The trial design of ORATORIO included MS patients with very heterogeneous disease characteristics, including a broad age range and distinct levels of disease activity as defined and measured by the presence of contrast-enhancing signal changes on brain MRI.[4] This is potentially problematic and obscures the true biological and clinical impact of this trial, especially given the background of anti-CD20 mAb in PPMS. Specifically, rituximab, a chimeric recombinant mAb with pharmacologic properties very similar to ocrelizumab[26] had already been tested against placebo in patients with PPMS in the phase II/III OLYMPUS trial. In OLYMPUS, there was no beneficial effect of rituximab on CDP at 12 weeks, which had been the primary endpoint.[27] One difference between ORATORIO and OLYMPUS was the age of the study participants, which likely affects the disease course of PPMS, and the response to pharmacologic interventions.[28,29] The entry criteria for OLYMPUS allowed the enrollment of patients aged between 18 and 65 years, with an average age of 49.9 years.[27] Perhaps, not surprisingly, based on our current understanding of immune-senescence and other age-associated factors that affect MS disease phenotypes, age was a relevant factor affecting rituximab efficacy: A preplanned analysis demonstrated that the primary endpoint was only met in patients aged younger than 51 years.[27]

In ORATORIO, the upper age limitation for inclusion was lower, enrolling patients with PPMS who are aged between 18 and 55 years.[4] This led to a study population that was approximately 5 years younger than in the OLYMPUS trial, and an enrichment of MS patients who still had contrast enhancement on MRI. Subanalyses between patients with active PPMS and those with nonactive PPMS could not detect a differential response to ocrelizumab in ORATORIO. However, the trial was not powered to show such a difference. Although long-term follow-up data from ORATORIO showed a sustained benefit for patients in the active treatment arm,[30] this could be explained by enrolling a mixed study population.

Interestingly, although age may not be the only pertinent factor to be considered in trial outcome in patients with MS, the main distinguishing feature between ORATORIO and INFORMS, another phase 3 trial in PPMS that compared the sphingosine 1-phosphate receptor modulator fingolimod to placebo, was the mean ago of participants. In INFORMS, inclusion criteria and the average age of participants was similar to those in the OLYMPUS study.

Given the above-mentioned study design of ORATORIO, it is currently unclear that its beneficial results apply to all patients with PPMS. Given the low bioavailability of therapeutic mAb behind the blood–brain barrier (BBB), and the recognition that the inflammation in progressive MS is mostly compartmentalized behind the BBB, a strong effect of ocrelizumab directly on central nervous system (CNS)-resident B lymphocytes is implausible. It does not seem to have a neuroprotective effect as determined by serum neurofilament light (NfL) levels in patients with PPMS who were included in ORATORIO, and who have no MS disease activity as defined above.[31] Specifically, NfL, a scaffolding protein that is abundantly expressed in the axons and dendrites of neurons in the CNS and peripheral nervous system,[32] and which has been demonstrated to track well with MS disease activity and treatment responses on a group level, is currently considered a meaningful marker of neurodegeneration in MS and other disorders. Unpublished data on every 12 weekly blood NfL assessments during ORATORIO[33] show that ocrelizumab had no effect on blood NfL levels in patients with PPMS who did not have gadolinium-enhancing lesions at study enrollment. These observations may suggest that beneficial effects demonstrated for ocrelizumab in PPMS were driven mostly by its anti-inflammatory properties on immune cells outside of the CNS, or that BBB breakdown (indicated by gadolinium enhancement) was required for CNS access. Consequently, ocrelizumab may benefit only PPMS patients with inflammatory activity, or its beneficial effects may occur over a slower timeframe in PPMS without inflammatory MS activity.

Ocrelizumab is widely used in patients with MS, including patients with PPMS. Based on all available clinical trial efficacy and safety data, this agent has a favorable benefit-to-risk profile. We recently assessed the prescription patterns of approved MS disease-modifying therapies (DMTs) by age.[34] Real-world data were obtained from the US Department of Veterans Affairs Multiple Sclerosis Surveillance Registry (MSSR), and the North American Research Committee on Multiple Sclerosis (NARCOMS) registry. A total of 1719 participants were surveyed from the MSSR, and NARCOMS had 6948 participants. Among patients with MS aged older than 60 years, in whom ocrelizumab has never been studied in a PPMS population, 239 (36.3%) in the MSSR, and 1575 (40.1%) in NARCOMS were prescribed DMTs. It is likely that the majority of the older patients with PPMS received ocrelizumab because it is currently the only approved DMT for that patient population, despite that it was not studied in their age group.

In summary, the remarkable success of anti-CD20 mAb therapies in RMS was not recapitulated in PPMS. Whether specific B cell subsets perpetuate disease progression in PPMS, and to what extent, is currently not entirely clear. Fenebrutinib, a Bruton tyrosine kinase (BTK) inhibitor is currently being evaluated in comparison to ocrelizumab as an active comparator in a Phase 3 clinical trial, FENtrepid (https://clinicaltrials.gov/ct2/show/NCT04544449). Patients aged 18 to 65 years are being enrolled, and the primary endpoint is 12-week CDP. Similar to other drugs of its class, fenebrutinib affects the activation, proliferation, maturation, and survival of B cells.[35] BTK inhibitors in clinical trials are small molecules that may have better CNS bioavailability than mAbs but at this time, there are no pertinent data in the public domain. Results from FENtrepid will hopefully be informative to MS patients and neurologists on the effectiveness of fenebrutinib and ocrelizumab in an older PPMS patient population and on the role of B cells in MS progression.

## PART 3. SAFETY AND LONG-TERM RISKS OF PERIPHERAL B CELL DEPLETION IN MULTIPLE SCLEROSIS

Previous studies have reported relatively favorable safety profile of anti-CD20 mAbs in MS although during the course of short-term clinical trials. Available short-term and medium-term real-world data pertaining to anti-CD20 mAbs seem to be mostly consistent with those from clinical trials; however, long-term postmarketing surveillance is critical to detect less common safety signals. In this section, we review the safety and side effects of anti-CD20 mAbs used in MS (**Table 2**) including infusion-related or injection-related reactions, infections, reduced immune response to vaccinations, and rare adverse events such as malignancy, progressive multifocal leukoencephalopathy (PML), immune-mediated colitis, and so forth. Pregnancy-related considerations are discussed elsewhere (see chapter 15 in this volume).

### *Infusion-Related or Injection-Related Reactions*

Infusion-related or injection-related reactions are common adverse events occurring with anti-CD20 mAbs used in MS, whether chimeric (rituximab and ublituximab), humanized (ocrelizumab), or fully human (ofatumumab). Infusion-related reactions were reported in 78.3% of patients treated with rituximab within 24 hours after first infusion in HERMES phase II trial,[36] 34.3% of ocrelizumab recipients in OPERA I and II,[1] 39.9% of ocrelizumab recipients in ORATORIO,[4] and 47.7% of patients treated with ublituximab in ULTIMATE I and II.[3] Injection-related reactions occurred in 20.2% in the ofatumumab group in ASCLEPIOS I and II.[2] These reactions can present as pyrexia, pruritis, rash or flushing, throat irritation, cough, headache, and influenza-like illness. Most of these reactions were reported as mild-to-moderate in severity. The higher rate of infusion-related reactions with ublituximab (compared with that of ocrelizumab) could be at least partially related to the more rapid maintenance infusion of ublituximab.[3,37] Of note, shortening the infusion time of ocrelizumab maintenance infusions from 3.5 hours to 2 hours did not show a significant difference in the rates and severity of infusion-related reactions.[38]

Acute infusion reactions are thought to be caused by B cell lysis and mast cell degranulation. Premedications, adjustments to infusion rate, and symptomatic treatment are helpful in reducing these reactions. Severe reactions such as life-threatening bronchospasms and angioedema, or other anaphylactoid reactions are rare. Kounis syndrome—also known as allergic angina—following ocrelizumab infusion has been reported.[39] Kounis syndrome is thought to be associated with mast-cell and platelet activation in the setting of allergic or anaphylactic insults resulting in coronary artery vasospasm.[40] Prompt recognition is crucial for the appropriate management of anaphylactic reactions.

### *Infections (Other than Progressive Multifocal Leukoencephalopathy)*

Infections were reported in 56.9% and 60.2% of patients with RMS in the ocrelizumab group (vs 54.3% and 52.5% in the interferon beta-1a group) in OPERA I and II trials, respectively.[1] The most common infections (reported in $\geq$10% of the patients in either group across both trials) were upper respiratory tract infection, nasopharyngitis, and urinary tract infection. The percentage of patients with PPMS who reported upper respiratory tract infections in the ORATORIO trial was 10.9% in the ocrelizumab group versus 5.9% in the placebo group.[4] Infections and infestations were reported in 51.6% of patients in the ofatumumab group and 52.7% in the teriflunomide group in ASCLEPIOS I and II trials.[2] These results are comparable to ULTIMATE I and II trials where infections occurred in 55.8% of ublituximab-treated patients and 54.4% of

**Table 2**
**Summary of adverse events reported in phase III trials of ocrelizumab, ofatumumab, and ublituximab**

| Anti-CD20 mAb | Ocrelizumab | | | | | | Ofatumumab | | | | Ublituximab | | | |
|---|---|---|---|---|---|---|---|---|---|---|---|---|---|---|
| Phase III Trials | OPERA I | | OPERA II | | ORATORIO | | ASCLEPIOS I | | ASCLEPIOS II | | ULTIMATE I | | ULTIMATE II | |
| Treatment arms[a] | Ocrelizumab (N = 408) | IFN-β1a (N = 409) | Ocrelizumab (N = 417) | IFN-β1a (N = 417) | Ocrelizumab (N = 486) | Placebo (N = 239) | Ofatumumab (N = 465) | Teriflunomide (N = 462) | Ofatumumab (N = 481) | Teriflunomide (N = 474) | Ublituximab (N = 273) | Teriflunomide (N = 275) | Ublituximab (N = 272) | Teriflunomide (N = 273) |
| Age—y, mean ± SD | 37.1 ± 9.3 | 36.9 ± 9.3 | 37.2 ± 9.1 | 37.4 ± 9.0 | 44.7 ± 7.9 | 44.4 ± 8.3 | 38.9 ± 8.8 | 37.8 ± 9.0 | 38.0 ± 9.3 | 38.2 ± 9.5 | 36.2 ± 8.2 | 37.0 ± 9.6 | 34.5 ± 8.8 | 36.2 ± 9.0 |
| Infusion/ injection-related reactions | 30.9% | 7.3% | 37.6% | 12.0% | 39.9% | 25.5% | 16.1% | 16.5% | 24.1% | 13.5% | 44.0% | 6.9% | 51.5% | 17.6% |
| Infections | 56.9% | 54.3% | 60.2% | 52.5% | 71.4% | 69.9% | 49.2% | 51.5% | 53.8% | 53.8% | 49.5% | 48.4% | 62.1% | 60.4% |
| Serious infections[b] | 1.2% | 2.9% | 1.4% | 2.9% | 6.2% | 5.9% | 2.6% | 1.5% | 2.5% | 2.1% | 5.5% | 2.2% | 4.4% | 3.7% |
| Neoplasms[c] | 0.7% | 0.2% | 0.2% | 0.2% | 2.3% | 0.8% | 0.6% | 0.6% | 0.4% | 0.2% | 0 | 0 | 0.7% | 0.4% |
| Deaths[d] | 0 | 0.2% | 0.2% | 0.2% | 0.8% | 0.4% | 0 | 0 | 0 | 0.2% | 0.7% | 0 | 0.4% | 0 |

[a] Number of patients included in safety analysis in each treatment arm.

[b] Cases of serious infections and infestations reported in the ocrelizumab group in OPERA I and II included appendicitis (3 patients), cellulitis (2 patients), pyelonephritis (2 patients), as well as individual cases of biliary sepsis, device-related infection, herpes simplex infection, pneumonia, and upper respiratory tract infection (1 patient each). In the interferon beta-1a group in OPERA I and II, serious infections and infestations included appendicitis (3 patients), limb abscess (2 patients), injection-site cellulitis (2 patients), pneumonia (2 patients), urinary tract infection (2 patients), and individual cases of acute tonsillitis, anal abscess, infective cholecystitis, cystitis, infectious enterocolitis, viral gastritis, gastroenteritis, perirectal abscess, staphylococcal septic arthritis, staphylococcal sepsis, tooth infection, viral infection, and viral pericarditis (1 patient each). In the ORATORIO trial, the proportion of patients experiencing serious infections, classified by system organ class, was comparable between the 2 groups (6.2% with ocrelizumab and 5.9% with placebo). The inclusion of nonserious infections treated with intravenous anti-infective agents in the broader definition of serious infections resulted in minimal changes. With this expanded definition, 7.6% of patients receiving ocrelizumab and 8.8% of patients receiving placebo were affected by serious infections in ORATORIO. In ASCLEPIOS I and II trials, among the group receiving ofatumumab, the following serious infections and infestations were reported: appendicitis (in 8 patients), gastroenteritis (in 3 patients), urinary tract infection (in 3 patients), influenza (in 2 patients), and individual cases of cystitis, *Escherichia* urinary tract infection, kidney infection, lower respiratory tract infection, neutropenic sepsis, osteomyelitis, pneumonia, upper respiratory tract infection, urosepsis, and viral respiratory tract infection (each in one patient). In the teriflunomide group in ASCLEPIOS I and II, serious infections and infestations reported were appendicitis (in 2 patients), urinary tract infection (in 2), and individual cases of abscess of the sweat glands, *Campylobacter* infection, cystitis, influenza pneumonia, osteomyelitis, paronychia, peritonitis, pneumonia, postoperative abscess, salpingo-oophoritis, sepsis, tickborne viral encephalitis, and viral infection (in 1 patient each). Regarding serious infections in ULTIMATE I and II trials, pneumonia was the most frequently reported in the ublituximab group, whereas urinary tract infections were more commonly reported in the teriflunomide group in both trials.

[c] The neoplasms reported in the OPERA I trial included ductal breast carcinoma (2 patients) and renal cancer (1 patient) in the ocrelizumab group, whereas the interferon beta-1a group had one case of mantle-cell lymphoma. In the OPERA II trial, one patient in the ocrelizumab group was reported to have malignant melanoma, while another patient in the interferon beta-1a group was diagnosed with squamous-cell carcinoma. Regarding neoplasms in ORATORIO, 2 events were classified as invasive ductal breast carcinoma and one each as breast cancer and invasive breast carcinoma. In ASCLEPIOS I and II trials, in patients treated with ofatumumab, the following neoplasms were reported: one case of malignant melanoma in situ, one case of invasive breast carcinoma, one case of recurrent non-Hodgkin's lymphoma, and 2 cases of basal-cell carcinoma. In patients receiving teriflunomide in ASCLEPIOS I and II trials, the reported neoplasms included one case of fibrosarcoma, one case of cervix carcinoma, and 2 cases of basal-cell carcinoma. No pattern or cluster of neoplasms was identified. In both ULTIMATE I and II trials, neoplasms observed in the ublituximab group included endometrial and uterine neoplasms. In the teriflunomide group in ULTIMATE II, a tongue neoplasm was reported.

[d] During OPERA I and II, deaths occurred due to suicide (1 patient in the ocrelizumab group in OPERA II and 1 in the interferon beta-1a group in OPERA I) and mechanical ileus (1 patient in the interferon beta-1a group in OPERA II). In ORATORIO, among the placebo group, 1 death resulted from a road-traffic accident. In the ocrelizumab group in ORATORIO, deaths were due to pulmonary embolism, pneumonia, pancreatic carcinoma, and aspiration pneumonia. During the ASCLEPIOS I and II trials, there was only one reported case of fatality, which occurred in a patient receiving teriflunomide in ASCLEPIOS II. The cause of death in this particular case was identified as aortic dissection. In ULTIMATE I and II trials, among the ublituximab group, the deaths that occurred were attributed to pneumonia (deemed possibly related to treatment), encephalitis (following measles infection), and salpingitis (after an ectopic pregnancy).

teriflunomide-treated patients[3] and also with that of the phase II trial of rituximab.[36] Most infections were respiratory tract–related.

Across OPERA I and II combined, the percentage of patients reporting herpesvirus-associated infection (herpes simplex or herpes zoster) was 5.9% in the ocrelizumab group versus 3.4% in the interferon beta-1a group.[1] Such slightly higher rate of herpesvirus-associated infections was also observed in the ORATORIO trial (4.7% with ocrelizumab vs 3.3% with placebo),[4] ASCLEPIOS trials (4.9% with ofatumumab vs 4.2% with teriflunomide),[2] and ULTIMATE trials (5.7% with ublituximab vs 4.6% with teriflunomide).[3] The vast majority of all infection-related adverse events was reported to be mild to moderate. Serious infections in phase III clinical trials of mAbs occurred in 1.3% of ocrelizumab-treated patients with RMS (vs 2.9% of those treated with interferon beta-1a),[1] 6.2% of ocrelizumab-treated patients with PPMS (vs 5.9% of those treated with placebo),[4] 2.5% of the ofatumumab group (vs 1.8% of the teriflunomide group),[2] and 5.0% of the ublituximab recipients (vs 2.9% of the teriflunomide recipients).[3]

A large observational study from Sweden where rituximab is extensively used off-label showed that rituximab was associated with the highest rate of serious infections compared with interferon beta, glatiramer acetate, fingolimod, and natalizumab.[41] There is however a paucity of literature on head-to-head real-world comparisons of the safety profiles of different anti-CD20 mAbs used for MS. Findings from the FDA Adverse Event Reporting System (FAERS) database showed that ocrelizumab was associated with an almost 2 times higher frequency of infections than rituximab (21.93% vs 11.05%, respectively).[42] Although speculative, a potentially differential or more extensive B cell depletion by ocrelizumab compared with rituximab might explain these observations.

It should be noted that infection risk is not uniform in all patients treated with anti-CD20 mAbs. Factors such as older age, hypogammaglobulinemia, comorbidities, higher EDSS scores, and longer duration of treatment can increase the risk of infections in patients treated with anti-CD20 mAbs.[43,44] Long-term pharmacovigilance studies are needed for further characterization of the adverse event profiles of individual anti-CD20 mAbs particularly the second-generation and third-generation mAbs.

#### *Hypogammaglobulinemia*

Even though anti-CD20 mAbs do not affect plasma cells that are responsible for producing antibodies in large quantities, they can still decrease immunoglobulin levels. This is most likely due to depleting memory B cells and B cell and plasma cell precursors. Moreover, follicular helper T cells, a subset of CD4+ helper T cells, which are essential for maturation and survival of B cells within germinal centers can be suppressed by anti-CD20 mAbs.[45]

The proportion of ocrelizumab-treated patients with immunoglobulin levels less than the normal limit at week 96 in OPERA I and II was 1.5%, 2.4%, and 16.5% for IgG, IgA, and IgM, respectively.[1] In the ORATORIO trial, the proportion of ocrelizumab-treated patients with IgG, IgA, and IgM less than the lower limit of normal was 1.1%, 0.5%, and 15.5%, respectively.[4] In ULTIMATE I and II, the proportion of ublituximab-treated patients with less than normal immunoglobulin levels at week 96 was 6.5%, 2.4%, and 20.9% for IgG, IgA, and IgM, respectively.[3] Overall, the greatest impact of B cell depletion on immunoglobulin levels in the above studies were on IgM; however, no specific association was found between low IgM levels and serious infections. In ASCLEPIOS I and II trials, a reduction from baseline in IgG levels was observed until week 36 of ofatumumab treatment, thereafter the IgG levels recovered. A reduction in IgM levels was found over time throughout the duration of ASCLEPIOS I and II (120 weeks); yet, both average IgG and IgM levels remained well within the normal range over time and no apparent association was found between decreased immunoglobulin levels and risk of infections.[46]

It should however be noted that evidence from long-term observational studies in patients treated with rituximab suggest that reduced IgG levels are associated with an increased risk of infections.[47,48] There is a need for similar long-term real-world studies for ocrelizumab, ofatumumab, and ublituximab. We recommend monitoring immunoglobulin levels both before and after treatment with anti-CD20 mAbs for earlier detection of potential infection risks and identification of patients who could benefit from immunoglobulin replacement or an alternative DMT strategy (eg, DMT switch or extend the dosing interval to reduce exposure to anti-CD20 therapy).

#### *Reduced Immune Response to Vaccination*

Anti-CD20 mAbs diminish humoral response to recall and novel vaccinations in MS and non-MS patient populations.[49,50] A phase 3b study to evaluate the effects of ocrelizumab on immune responses showed that patients with RMS who were peripherally B cell depleted after treatment with ocrelizumab could mount humoral responses, although attenuated, to inactivated clinically relevant vaccines.[49] Humoral responses to both T cell–dependent antigens such as tetanus toxoid-containing vaccine and T cell-independent antigens such as 23-valent pneumococcal polysaccharide vaccine were attenuated in ocrelizumab-treated patients.[49] The use of anti-CD20 mAbs has also been associated with lower seroconversion following the SARS-CoV-2 vaccine.[51] Both time since last anti-CD20 mAb treatment and total time on treatment were significantly associated with the humoral response to the vaccination. A subpopulation of seronegative subjects showed measurable anti-SARS-CoV-2 T cell responses.[51] Whenever possible, vaccinations should be administered before starting anti-CD20 mAbs.

#### *Progressive Multifocal Leukoencephalopathy*

Based on the data from Genentech, as of March 2022, there have been 12 confirmed cases of PML in more than 250,000 patients treated with ocrelizumab worldwide.[52] Of these, 10 cases were carry-over cases attributed to a prior DMT such as natalizumab and fingolimod. Only 2 noncarry-over cases were reported with ocrelizumab. These occurred in a 78-year-old patient and a 57-year-old patient, both previously untreated, after approximately 2 years and 4.5 years of ocrelizumab treatment, respectively. Both patients died within a few months following PML diagnosis.[52]

No cases of PML have yet been reported in patients with MS treated with ofatumumab and ublituximab as of April 2023; however, this is not unexpected given that these DMTs have been on the market for a shorter time compared with ocrelizumab. PML has been reported in a patient treated with ofatumumab for chronic lymphocytic leukemia (CLL).[53] PML has also been described in association with rituximab in non-MS populations such as those with non-Hodgkin lymphoma or CLL, and rheumatoid arthritis.[54,55] Even though overall very rare, PML risk might be a class effect of anti-CD20 mAbs. Ongoing vigilance and monitoring is recommended with long-term use of anti-CD20 mAbs particularly in those with advanced age and/or CD4+ T cell lymphopenia.[55–57]

#### *Malignancy*

There was a reported numerical imbalance of malignancies in the ocrelizumab group compared with control groups in phase 3 trials of ocrelizumab. Breast cancer occurred in 2 out of 408 patients in the ocrelizumab group versus none in the interferon beta-1a group (n = 409) in OPERA I,[1] and 4 out of 486 ocrelizumab-treated patients versus none in the placebo group (n = 239) in ORATORIO.[4] Such numerical imbalances were not observed in phase 3 trials of ofatumumab and ublituximab. There have also been reports of skin cancers such as malignant melanoma and basal cell carcinoma with anti-CD20 mAbs.[1,2,4,42,58] A safety analysis of continuous administration of ocrelizumab for up to 7 years in patients participating in ocrelizumab phase 2 and 3 trials and the relevant open label extension studies did not indicate an increased risk of cancer compared with matched reference populations.[58,59] Even though there is currently no specific risk mitigation program for cancer in patients treated with anti-CD20 mAbs, it is recommended that these patients adhere to age-appropriate cancer screening guidelines including but not limited to skin surveys and breast cancer screening.

### *Immune-Mediated Colitis*

Cases of inflammatory colitis including immune-mediated colitis have been reported in patients receiving ocrelizumab in the postmarketing setting without obvious contributory risk factors or alternate explanations.[60–62] Inflammatory bowel disease has also been reported with rituximab in the non-MS population[63] and in patients with MS.[64] The exact mechanism of anti-CD20-induced colitis is not known. Depletion of regulatory B cells, dysregulation of the gastrointestinal immune system via B cell depletion, reduced production of anti-inflammatory cytokines such as IL-10, upregulation of proinflammatory cytokines such as IL-17, and inadequate regulation of pathogenic T cells may play a role.[61] In 2022, FDA added an update to the drug label for ocrelizumab indicating that health-care providers should monitor patients for immune-mediated colitis during ocrelizumab treatment and evaluate promptly if new or persistent diarrhea or other gastrointestinal symptoms suggestive of immune-mediated colitis occur.

### *Psoriasis*

Case reports of the possible association between psoriasis and anti-CD20 mAbs have been published.[65,66] A disproportionate increase in psoriasis reports in association with anti-CD20 mAbs in patients with MS has been described using the FAERS and OpenFDA databases (reporting odds ratios: 7.14 [95% CI: 3.92–13.00] for rituximab and 3.79 [95% CI: 2.74–5.23] for ocrelizumab).[67] The mechanism linking B cell depletion and psoriasis is not fully known; however, it is thought that a B cell-depleted environment may induce abnormal T cell activation and T cell responses. This can be provoked by depletion of regulatory B cells resulting in unrestrained activation of T cells, or by subclinical infection.[68,69] B cell-depleting mAbs are not contraindicated in psoriasis; however, clinicians should be aware of the possible risk of psoriasis worsening in patients with coexisting MS. The decision to avoid or stop anti-CD20 mAbs in these patients needs to be made on an individual basis.

### *Serum Sickness*

Serum sickness—a type III hypersensitivity reaction—has been reported with rituximab.[70,71] It is thought that immune complexes between the chimeric mAb and antidrug antibodies (ADAs) activate complement, and the deposition of these complexes in different tissues causes an inflammatory reaction presented with symptoms such as fever, arthralgia, rash, myalgia, malaise, fatigue, conjunctival hyperemia, and so forth. Serum sickness is much less likely with humanized or fully human mAbs. In patients with rituximab-induced serum sickness and high levels of ADAs against rituximab, switching to a humanized or fully human mAbs is advised.[70]

Doubts have been cast on a reported possible case of serum sickness after ocrelizumab infusion[72] due to lack of typical clinical and laboratory features.[73] It is still important for clinicians to be vigilant of the possibility of serum sickness when prescribing anti-CD20 mAbs because exposure after a first event may result in more severe reactions.

## SUMMARY

In summary, anti-CD20 mAbs have shown clear reduction of inflammatory activity in people with RMS but only blunted reduction of progression in people with nonrelapsing progressive MS. The exact mechanisms by which anti-CD20 mAbs achieve reduction of MRI and clinical relapse activity in people with RMS remains to be clarified. Why anti-CD20 agents do not fully protect from disease progression is not known but likely relates to inability of mAbs to cross the BBB, as well as lack of effect on the full extent of biology of MS progression, which is under intense study but as of yet not fully understood. Fortunately, anti-CD20 mAbs seem to have a relatively favorable safety profile; however, further long-term safety studies with a focus on comparing the safety profiles of different anti-CD20 mAbs are warranted. This is particularly important because with the broad and early use of anti-CD20 mAbs as high-efficacy DMTs, it is anticipated that in future, there will be a significant number of patients with decades of exposure to anti-CD20 mAbs. Better understanding of the risks associated with long-term use of anti-CD20 mAbs will help better position these therapies within the rapidly growing landscape of DMTs for MS.

## CLINICS CARE POINTS

- Clinicians should consider anti-CD20 monoclonal antibodies as a highly effective treatment option for patients with relapsing forms of MS, when appropriate.
- Careful consideration should be given to the potential risk-benefit ratio of anti-CD20 monoclonal antibodies in patients with progressive forms of MS, as the evidence for its efficacy in this population is limited.
- Clinicians should be aware of the potential risk of infections associated with anti-CD20 monoclonal antibodies in patients with MS. Appropriate screening and preventive measures should be implemented.

## DISCLOSURE

A. Shirani has no disclosures to report. O. Stuve serves on the editorial boards of Therapeutic Advances in Neurological Disorders, has served on data monitoring committees for Genentech-Roche, Pfizer, Novartis, and TG Therapeutics without monetary compensation, has advised EMD Serono and VYNE, receives grant support from EMD Serono, is a 2021 recipient of a Grant for Multiple Sclerosis Innovation (GMSI), Merck KGaA, is funded by a Merit Review grant federal award document number (FAIN) BX005664-01 from the United States (U.S.) Department of Veterans Affairs, Biomedical Laboratory Research and Development, is funded by RFA-2203-39314 (PI) and RFA-2203-39305 (co-PI) grants from the National Multiple Sclerosis Society, United States (NMSS). A.H. Cross was supported in part by the Manny & Rosalyn Rosenthal—Dr John L. Trotter Chair in Neuroimmunology. A.H. Cross has received honoraria for consulting or serving on scientific advisory boards from Biogen, Bristol Myers Squibb, EMD Serono, United States, Genentech, Horizon, Janssen (J&J),

Novartis, Octave, Roche, Switzerland, and TG Therapeutics. A.H. Cross has received contracted grants from Genentech, United States, EMD Serono, and Roche.

## REFERENCES


1. Hauser SL, Bar-Or A, Comi G, et al. Ocrelizumab versus Interferon Beta-1a in Relapsing Multiple Sclerosis. N Engl J Med 2017;376(3):221–34.
2. Hauser SL, Bar-Or A, Cohen JA, et al. Ofatumumab versus Teriflunomide in Multiple Sclerosis. N Engl J Med 2020;383(6):546–57.
3. Steinman L, Fox E, Hartung HP, et al. Ublituximab versus Teriflunomide in Relapsing Multiple Sclerosis. N Engl J Med 2022;387(8):704–14.
4. Montalban X, Hauser SL, Kappos L, et al. Ocrelizumab versus Placebo in Primary Progressive Multiple Sclerosis. N Engl J Med 2017;376(3):209–20.
5. Cross AH, Stark JL, Lauber J, et al. Rituximab reduces B cells and T cells in cerebrospinal fluid of multiple sclerosis patients. J Neuroimmunol 2006;180(1–2):63–70.
6. Piccio L, Naismith RT, Trinkaus K, et al. Changes in B- and T-lymphocyte and chemokine levels with rituximab treatment in multiple sclerosis. Arch Neurol 2010;67(6):707–14.
7. Barr TA, Shen P, Brown S, et al. B cell depletion therapy ameliorates autoimmune disease through ablation of IL-6-producing B cells. J Exp Med 2012;209(5):1001–10.
8. Schuh E, Berer K, Mulazzani M, et al. Features of Human CD3+CD20+ T Cells. J Immunol 2016;197(4):1111–7.
9. von Essen MR, Ammitzboll C, Hansen RH, et al. Proinflammatory CD20+ T cells in the pathogenesis of multiple sclerosis. Brain 2019;142(1):120–32.
10. Gingele S, Jacobus TL, Konen FF, et al. Ocrelizumab Depletes CD20(+) T Cells in Multiple Sclerosis Patients. Cells 2018;8(1). https://doi.org/10.3390/cells8010012.
11. Sabatino JJ Jr, Wilson MR, Calabresi PA, et al. Anti-CD20 therapy depletes activated myelin-specific CD8(+) T cells in multiple sclerosis. Proc Natl Acad Sci U S A 2019;116(51):25800–7.
12. Lovett-Racke AE, Gormley M, Liu Y, et al. B cell depletion with ublituximab reshapes the T cell profile in multiple sclerosis patients. J Neuroimmunol 2019;332:187–97.
13. Jelcic I, Al Nimer F, Wang J, et al. Memory B Cells Activate Brain-Homing, Autoreactive CD4(+) T Cells in Multiple Sclerosis. Cell 2018;175(1):85–100 e23.
14. Bar-Or A, Calabresi PA, Arnold D, et al. Rituximab in relapsing-remitting multiple sclerosis: a 72-week, open-label, phase I trial. Ann Neurol 2008;63(3):395–400.
15. Juto A, Fink K, Al Nimer F, et al. Interrupting rituximab treatment in relapsing-remitting multiple sclerosis; no evidence of rebound disease activity. Mult Scler Relat Disord 2020;37:101468.
16. Kappos L, Hartung HP, Freedman MS, et al. Atacicept in multiple sclerosis (ATAMS): a randomised, placebo-controlled, double-blind, phase 2 trial. Lancet Neurol 2014;13(4):353–63.
17. Howell OW, Reeves CA, Nicholas R, et al. Meningeal inflammation is widespread and linked to cortical pathology in multiple sclerosis. Brain 2011;134(Pt 9):2755–71.
18. Magliozzi R, Howell O, Vora A, et al. Meningeal B-cell follicles in secondary progressive multiple sclerosis associate with early onset of disease and severe cortical pathology. Brain 2007;130(Pt 4):1089–104.

19. Ansel KM, Ngo VN, Hyman PL, et al. A chemokine-driven positive feedback loop organizes lymphoid follicles. Nature 2000;406(6793):309–14.
20. Serafini B, Rosicarelli B, Magliozzi R, et al. Detection of ectopic B-cell follicles with germinal centers in the meninges of patients with secondary progressive multiple sclerosis. Brain Pathol 2004;14(2):164–74.
21. Alvarez E, Piccio L, Mikesell RJ, et al. CXCL13 is a biomarker of inflammation in multiple sclerosis, neuromyelitis optica, and other neurological conditions. Mult Scler 2013;19(9):1204–8.
22. Choi SR, Howell OW, Carassiti D, et al. Meningeal inflammation plays a role in the pathology of primary progressive multiple sclerosis. Brain 2012;135(Pt 10): 2925–37.
23. Absinta M, Vuolo L, Rao A, et al. Gadolinium-based MRI characterization of leptomeningeal inflammation in multiple sclerosis. Neurology 2015;85(1):18–28.
24. Zivadinov R, Jakimovski D, Ramanathan M, et al. Effect of ocrelizumab on leptomeningeal inflammation and humoral response to Epstein-Barr virus in multiple sclerosis. A pilot study. Mult Scler Relat Disord 2022;67:104094.
25. Lucchinetti CF, Popescu BF, Bunyan RF, et al. Inflammatory cortical demyelination in early multiple sclerosis. N Engl J Med 2011;365(23):2188–97.
26. Klein C, Lammens A, Schafer W, et al. Epitope interactions of monoclonal antibodies targeting CD20 and their relationship to functional properties. MAbs 2013;5(1):22–33.
27. Hawker K, O'Connor P, Freedman MS, et al. Rituximab in patients with primary progressive multiple sclerosis: results of a randomized double-blind placebo-controlled multicenter trial. Ann Neurol 2009;66(4):460–71.
28. Manouchehri N, Stuve O. Should ocrelizumab be used in non-active primary progressive multiple sclerosis? Time for a re-assessment. Ther Adv Neurol Disord 2021;14. 1756286421990500.
29. Manouchehri N, Salinas VH, Rabi Yeganeh N, et al. Efficacy of Disease Modifying Therapies in Progressive MS and How Immune Senescence May Explain Their Failure. Front Neurol 2022;13:854390.
30. Wolinsky JS, Arnold DL, Brochet B, et al. Long-term follow-up from the ORATORIO trial of ocrelizumab for primary progressive multiple sclerosis: a post-hoc analysis from the ongoing open-label extension of the randomised, placebo-controlled, phase 3 trial. Lancet Neurol 2020;19(12):998–1009.
31. Lublin F, Miller DH, Freedman MS, et al. Oral fingolimod in primary progressive multiple sclerosis (INFORMS): a phase 3, randomised, double-blind, placebo-controlled trial. Lancet 2016;387(10023):1075–84.
32. Berger T, Stuve O. Neurofilament light chain: An important step toward a disease biomarker in multiple sclerosis. Neurology 2019;92(10):451–2.
33. Blood Neurofilament Light Levels are Lowered to a Healthy Donor Range in Patients with RMS and PPMS Following Ocrelizumab Treatment. 35th Congress of the European Committee for Treatment and Research in Multiple Sclerosis (ECTRIMS); 2019; Stockholm, Sweden.
34. Zhang Y, Salter A, Jin S, et al. Disease-modifying therapy prescription patterns in people with multiple sclerosis by age. Ther Adv Neurol Disord 2021;14. 17562864211006499.
35. Kramer J, Bar-Or A, Turner TJ, et al. Bruton tyrosine kinase inhibitors for multiple sclerosis. Nat Rev Neurol 2023;1–16.
36. Hauser SL, Waubant E, Arnold DL, et al. B-cell depletion with rituximab in relapsing-remitting multiple sclerosis. N Engl J Med 2008;358(7):676–88.

37. Oh J, Bar-Or A. Ublituximab: a new anti-CD20 agent for multiple sclerosis. Lancet Neurol 2022;21(12):1070–2.
38. Hartung HP, members ESC, study i. Ocrelizumab shorter infusion: Primary results from the ENSEMBLE PLUS substudy in patients with MS. Neurol Neuroimmunol Neuroinflamm 2020;7(5). https://doi.org/10.1212/NXI.0000000000000807.
39. Din MTU GK, Ivanova V. Ocrelizumab induced Kounis syndrome. Abstract. Circulation 2021;144.
40. Alblaihed L, Huis In 't Veld MA. Allergic acute coronary syndrome-Kounis syndrome. Emerg Med Clin North Am 2022;40(1):69–78.
41. Luna G, Alping P, Burman J, et al. Infection risks among patients with multiple sclerosis treated with fingolimod, natalizumab, rituximab, and injectable therapies. JAMA Neurol 2020;77(2):184–91.
42. Caldito NG, Shirani A, Salter A, et al. Adverse event profile differences between rituximab and ocrelizumab: Findings from the FDA Adverse Event Reporting Database. Mult Scler 2021;27(7):1066–76.
43. Oksbjerg NR, Nielsen SD, Blinkenberg M, et al. Anti-CD20 antibody therapy and risk of infection in patients with demyelinating diseases. Mult Scler Relat Disord 2021;52:102988.
44. Seery N, Sharmin S, Li V, et al. Predicting infection risk in multiple sclerosis patients treated with ocrelizumab: a retrospective cohort study. CNS Drugs 2021; 35(8):907–18.
45. Ise W. Development and function of follicular helper T cells. Biosci Biotechnol Biochem 2016;80(1):1–6.
46. Bar-Or A, DeSeze J, Correale J, et al. Effect of ofatumumab on serum immunoglobulin levels and infection risk in relapsing multiple sclerosis (RMS) patients from the phase 3 ASCLEPIOS I and II trials. Neurology 2021;96(15 Supplement).
47. Barmettler S, Ong MS, Farmer JR, et al. Association of immunoglobulin levels, infectious risk, and mortality with rituximab and hypogammaglobulinemia. JAMA Netw Open 2018;1(7):e184169.
48. Perriguey M, Maarouf A, Stellmann JP, et al. Hypogammaglobulinemia and infections in patients with multiple sclerosis treated with rituximab. Neurol Neuroimmunol Neuroinflamm 2022;9(1). https://doi.org/10.1212/NXI.0000000000001115.
49. Bar-Or A, Calkwood JC, Chognot C, et al. Effect of ocrelizumab on vaccine responses in patients with multiple sclerosis: The VELOCE study. Neurology 2020;95(14):e1999–2008.
50. Ciotti JR, Valtcheva MV, Cross AH. Effects of MS disease-modifying therapies on responses to vaccinations: A review. Mult Scler Relat Disord 2020;45:102439.
51. Tallantyre EC, Vickaryous N, Anderson V, et al. COVID-19 Vaccine Response in People with Multiple Sclerosis. Ann Neurol 2022;91(1):89–100.
52. Genentech. Ocrelizumab and PML. Available at: https://www.ocrelizumabinfo.com/content/dam/gene/ocrelizumabinfo/pdfs/progressive-multifocal-leukoencephalopathy.pdf. accessed: April 23, 2023.
53. Avila JD. Alexia without agraphia as the initial manifestation of progressive multifocal leukoencephalopathy in chronic lymphocytic leukemia. Neurohospitalist 2020;10(1):71–2.
54. Berger JR, Malik V, Lacey S, et al. Progressive multifocal leukoencephalopathy in rituximab-treated rheumatic diseases: a rare event. J Neurovirol 2018;24(3):323–31.
55. Focosi D, Tuccori M, Maggi F. Progressive multifocal leukoencephalopathy and anti-CD20 monoclonal antibodies: What do we know after 20 years of rituximab. Rev Med Virol 2019;29(6):e2077.

56. Mills EA, Mao-Draayer Y. Aging and lymphocyte changes by immunomodulatory therapies impact PML risk in multiple sclerosis patients. Mult Scler 2018;24(8): 1014–22.
57. Prosperini L, Scarpazza C, Imberti L, et al. Age as a risk factor for early onset of natalizumab-related progressive multifocal leukoencephalopathy. J Neurovirol 2017;23(5):742–9.
58. Melamed E, Lee MW. Multiple sclerosis and cancer: the ying-yang effect of disease modifying therapies. Front Immunol 2019;10:2954.
59. Hauser SL, Kappos L, Montalban X, et al. Safety of ocrelizumab in patients with relapsing and primary progressive multiple sclerosis. Neurology 2021;97(16): e1546–59.
60. Barnes A, Hofmann D, Hall LA, et al. Ocrelizumab-induced inflammatory bowel disease-like illness characterized by esophagitis and colitis. Ann Gastroenterol 2021;34(3):447–8.
61. Lee HH, Sritharan N, Bermingham D, et al. Ocrelizumab-induced severe colitis. Case Rep Gastrointest Med 2020;2020:8858378.
62. Sunjaya DB, Taborda C, Obeng R, et al. First case of refractory colitis caused by ocrelizumab. Inflamm Bowel Dis 2020;26(6):e49.
63. Eckmann JD, Chedid V, Quinn KP, et al. De novo colitis associated with rituximab in 21 patients at a tertiary center. Clin Gastroenterol Hepatol 2020;18(1):252–3.
64. Shahmohammadi S, Sahraian MA, Shahmohammadi A, et al. A presentation of ulcerative colitis after rituximab therapy in a patient with multiple sclerosis and literature review. Mult Scler Relat Disord 2018;22:22–6.
65. Darwin E, Romanelli P, Lev-Tov H. Ocrelizumab-induced psoriasiform dermatitis in a patient with multiple sclerosis. Dermatol Online J 2018;24(7).
66. Diebold M, Muller S, Derfuss T, et al. A case of concomitant psoriasis and multiple sclerosis: Secukinumab and rituximab exert dichotomous effects in two autoimmune conditions. Mult Scler Relat Disord 2019;31:38–40.
67. Porwal MH, Patel D, Maynard M, et al. Disproportional increase in psoriasis reports in association with B cell depleting therapies in patients with multiple sclerosis. Mult Scler Relat Disord 2022;63:103832.
68. Darabi K, Jaiswal R, Hostetler SG, et al. A New Kid on the Block: IL-10+ Regulatory B Cells and a Possible Role In Psoriasis. J Pediatr Pharmacol Ther 2009; 14(3):148–53.
69. Dass S, Vital EM, Emery P. Development of psoriasis after B cell depletion with rituximab. Arthritis Rheum 2007;56(8):2715–8.
70. Holmoy T, Fogdell-Hahn A, Svenningsson A. Serum sickness following rituximab therapy in multiple sclerosis. Neurol Clin Pract 2019;9(6):519–21.
71. Karmacharya P, Poudel DR, Pathak R, et al. Rituximab-induced serum sickness: A systematic review. Semin Arthritis Rheum 2015;45(3):334–40.
72. Moreira Ferreira VF, Kimbrough DJ, Stankiewicz JM. A possible case of serum sickness after ocrelizumab infusion. Mult Scler 2021;27(1):155–8.
73. Al-Araji S, Ciccarelli O. A possible case of serum sickness after ocrelizumab infusion - Commentary. Mult Scler 2021;27(1):158–9.

# Bruton's Tyrosine Kinase Inhibitors for Multiple Sclerosis Treatment: A New Frontier

Benjamin M. Greenberg, MD, MHS,

**KEYWORDS**

• BTK inhibitor • Multiple sclerosis • Clinical trial • Microglia • B cell

**KEY POINTS**

- Although there have been significant advances in multiple sclerosis therapeutics, there remains a need to safely suppress pathologic processes that may cause progression independent of relapses.
- Bruton's tyrosine kinase (BTK) represents a unique drug target based on its biology in both B cells and microglia.
- Each BTK inhibitor will need to be assessed for safety and efficacy individually due to the potential for dramatically different pharmacologic profiles.

## INTRODUCTION

Multiple sclerosis (MS) has had a revolution in therapeutics during the last 30 years. Since the Federal Drug Administration (FDA) approval of interferon beta 1b in 1993, more than 20 subsequent therapies have been approved for relapsing remitting MS and multiple therapies have acquired indications for progressive disease.[1] Additionally, the field advanced beyond injectable therapies as the only option to an environment that provides injectable, infusible, and oral therapies to patients. Additionally, the relative efficacy of therapeutics has increased over time. The impact of these changes has been a significant reduction in the frequency of relapses and the disability that accrues from those events.[2] The most effective of these therapies, however, do come with a variety of risks including increased rates of common and opportunistic infections.

There remain multiple critical unmet needs in MS therapeutics. These include high efficacy but low-risk immunotherapies, therapies that prevent neurodegeneration independent of the immune system (ie, neuroprotection therapies) and therapies that induce neurologic repair and functional improvement. Additionally, there are no MS therapeutics that have biomarkers correlating dose-to-drug efficacy. Having a variety

Department of Neurology, The University of Texas Southwestern Medical Center, 5323 Harry Hines Boulevard, Dallas, TX 75390, USA
*E-mail address:* Benjamin.greenberg@utsouthwestern.edu

Neurol Clin 42 (2024) 155–163
https://doi.org/10.1016/j.ncl.2023.07.006

of therapies with unique mechanisms of action allows for a diversity of options for patients and clinicians when and if they are found to be a nonresponder to an existing therapy.

Despite our ability to suppress relapses, patients with MS can still experience progression of disability. This process is now recognized in both progressive patients with MS and in early patients with MS.[3] Multiple studies have implicated various pathogenic processes that could cause progression independent of relapse activity via neurodegeneration. Two of the potential processes involve B cells or microglia. It is known that B cells can increase MS pathologic condition via antibody-independent pathways.[4] Clinical-pathologic correlations have implicated meningeal follicles with activated B cells as a potential contributor to neurodegeneration in MS.[5] Additionally, multiple animal and human studies have implicated activated microglia in the pathogenesis of neurodegeneration.[6]

## *Biology of Bruton's Tyrosine Kinase*

Recurrent bacterial infections in a child with low immunoglobulins was described by Dr Ogdon Bruton in 1952.[7] This was the first description of children with X-linked agammaglobulinemia, which was ultimately proven to be related to a mutation in a tyrosine kinase.[8] This pediatric immunodeficiency disease caused children to have low numbers of circulating B cells, low immunoglobulin levels, and recurrent bacterial infections. After the discovery of this mutated tyrosine kinase, basic science studies outlined its role in B cell activation, differentiation and antibody production. Bruton's tyrosine kinase (BTK) activates proteins downstream of the B cell receptor and is instrumental for B cell maturation from pre-B cells to immature B cells and ultimately to mature B cells and plasma cells (**Fig. 1**).[9] Overexpression and increased activation of BTK in B cells is associated with autoimmune disease.[10]

BTK is also active in monocyte and macrophage lineage cells. Importantly, this includes microglial cells. Activation of BTK occurs via Fc receptor signaling.[11] Microglia have the potential to adopt various profiles including an M1 "proinflammatory" phenotype and an M2 "anti-inflammatory" phenotype (see **Fig. 1**).[12] Although in reality, these

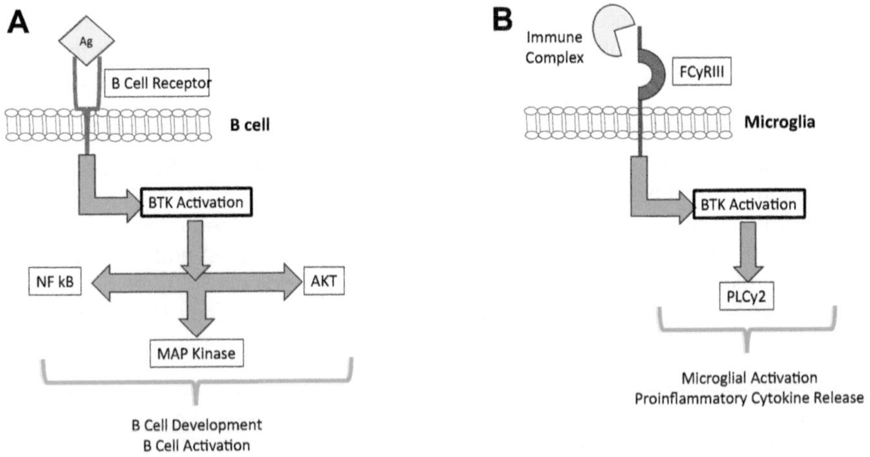


**Fig. 1.** BTK activation in B cells (*A*) and microglia (*B*). Created with Biorender.com. Ag, antigen; BTK, Bruton's tyrosine kinase; NF kB, Nuclear factor kappa-light-chain-enhancer of activated B cells; AKT, protein kinase B; MAP, mitogen-activated protein; PLCy2, Phosphatidylinositol-specific phospholipase Cγ2.

phenotypes are not dichotomous and exist on a spectrum, an imbalance of these phenotypes, with a prevalence of M1 type microglia, is associated with neurodegenerative conditions including MS.[12] The slowly expanding lesions (SELs) and paramagnetic rim lesions associated with progressive MS have an accumulation of the M1 microglia phenotype.[13]

There are a multitude of physiologic changes in microglia that occur with BTK inhibition, including decreased phagocytosis, prevention of microglial activation, and reduction in proinflammatory cytokine secretion.[14,15] Additionally, in vitro studies have suggested that microglial inhibition via Bruton's Tyrosine Kinase inhibitors (BTKi therapies may promote remyelination.[16,17] Inhibiting microglia presents a unique therapeutic target for MS.[18]

The BTK is a member of the Tec family of kinases. Tec family kinases (TFKs) are the second largest of the cytoplasmic tyrosine kinase families and are critical for many immunoreceptor-mediated intracellular signaling pathways. Mammalian members of the Tec kinase family include BTK, Interleukin-2 tyrosine kinase, tyrosine protein kinase (Tec), resting lymphocyte kinase, and bone marrow tyrosine kinase on chromosome X (Bmx). They share analogous Pleckstrin homology domain at the N-terminus, a Tec homology domain, a Src Homology 3 domain, a Src Homology 2 domain, and the kinase domain. Although the Tec family of protein tyrosine kinases has been extensively studied in the hematopoietic system, there is a growing body of evidence implicating TFKs in cardiovascular physiology and disease.[19] Understanding the diversity of cells and tissues that are affected by TFKs, including BTK, is critical for understanding the potential impacts of altering protein function.

### *History of Bruton's Tyrosine Kinase Inhibition*

BTK was identified as a potential therapeutic target in multiple hematopoietic cell malignancies and achieved FDA approval for mantle cell lymphoma after a successful phase 3 clinical trial.[20] Ibrutinib is considered a first-generation BTK inhibitor that had notable off-target effects associated with adverse events including cardiotoxicity. Second-generation BTK inhibitors were designed to have fewer off-target effects.[21] To date, there are 4 FDA-approved BTK inhibitors for various hematologic malignancies, including ibrutinib, acalabrutinib, zanubrutinib, and pirtobrutinib.[22]

The approved BTK inhibitors have indications for various hematologic malignancies but none is FDA approved for autoimmune disorders as of yet. Although data from the oncology clinical trials identified an increased risk of cardiovascular adverse events with first-generation BTK inhibitors when compared with second-generation BTK inhibitors, there was a higher prevalence of hematologic and gastrointestinal side effects with second-generation BTK inhibitors.[23] These adverse events are thought to be related to off-target binding of the inhibitors to various members of the Tec family of kinases. BTK inhibitors are currently under study for multiple neoplastic indications and multiple autoimmune diseases including rheumatoid arthritis, systemic lupus erythematosus, and MS.[24]

### *Pharmacologic Considerations with Bruton's Tyrosine Kinase Inhibition*

Inhibiting BTK is achieved by the binding of small molecules to various sites on the enzyme. Enzymatic inhibitors can be classified based on the type of bond that is formed with the target: covalent versus noncovalent and whether the inhibition is reversible or irreversible. Irreversible inhibitors cause chemical reactions on their enzymatic target so that the enzyme cannot reactivate. Covalent inhibitors form chemical bonds with their target enzymes. Noncovalent inhibitors will associate or dissociate with their target based on the surrounding environment. Although most covalent inhibitors cause irreversible inactivation of enzymes, there are some covalent reversible inhibitors whose bond can be cleaved causing reactivation of the enzyme.[25]

The implications of the various mechanisms of enzyme inhibition are significant for MS therapeutics. Enzymes that are inhibited by an irreversible inhibitor have to be replaced by new protein expression, whereas enzyme activity blocked by reversible inhibitors can activate when steady state concentrations are low. Thus, based on the mechanism of binding, the Half-maximal inhibitory concentration (IC50) of an agent does not carry the same significance. A low IC50 may be needed for a reversible enzyme but less necessary for irreversible inhibitors.

Additionally, specific to neurologic conditions such as MS, the relative amount of Central Nervous System (CNS) penetration will be important for increasing pharmacologic effects on CNS resident microglia and B cells. CNS penetration is often considered critical for neurodegenerative therapeutics, and agents with higher penetrance are thought to have greater likelihood of clinical success. In the case of BTK inhibitors, however, this may not be the case. The CNS penetration data must also be put into context with enzyme-binding characteristics such as covalent versus noncovalent binding and reversible versus irreversible inhibition. A covalent binding inhibitor or irreversible inhibitor that has low CNS penetration may achieve a similar efficacy to a noncovalent binding, reversible inhibitor with high CNS penetration. Similarly, drug half-life has distinctly different implications in the setting of enzyme inhibition compared with other small molecule therapeutics.

Finally, in the setting of oncology indications, there has been the recognition of BTKi resistance developing in some neoplasms.[26] Although this phenomena may be restricted to the environment of mutating, dividing malignant cells, its implications for treating autoimmune disorders such as MS remain unknown.

### *Opportunities for Bruton's Tyrosine Kinase Inhibition in Multiple Sclerosis*

The current landscape of MS therapeutics includes a variety of medications that induce immune modulations, immunosuppression, and/or immune remodeling.[1] The higher efficacy therapies are associated with variable levels of immunosuppression and risks of infections.[27] Additionally, there are no therapies with proven alterations of microglia that lead to a quantifiable benefit for patients with MS. BTK inhibition in MS could benefit patients with MS via 2 critical paths. First, BTKi medications modulate B cell physiology without inducing death of this cell population. Altering B cells via BTK inhibition may lead to therapeutic benefits without the level of immunosuppression observed with B cell-depleting therapies. This remains to be proven in prospective clinical trials. Second, inhibiting microglial activation may provide a novel mechanism of action for preventing neurodegeneration. Considered together, having 2 cellular drug targets with independent mechanisms of clinical benefit from one medication is a unique opportunity for MS therapeutics.

Beyond the cellular targeting of BTKi therapeutics and the potential for benefit this provides to patients with MS, there are additional opportunities to advance MS care with incorporation of BTKi drugs into the MS therapeutic arsenal. Assays to quantify BTK occupancy by an inhibitor have been used in some clinical trials.[28] To date, these data have been used to optimize dose-finding studies at the population level but could be applied to MS in 2 novel fashions. First, using enzyme occupancy data to guide dosing would allow for personalized approaches to dose selection that maximize efficacy and limit opportunities for off-target effects. Second, personalized dosing strategies would potentially allow clinicians to understand breakthrough disease events in more detail. Separating a breakthrough event as representing a lack of response to a therapy versus a lack of therapeutic dosing strategies has been absent in MS care.

Using enzyme occupancy as a biomarker of dosing efficacy could change how we manage MS therapeutics in profound ways. Until now, treatment approaches to MS have mostly adopted a "one-size fits all" approach to dosing with few exceptions. Using assays to quantify enzyme occupancy relative to BTKi therapeutics could allow the MS field to usher in the era of personalized medicine. Additionally, tracking enzyme occupancy could provide a surrogate measure of compliance and adherence.

### *Clinical Trials of Bruton's Tyrosine Kinase Inhibitors in Multiple Sclerosis*

Two phase 2 trials of BTKi therapeutics in patients with MS have been completed and published including 1 for evobrutinib and 1 for tolebrutinib.[29,30] The evobrutinib study was a double-blind, randomized trial with 5 arms, including placebo, evobrutinib 25 mg po qd, evobrutinib 75 mg qd, evobrutinib 75 mg bid, or open-label dimethyl fumarate. The primary endpoint of the trial was cumulative number of gadolinium-enhancing lesions on T1-weighted MRI at week 12, 16, 20, and 24.[29] After the 24-week double-blind, placebo-controlled period, patients were entered into a 24-week blinded extension study with placebo patients transitioned to active therapy with evobrutinib 25 mg qd. 267 patients were randomized and 244 completed the first portion of the placebo-controlled phase. Of the 244 patients who entered the second 24-week double-blind extension phase, 227 completed the study. Based on the primary endpoint of the study, both the 75 mg qd and 75 mg bid dose showed a statistically significant lower number of cumulative gadolinium-enhancing lesions on T1-weighted imaging as compared with placebo.[29] Using SELs as a surrogate for microglia-associated smoldering disease, principal investigators reviewed the impact of evobrutinib on SEL volumes and noted a dose-dependent reduction.[31] Annualized relapse rate data through 48 weeks of study favored the 75 mg bid dosing arm with overall similar adverse event rates between the 75 mg qd and bid dosing but slightly more serious adverse events in the bid dosing arm including one "toxic hepatits."[29]

Tolebrutinib was studied in a phase 2, double-blind, placebo-controlled, randomized, crossover study of 16 weeks duration. In this novel study design, a 2-step randomization schema was used. Patients were randomized 1:1 into 2 cohorts and then 1:1:1:1 within each group to receive 5, 15, 30, or 60 mg po daily of tolebrutinib. Cohort 1 began active treatment immediately, for 12 weeks, followed by a 4-week washout period, whereas cohort 2 delayed initiating treatment for 4 weeks before starting their assigned tolebrutinib dose. MRIs were acquired every 4 weeks and the primary efficacy endpoint of the study was number of new gadolinium-enhancing lesions at week 12 of treatment.[30] Of the 130 participants enrolled, 129 completed the study. There was a dose-dependent trend relative to preventing new gadolinium-enhancing lesions favoring the 60-mg daily dose of tolebrutinib.[30] Rates of adverse events were similar across the study arms, with 3 treated patients experiencing elevations in alanine aminotransferase, 2 of whom had levels higher than 3 times the upper limit of normal.[30]

There are 4 BTK inhibitors currently being studied in 11 different phase 3 trials in MS. These include evobrutinib, tolebrutinib, fenebrutinib, and remibrutinib. These therapies vary in their enzyme binding and inhibition characteristics, half-life, CNS penetration, IC50, binding selectivity, and phase 3 trial portfolio. These differences are summarized in **Table 1**. Evobrutinib and remibrutinib are each being studied in two phase 3 trials versus teriflunomide in relapsing MS (NCT05156281, NCT 05147220, NCT04338061, and NCT04338022). Tolebrutinib is being studied in 2 studies versus teriflunomide in relapsing patients (NCT 04410991 and NCT04410978). Tolebrutinib is also being studied against placebo in a trial of nonrelapsing secondary progressive MS (SPMS) and a placebo-controlled trial of primary progressive MS (PPMS)

**Table 1**
**Features of BTKi therapeutics currently in phase 3 clinical trials**

| | Evobrutinib | Fenebrutinib | Remibrutinib | Tolebrutinib |
|---|---|---|---|---|
| Current Relapsing Remitting Multiple Sclerosis (RRMS) trials | RRMS vs Teriflunomide | RRMS vs Teriflunomide | RRMS vs Teriflunomide | RRMS vs Teriflunomide |
| Current SPMS trials | N/A | N/A | N/A | SPMS vs Placebo |
| Current PPMS trials | N/A | PPMS vs Ocrelizumab | N/A | PPMS vs Placebo |
| Dosing regimen used in phase 3 studies | 75 mg po bid | 200 mg po bid | 100 mg po bid | 60 mg po qd |
| Enzyme inhibition characteristics | Covalent Irreversible | Noncovalent Reversible | Covalent Irreversible | Covalent Irreversible |
| Half-life | 2.29 h (75 mg dose) | 10.9 h (400 mg dose) | 1.41 h (100 mg dose) | 1.67 h (60 mg dose) |
| $T_{max}$, h | 0.5 | 1.26 | 0.867 | 1.5 |
| *References* | Becker et al,[32] 2020 | Herman et al,[33] 2018 | Kaul et al,[34] 2021 | Owens et al,[35] 2022 |

(NCT04411641 and NCT04458051). Fenebrutinib is completing two phase 3 trials versus teriflunomide in relapsing MS and one phase 3 trial versus ocrelizumab in patients with PPMS (NCT04586023, NCT04586010, and NCT04544449). Of note, 2 of the BTK inhibitors in MS phase 3 trials have had holds or partial holds placed by the FDA (evobrutinib and tolebrutinib) and one BTKi, orelabrutinib, in phase 2 trials, for liver enzyme abnormalities. These abnormalities have reportedly been reversible with drug cessation.

## DISCUSSION

Based on the current understanding of relapsing remitting MS and progressive disease, inhibiting BTK presents an exciting therapeutic target in MS. Simultaneously reducing the activation of autoreactive B cells and suppressing proinflammatory microglia may provide patients a mechanism for preventing relapses and progressive symptoms via a singular therapy. Additionally, BTKi therapies offer the potential for individualized dosing strategies and biomarkers of adequate dosing that are not available with current therapies. Thus, BTKi therapeutics remain a promising and exciting group of potential therapies.

Beyond the notable contributions to MS therapeutics that BTKi therapies bring to the field, the class of drugs will contain entirely unique molecules with variable impacts on the target enzyme. As such, each of the potential therapeutics has the potential to display unique efficacy and safety profiles. Just because one agent is successful in either relapsing or progressive patients will not predict the relative success of another BTKi in the same patient population. Clinical trials for each therapy in any given target population will be required to quantify the potential benefit of a given medication.

## SUMMARY

BTK presents a novel and exciting therapeutic target in MS. Based on its role in the activation of autoreactive B cells, inhibition of BTK may result in fewer relapses and potentially less progression independent of relapse activity. Additionally, inhibition of BTK results in blunting of the proinflammatory phenotype of microglia. This alteration of microglia may therapeutically benefit patients by preventing neurodegeneration. Although multiple agents are undergoing study in phase 3 trials, practitioners should be wary of lumping these medications into a "class" with shared efficacy and/or safety experiences. The profoundly unique pharmacologic characteristics of the medications, including binding site specificity, CNS penetration, half-life, and enzyme inhibition properties will mandate that each agent be judged on its own data. If one agent achieves therapeutic success for progressive disease, it does not mean that all will. Similarly, if one agent is associated with certain adverse events or side effects, it does not mean that all will. Regardless of these caveats, the potential addition of new medications with novel mechanisms of action to the therapeutic arsenal in MS is an exciting and welcome milestone.

## DISCLOSURE

Dr B.M. Greenberg has received consulting fees from Alexion, Novartis, EMD Serono, Horizon Therapeutics, Genentech/Roche, Signant, IQVIA, Sandoz, Genzyme, Immunovant, TG Therapeutics, Cycle Pharma, PHAR, Intervenn, Arialys, Bayer, Janssen, Clene, Syneos, and PRIME Education. He has received grant funding from NIH, United States, Anokion, and Regeneron, United States. He serves as an unpaid member of the board of the Siegel Rare Neuroimmune Association. He has equity in Clene and GenrAb. He receives royalties from UpToDate.

## CLINICS CARE POINTS

- BTK inhibitors represent a new class of drug for MS specialists that, if proven in phase 3 trials, will provide a novel mechanism for treating patients.
- BTK inhibition has the potential to alter both B cell and microglial activation, potentially benefiting both relapsing and progressive MS.
- BTK inhibitors each have unique binding characteristics, which will prevent extrapolation of clinical trial data from one agent to predict the impact of another therapeutic.

## REFERENCES

1. Amin M, Hersh CM. Updates and advances in multiple sclerosis neurotherapeutics. Neurodegener Dis Manag 2023;13(1):47–70.
2. Peterson S, Jalil A, Beard K, et al. Updates on efficacy and safety outcomes of new and emerging disease modifying therapies and stem cell therapy for Multiple Sclerosis: A review. Mult Scler Relat Disord 2022;68:104125.
3. Tur C, Carbonell-Mirabent P, Cobo-Calvo Á, et al. Association of Early Progression Independent of Relapse Activity With Long-term Disability After a First Demyelinating Event in Multiple Sclerosis. JAMA Neurol 2023;80(2):151–60.
4. Ireland SJ, Blazek M, Harp CT, et al. Antibody-independent B cell effector functions in relapsing remitting multiple sclerosis: clues to increased inflammatory and reduced regulatory B cell capacity. Autoimmunity 2012;45(5):400–14.
5. Zhan J, Kipp M, Han W, et al. Ectopic lymphoid follicles in progressive multiple sclerosis: From patients to animal models. Immunology 2021;164(3):450–66.

6. Distéfano-Gagné F, Bitarafan S, Lacroix S, et al. Roles and regulation of microglia activity in multiple sclerosis: insights from animal models. Nat Rev Neurosci 2023. https://doi.org/10.1038/s41583-023-00709-6.
7. BRUTON OC. Agammaglobulinemia. Pediatrics 1952;9(6):722–8.
8. Tsukada S, Saffran DC, Rawlings DJ, et al. Deficient expression of a B cell cytoplasmic tyrosine kinase in human X-linked agammaglobulinemia. Cell 1993;72(2):279–90.
9. Rawlings DJ. Bruton's tyrosine kinase controls a sustained calcium signal essential for B lineage development and function. Clin Immunol 1999;91(3):243–53.
10. Kil LP, de Bruijn MJ, van Nimwegen M, et al. Btk levels set the threshold for B-cell activation and negative selection of autoreactive B cells in mice. Blood 2012;119(16):3744–56.
11. Jongstra-Bilen J, Puig Cano A, Hasija M, et al. Dual functions of Bruton's tyrosine kinase and Tec kinase during Fcgamma receptor-induced signaling and phagocytosis. J Immunol 2008;181(1):288–98.
12. Guo S, Wang H, Yin Y. Microglia Polarization From M1 to M2 in Neurodegenerative Diseases. Front Aging Neurosci 2022;14:815347.
13. Jäckle K, Zeis T, Schaeren-Wiemers N, et al. Molecular signature of slowly expanding lesions in progressive multiple sclerosis. Brain 2020;143(7):2073–88.
14. Nam HY, Nam JH, Yoon G, et al. Ibrutinib suppresses LPS-induced neuroinflammatory responses in BV2 microglial cells and wild-type mice. J Neuroinflammation 2018;15(1):271.
15. Keaney J, Gasser J, Gillet G, et al. Inhibition of Bruton's Tyrosine Kinase Modulates Microglial Phagocytosis: Therapeutic Implications for Alzheimer's Disease. J Neuroimmune Pharmacol 2019;14(3):448–61.
16. Martin E, Aigrot MS, Grenningloh R, et al. Bruton's Tyrosine Kinase Inhibition Promotes Myelin Repair. Brain Plast 2020;5(2):123–33.
17. Mangla A, Khare A, Vineeth V, et al. Pleiotropic consequences of Bruton tyrosine kinase deficiency in myeloid lineages lead to poor inflammatory responses. Blood 2004;104(4):1191–7.
18. Wang J, Yang B, Weng Q, et al. Targeting Microglia and Macrophages: A Potential Treatment Strategy for Multiple Sclerosis. Front Pharmacol 2019;10:286.
19. Yin Z, Zou Y, Wang D, et al. Regulation of the Tec family of non-receptor tyrosine kinases in cardiovascular disease. Cell Death Discov 2022;8(1):119.
20. Dreyling M, Jurczak W, Jerkeman M, et al. Ibrutinib versus temsirolimus in patients with relapsed or refractory mantle-cell lymphoma: an international, randomised, open-label, phase 3 study. Lancet 2016;387(10020):770–8.
21. Thompson PA, Burger JA. Bruton's tyrosine kinase inhibitors: first and second generation agents for patients with Chronic Lymphocytic Leukemia (CLL). Expert Opin Investig Drugs 2018;27(1):31–42.
22. Hatashima A, Karami M, Shadman M. Approved and emerging Bruton's tyrosine kinase inhibitors for the treatment of chronic lymphocytic leukemia. Expert Opin Pharmacother 2022;23(13):1545–57.
23. Arustamyan M, Kibrik P, Hatipoglu D, et al. The safety of Bruton's tyrosine kinase inhibitors in B-cell malignancies: A systematic review. Eur J Haematol 2022;109(6):696–710.
24. Garg N, Padron EJ, Rammohan KW, et al. Bruton's Tyrosine Kinase Inhibitors: The Next Frontier of B-Cell-Targeted Therapies for Cancer, Autoimmune Disorders, and Multiple Sclerosis. J Clin Med 2022;11(20). https://doi.org/10.3390/jcm11206139.

25. Tuley A, Fast W. The Taxonomy of Covalent Inhibitors. Biochemistry 2018;57(24): 3326–37. https://doi.org/10.1021/acs.biochem.8b00315.
26. Nakhoda S, Vistarop A, Wang YL. Resistance to Bruton tyrosine kinase inhibition in chronic lymphocytic leukaemia and non-Hodgkin lymphoma. Br J Haematol 2023;200(2):137–49.
27. Tur C, Dubessy AL, Otero-Romero S, et al. The risk of infections for multiple sclerosis and neuromyelitis optica spectrum disorder disease-modifying treatments: Eighth European Committee for Treatment and Research in Multiple Sclerosis Focused Workshop Review. April 2021. Mult Scler 2022;28(9):1424–56.
28. Skånland SS, Tjønnfjord GE. Determining drug dose in the era of targeted therapies: playing it (un)safe′. Blood Cancer J 2022;12(8):123.
29. Montalban X, Arnold DL, Weber MS, et al. Placebo-Controlled Trial of an Oral BTK Inhibitor in Multiple Sclerosis. N Engl J Med 2019;380(25):2406–17.
30. Reich DS, Arnold DL, Vermersch P, et al. Safety and efficacy of tolebrutinib, an oral brain-penetrant BTK inhibitor, in relapsing multiple sclerosis: a phase 2b, randomised, double-blind, placebo-controlled trial. Lancet Neurol 2021;20(9): 729–38.
31. Arnold D, Elliott C, Montalban X, Martin E, Hyvert Y, Tomic D. Effects of evobrutinib, a Bruton's tyrosine kinase inhibitor, on slowly expanding lesions: An emerging imaging marker of chronic tissue loss in multiple sclerosis CMSC; Poster, DMT17, 2022.
32. Becker A, Martin EC, Mitchell DY, et al. Safety, Tolerability, Pharmacokinetics, Target Occupancy, and Concentration-QT Analysis of the Novel BTK Inhibitor Evobrutinib in Healthy Volunteers. Clin Transl Sci 2020;13(2):325–36.
33. Herman AE, Chinn LW, Kotwal SG, et al. Safety, Pharmacokinetics, and Pharmacodynamics in Healthy Volunteers Treated With GDC-0853, a Selective Reversible Bruton's Tyrosine Kinase Inhibitor. Clin Pharmacol Ther 2018;103(6):1020–8.
34. Kaul M, End P, Cabanski M, et al. Remibrutinib (LOU064): A selective potent oral BTK inhibitor with promising clinical safety and pharmacodynamics in a randomized phase I trial. Clin Transl Sci 2021;14(5):1756–68.
35. Owens TD, Smith PF, Redfern A, et al. Phase 1 clinical trial evaluating safety, exposure and pharmacodynamics of BTK inhibitor tolebrutinib (PRN2246, SAR442168). Clin Transl Sci 2022;15(2):442–50.

# Autologous Hematopoietic Stem Cell Transplantation to Treat Multiple Sclerosis

Lindsay A. Ross, MD, MSc[1], Lisa M. Stropp, MD[1],
Jeffrey A. Cohen, MD*

**KEYWORDS**

• Multiple sclerosis • Therapeutics • Stem cell transplantation • Clinical trials
• Immune reconstitution

**KEY POINTS**

- In aggregate, the available data suggest autologous hematopoietic stem cell transplantation (AHSCT) has potent, durable efficacy.
- Safety issues and financial costs are significant but largely "front-loaded."
- The published data have several caveats. The overall published experience is relatively modest. The studies had different patient populations, therapeutic protocols, outcome measures. The 2 randomized controlled trials had suboptimal control groups.
- AHSCT is a reasonable option for patients with highly active relapsing multiple sclerosis (MS) and an inadequate response to the available disease therapies.
- The key question is where to place AHSCT in the overall relapsing MS algorithm relative to other high-efficacy therapies.

## INTRODUCTION

Multiple sclerosis (MS) is a chronic neurologic disorder, which often leads to disability due to cumulative inflammatory demyelination, neuronal damage, and neurodegeneration in the central nervous system. The therapeutic landscape for MS has greatly expanded during the past 3 decades and now includes more than 20 disease-modifying therapies (DMTs) with regulatory approval. Despite these advances, there remains a small but substantial proportion of people with MS with highly active disease that is inadequately controlled by the available DMTs. The role of immune system ablation followed by autologous hematopoietic stem cell transplantation (AHSCT) as a treatment of MS has been studied since the 1990s. The available evidence

Mellen Center, Neurological Institute, Cleveland Clinic, 9500 Euclid Avenue, Cleveland, OH 44195, USA
[1] Contributed equally.
* Corresponding author.
*E-mail address:* cohenj@ccf.org

Neurol Clin 42 (2024) 165–184
https://doi.org/10.1016/j.ncl.2023.06.002
0733-8619/24/

indicates that AHSCT is a highly efficacious treatment of relapsing MS with long-lasting benefit on clinical and radiographic disease activity, often with stabilization and in some cases improvement in disability.[1] Although initial data raised caution regarding mortality rate associated with treatment, more recent trials with improved patient selection and conditioning regimens have demonstrated improved safety profile of treatment with lower mortality rates.[2] Several organizations have published position statements supporting use of AHSCT in treatment-refractory patients with highly active relapsing MS.[3–5] However, the optimal AHSCT protocol and where to place AHSCT in the treatment sequence in relapsing MS remain uncertain. Ongoing clinical trials and future studies will explore these questions. This article will review the current status of AHSCT to treat MS.

## OVERVIEW OF AUTOLOGOUS HEMATOPOIETIC STEM CELL TRANSPLANTATION PROCEDURE

AHSCT is a multistep process: mobilization, harvesting, conditioning, transplantation, and recovery (**Fig. 1**). First, hematopoietic stem cells (HSCs) are mobilized from the bone marrow to the peripheral blood by administration of granulocyte colony-stimulating factor (G-CSF). Often, cyclophosphamide is given in conjunction to mitigate the risk of disease flare during this time.[6] To harvest the HSCs a large double lumen catheter is placed to minimize trauma to the cells and collection occurs by leukapheresis. Mobilization and harvesting are commonly done as outpatient procedures and together take between 5 and 15 days. After harvesting, the collected cells may undergo optional manipulation with selection for CD34+ cells (an HSC marker) and/or ex vivo T cell depletion to limit potential contamination of the graft with autoreactive lymphocytes.[1] The cells are then cryopreserved until ready for use. Two to 4 weeks later, the patient undergoes conditioning comprising chemotherapeutic agents with or without antibody therapy, for example, antithymocyte globulin (ATG). Conditioning

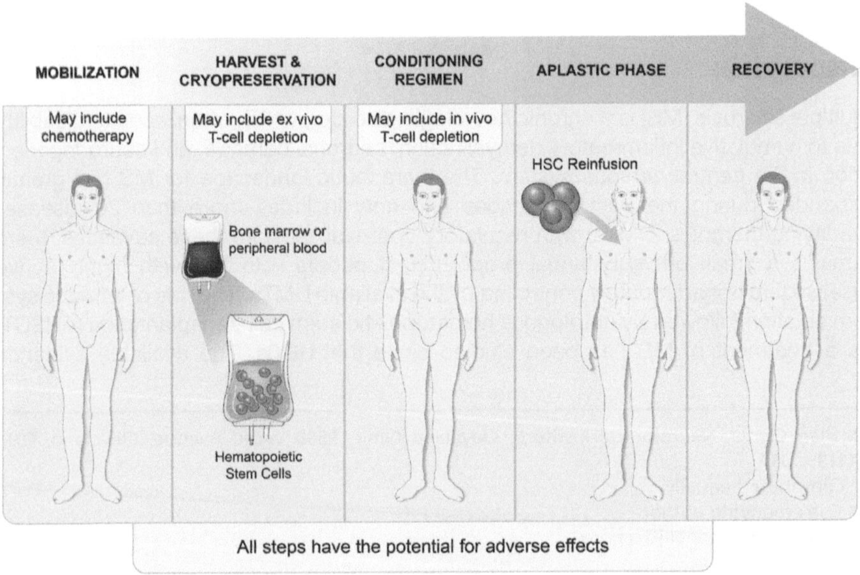


**Fig. 1.** Overview of the multistep AHSCT procedure. Details are provided in the text. (Reprinted with permission, Cleveland Clinic Foundation ©2023. All Rights Reserved.)

regimens are categorized based on their intensity and whether in addition to being lymphoablative they also are myeloablative. High-intensity regimens, for example, busulfan plus ATG as used in the Canadian phase 2 study,[7] may have more potent and durable efficacy but have the highest toxicity. Low-intensity (nonmyeloablative) regimens, for example, cyclophosphamide plus ATG used in the MIST phase 3 trial,[8] are better tolerated but may have less consistent and durable efficacy. The intermediate intensity BEAM (BCNU/carmustine, etoposide, cytarabine, melphalan) plus ATG regimen, as used in the HALT-MS phase 2 trial,[9,10] has been the most common conditioning regimen. After conditioning, the patient receives the graft of previously stored cells, which shortens the aplastic phase. Before reconstitution, the patient is pancytopenic for 10 to 14 days and during this time receives anti-infective agents.[11] For conditioning and transplantation, patients typically are hospitalized for myeloablative regimens for approximately several weeks for monitoring and supportive care.[1] Following this, the patient moves into the recovery stage where the immune system continues to rebuild over several years, which is further detailed below.

## SUMMARY OF EFFICACY RESULTS IN PREVIOUS STUDIES

This review summarizes 5 single-arm phase 2 trials and 2 randomized controlled phase 3 trials of AHSCT in MS (**Table 1**), as well as observational case series.

### *Single-Arm Phase 2 Trials*

A single-center phase 1/2 single-arm trial published in 2009 by Burt and colleagues[12] enrolled 21 participants with relapsing-remitting MS (RRMS) who had failed treatment with interferon beta, defined as either 2 intravenous steroid-treated relapses in the preceding year or one intravenous steroid-treated relapse in addition to 1 or more gadolinium-enhancing (GdE) MRI lesion (on a separate occasion) in the preceding year. The transplantation protocol included mobilization with cyclophosphamide and G-CSF followed by conditioning with cyclophosphamide in combination with either alemtuzumab or rabbit ATG. There were no transplant-related deaths. The first primary outcome of the trial was progression-free survival (with progression defined as increase of Expanded Disability Status Scale [EDSS] by $\geq$ 1.0 posttransplant), which was achieved by 100% of participants at 3 years follow-up. The second primary outcome was reversal of neurologic disability (defined as decreased EDSS of $\geq$1.0 posttransplant), which 81% of participants achieved at 3 years follow-up.

The single-center phase 2 single-arm trial published in 2012 by Shevchenko and colleagues[13] enrolled 95 participants, including RRMS (n = 42), secondary progressive MS (SPMS) (n = 35), and primary progressive MS (PPMS) (n = 15) refractory to DMT treatment. The transplantation protocol included mobilization with G-CSF followed by conditioning with modified BEAM regimen $\pm$ horse ATG. The primary outcome was overall clinical response (defined as disease stabilization or improvement by EDSS), which was achieved by 80% of participants at long-term follow-up (mean 46 months). A secondary outcome was the 36-item Short Form (SF-36) questionnaire, demonstrating significant improvement in several parameters of quality of life at 12 months posttransplant, which was sustained at long-term follow-up. No transplant-related deaths were reported.

A single-arm phase 2 trial of AHSCT in MS was published in 2016 by Atkins and colleagues.[7] The study enrolled 26 participants, 24 of which underwent transplantation (RRMS n = 12, SPMS n = 12). Participants enrolled had disease course notable for early development of sustained disability (EDSS $\geq$3.0 within 5 years of disease onset) as well as disease activity while on DMT. Transplantation protocol included

Table 1
Summary of phase 2 and phase 3 clinical trials of autologous hematopoietic stem cell transplantation in multiple sclerosis

| Study | Northwestern Trial (2009)[12] | Russian Trial (2012)[13] | Canadian Trial (2016)[7] | HALT-MS (2015, 2017)[9,10] | Australian Trial (2018)[14] | ASTIMS (2015)[21] | MIST (2018)[22] |
|---|---|---|---|---|---|---|---|
| **Identifier** | **NCT00278655** | **NA** | **NCT01099930** | **NCT00288626** | **ACTRN 12613000339752** | **EUDRACT 2007–000064–24** | **NCT00273364** |
| Study Design | | | | | | | |
| Protocol | Phase 1/2 clinical trial, single arm | Phase 2 clinical trial, single arm | Phase 2 clinical trial, single arm | Phase 2 clinical trial, single arm | Phase 2 clinical trial, single arm | Phase 2 RCT, AHSCT vs mitoxantrone | Phase 3 RCT, AHSCT vs DMT |
| Recruitment period | 2003–2005 | 2006–2011 | 2001–2009 | 2006–2009 | 2010–2016 | 2004–2009 | 2005–2016 |
| Sample size (n) | 21 | 95 | 26 enrolled, 24 underwent transplant | 25 enrolled, 24 underwent transplant | 35 | 21 (9 to AHSCT, 12 to control) | 110 (55 to AHSCT, 52 to control) |
| Inclusion criteria | RRMS, age 18–55 y, EDSS 2.0–5.5, failure of IFNβ treatment with either 2 relapses in prior year or 1 relapse and 1 GdE lesion at separate time over prior year | MS diagnosis, EDSS 1.5–8.0, disease refractory to DMT | RRMS or SPMS, age 18–50 y, early sustained disability (EDSS ≥3.0 within 5 y of disease onset) and disease activity while on DMT | RRMS, age 18–60 y, EDSS 3.0–5.5, failure of DMT in prior 18 mo (2 or more clinical relapses with EDSS increase of ≥1.0) | Age 8–60 y, EDSS 2.0–7.0, for RRMS: either ≥1 relapse in the prior year while on DMT or ≥1 GdE lesions in the prior year, for SPMS: worsening while on DMT over prior year and ≥1 GdE lesion in the prior year | RRMS or SPMS, EDSS worsening 0.5–1.0 point in prior year while on DMT, ≥1 GdE lesions | RRMS, age 18–55 y, EDSS 2.0–6.0, 2 clinical relapses or 1 relapse with GdE lesion at different time the prior year while on DMT |

| | | | | | | | |
|---|---|---|---|---|---|---|---|
| Primary outcome | Progression free survival (defined as increase of EDSS by ≥ 1.0 posttransplant) | Clinical response defined as disease stabilization or improvement by EDSS | Absence of disease activity at 3 y posttransplant | Time to treatment failure (death or MS disease activity—either EDSS progression by ≥ 1.0, clinical relapse, or new MRI lesions) | NEDA—absence of clinical relapse, radiographic progression, or disability progression | Cumulative number of new T2 lesions over 4 year period | 6 month-confirmed EDSS worsening >1.0 after at least 1 y of treatment or post-AHSCT |
| Patient Selection (for AHSCT group) | | | | | | | |
| Median age (range) | 33 (20–53) | 34.5 (Mean) | 34 (24–45) | 38 (27–53) | 37 (21–55) | 35.5 (19–46) (Mean) | 34 (18–54), for AHSCT participants |
| Median EDSS (range) | 3.1 (2.0–5.5) | 3.5 (1.5–8.0) | Median NA (3.0–6.0) | 4.5 (3.0–5.5) | Median NA; n = 6 < 4, n = 16 4–6, n = 13 > 6 | 6.0 (5.5–6.5) | 3.0 (1.5–6.5), for AHSCT participants |
| Median Disease duration, years (range) | Median 5 (1.6–10) | NA | Mean 6.1 ± 2.5 | Median 4.9 (0.6–12) | Median 6.9 (0.7–21.6) | 10.2 (2–23) | 4.7 (0.8–14), for AHSCT participants |
| % of participants with RRMS | 100 | 44 | 50 | 100 | 57 | 22, for AHSCT participants | 100 |
| AHSCT protocol | | | | | | | |
| Mobilization regimen | Cy (2 g/m²) and filgrastim (10 μg/kg/d) | Filgrastim (10 μg/kg/d) | Cy (4.5 g/m²) and filgrastim (10 μg/kg/d) | Filgrastim (16 μg/kg/d) and prednisone (1 mg/kg/d × 10 d, initiated 1 d before filgrastim) | Cy (2 g/m²) and filgrastim (10 μg/kg/d) | Cy (4 g/m²) + filgrastim (5 μg/kg/d) | Cy (2 g/m²) + filgrastim (5–10 μg/kg/d) |

(continued on next page)

**Table 1 (*continued*)**

| Study | Northwestern Trial (2009)[12] | Russian Trial (2012)[13] | Canadian Trial (2016)[7] | HALT-MS (2015, 2017)[9,10] | Australian Trial (2018)[14] | ASTIMS (2015)[21] | MIST (2018)[22] |
|---|---|---|---|---|---|---|---|
| **Identifier** | **NCT00278655** | **NA** | **NCT01099930** | **NCT00288626** | **ACTRN 12613000339752** | **EUDRACT 2007–000064–24** | **NCT00273364** |
| CD34+ selection | No | No | Yes | Yes | No | No | No |
| Conditioning regimen | Cy 200 mg/kg and either alemtuzumab (20 mg) or rabbit ATG (6 mg/kg) | Modified BEAM ± horse ATG | Busulfan (mean dose 10.9 mg/kg), Cy 200 mg/kg, and rabbit ATG 5 mg/kg | BEAM and rabbit ATG 5 mg/kg | BEAM and horse ATG 40 mg/kg | BEAM, rabbit ATG 7.5 mg/kg | Cy 200 mg/kg, rabbit ATG 6 mg/kg |
| Results | | | | | | | |
| Follow-up duration, years | Mean, 3.1 (range, 2–4) | Mean, 3.8 (range, 0.8–5.5) | Median, 6.7 (range, 3.9–12.7) | Mean, 5.2 (range, 1–6) | Median, 3 (range, 1–5.5) | 4 y | Up to 5 y |
| Result on primary outcome | 100% of participants achieved progression-free survival at 3 y follow-up posttransplant | 82% of participants achieved stability or improvement of EDSS at 5 y posttransplant | 69.6% of participants achieved absence of disease activity at 3 y posttransplant | 69.2% of participants achieved NEDA at 5 y posttransplant | NEDA was achieved in 82% of participants at 1 y, 65% at 2 y, and 60% at 3 y | AHSCT cohort had median of 2.5 new T2 MRI lesions, compared with 8 in mitoxantrone group | Disability worsening in 5.8% of AHSCT vs 66.7% of DMT |
| Transplant-related mortality | 0 | 0 | 1 | 0 | 0 | 0 | 0 |

*Abbreviations:* AHSCT, autologous hematopoietic stem cell transplantation; ATG, antithymocyte globulin; BEAM, carmustine/etoposide/cytarabine/melphalan; Cy, cyclophosphamide; DMT, disease modifying therapy; EDSS, expanded disability status scale; GdE, gadolinium-enhancing; IFNβ, interferon beta; MRI, magnetic resonance imaging; NA, not available; NEDA, no evidence of disease activity; RCT, randomized controlled trial; RRMS, relapsing-remitting multiple sclerosis; SPMS, secondary progressive multiple sclerosis.

mobilization with cyclophosphamide and G-CSF, CD34 selection, and conditioning with busulfan, cyclophosphamide, and rabbit ATG. The primary outcome was absence of disease activity at 3 years posttransplant, which was achieved in 69.6% (95%CI 46.6–84.2) of participants. Participants were followed for 13 years posttransplant and no participants experienced clinical relapses or radiographic activity (defined as presence of GdE or new T2 lesions). This trial also assessed rate of brain atrophy compared with healthy controls and found progressive slowing of atrophy rates in AHSCT participants, ultimately reaching the range of normal aging. There was one treatment-related death following transplantation in a patient who developed bacterial sepsis and sinusoid obstruction syndrome complicated by massive hepatic necrosis.

The interim results of the HALT-MS multicenter single arm phase 2 trial of AHSCT in MS were published in 2015 by Nash and colleagues[9] and the final results in 2017.[10] The study enrolled 25 participants and 24 participants underwent AHSCT. Participants enrolled had diagnosis of RRMS with failure of DMT, defined as 2 or greater clinical relapses in the preceding 18 months with associated sustained EDSS worsening. The transplantation protocol included mobilization with G-CSF and prednisone, CD34 selection, and conditioning with BEAM and rabbit ATG. At 5 years posttransplant, 69.2% (90% CI 50.2–82.1) of participants achieved no evidence of disease activity (NEDA)-free survival. NEDA was defined as absence of relapse, progression of disability measured by EDSS, or brain MRI lesion activity. The trial also found that there was improvement in EDSS by median of 0.5 points (interquartile range 0.0–1.5). No transplant-related deaths were reported.

The most recent single-arm phase 2 trial of AHSCT in MS was a single-center study published in 2018 by Moore and colleagues.[14] The trial enrolled 35 participants. Participants with RRMS (n = 20) met the criteria of either having 1 or greater relapses in the year prior while on DMT or having 1 or greater GdE lesions in the prior year. Participants with SPMS (n = 15) met criteria of worsening over the prior year while on DMT and evidence of 1 or greater GdE lesions in the year prior. The transplantation protocol included mobilization with cyclophosphamide and G-CSF followed by conditioning with BEAM and ATG. The primary outcome assessed in this trial was disease activity-free survival. The trial found that NEDA was achieved in 82% (95% CI 65% to 92%) at 1 year, 65% (95% CI 45% to 79%) at 2 years, and 60% (95% CI 40%–75%) at 3 years. Additionally, 44% of participants demonstrated sustained improvement in disability as measured by EDSS at 3 years posttransplant. No transplant-related deaths were reported.

### *Observational Studies*

Several uncontrolled case series have reported potent, long-lasting efficacy of AHSCT in relapsing MS.[8,15–17] In a nonrandomized single-center study, AHSCT had superior efficacy in maintaining efficacy and cognitive function measured by a comprehensive neuropsychological test battery compared with alemtuzumab.[18] In a comparative analysis, substantially higher rates of NEDA were reported in several studies of AHSCT (70%–92%) compared with that reported in phase 3 trials of approved DMTs: 7% to 16% for those receiving placebo, 13% to 27% receiving interferon-beta, and 22% to 48% receiving oral and infusion therapies (20%–50%).[1] A meta-analysis of AHSCT trials completed from 1995 to 2016 came to a similar conclusion.[19] The pooled proportion of NEDA patients was 83% (70%-92%) at 2 years and 67% (range 59%–70%) at 5 years.

In contrast, Kalincik and colleagues recently reported emulated clinical trials comparing the efficacy of AHSCT versus fingolimod, natalizumab, and ocrelizumab measured by annualized relapse rate (ARR), EDSS worsening, and EDSS improvement using data from participants from 6 AHSCT centers and the MSBase registry.[20] The sample sizes were relatively large, and propensity score techniques were applied to make the comparison groups comparable. AHSCT was more efficacious compared with fingolimod, a DMT considered to have moderate efficacy. When compared with DMTs with high efficacy, AHSCT was marginally superior to natalizumab and yielded similar results compared with ocrelizumab.

### *Randomized Controlled Phase 3 Trials*

The ASTIMS multicenter phase 2 randomized controlled trial (RCT) was published in 2015 by Mancardi and colleagues.[21] The study enrolled 21 participants from 2004 to 2009, with participants randomized to AHSCT (n = 9) or mitoxantrone (MTX, n = 12). Participants enrolled included RRMS (n = 7), SPMS (n = 13), and PPMS (n = 1) phenotypes classified as aggressive based on criteria of having exhibited EDSS worsening by 0.5 to 1.0 points per year while on DMT as well as 1 or greater GdE lesions. This trial found that AHSCT led to significantly fewer new T2 lesions as compared with MTX (rate ratio 0.21, $P = .00016$). During 4-year follow-up, no participants treated with AHSCT developed GdE lesions compared with 56% of MTX-treated participants ($P = .029$). Clinically, ARR was significantly lower in the AHSCT arm (0.19) compared with the MTX arm (0.6), (rate ratio = 0.36, 95% CI 0.15–0.88, $P = .026$). However, there was no significant difference between groups in EDSS change at annual evaluations during 4 years. No transplant-related deaths were reported.

The MIST multicenter phase 3 RCT comparing treatment with AHSCT versus conventional DMT was published in 2019 by Burt and colleagues.[22] The study enrolled 110 participants from 2005 to 2016, with 55 randomized to the AHSCT and DMT arms. Participants had RRMS and either 2 clinical relapses over the preceding year while on DMT or 1 clinical relapse in the preceding year with a GdE lesion at a different time during the year, while on DMT. The transplantation protocol included mobilization with cyclophosphamide and G-CSF followed by a nonmyeloablative conditioning regimen with high-dose cyclophosphamide and rabbit ATG. The control group treatment was a DMT of higher efficacy or a different class than DMT taken during the previous year and included natalizumab, dimethyl fumarate, fingolimod, glatiramer acetate, interferon beta-1a, mitoxantrone, and teriflunomide. In addition to regulatory approved DMT, 38 participants received methylprednisolone, rituximab, plasmapheresis, intravenous cyclophosphamide, or intravenous immunoglobulin. The trial found that 5.8% of participants treated with AHSCT experienced disability worsening as compared with 69.2% of controls (hazard ratio 0.07, 95% CI, 0.02–0.24, $P < .001$). Median time to progression could not be calculated for the AHSCT group due to the small number of events. In the DMT group, median time to progression (defined as EDSS score increase of $\geq 1$) was 24 months (interquartile range 18–48 months). There was also a statistically significant difference in EDSS change during the first year with improvement following AHSCT from 3.38 to 2.36, and worsening from 3.31 to 3.98 in the DMT group (between-group mean difference, −1.7, 95% CI −2.03 to −1.29; $P < .001$). No transplant-related deaths were reported.

## SAFETY AND TOLERABILITY

### *Adverse Effects Associated with the Autologous Hematopoietic Stem Cell Transplantation Procedure*

Improvements have been made in safety and tolerability over time as the field has learned more about AHSCT for MS. However, this remains a key area of concern. Overall complications rates are difficult to delineate given variations in the procedure and patient populations studied across reports. However, in a recent study of more than 100 patients with MS receiving AHSCT at 2 centers in the United Kingdom with a conditioning regimen of cyclophosphamide and ATG, 90% had at least one complication.[23] Adverse effects of the conditioning agents include nausea, alopecia, mucositis, fluid overload, and allergic reactions to ATG. Indirect adverse effects relate to effects, for example, infection, hemorrhage. The transplant can be associated with so-called engraftment syndrome, with potential manifestations including fever, rash, pulmonary edema, liver or renal impairment, and encephalopathy. Further discussion of safety is broken down by individual risks.

### *Treatment-Related Mortality*

The rate of treatment-related mortality (TRM) has been quite variable ranging from 0% to 4% across studies.[24] This variation may be attributable to patient level factors and choice of conditioning regimen. TRM has decreased in more recent studies, coinciding with the increased proportion of patients with RRMS (as opposed to progressive disease) included.[25] TRM is also significantly associated with a higher baseline level of disability.[2] There has also been less use of the high-intensity conditioning regimens recently but 2 meta-analyses came to differing conclusions as to whether this was associated with TRM.[2,25] A recent analyses estimated the rate of TRM at 0.2% to 0.3%.[1]

### *Infection*

In a review of studies published between 2016 and 2020 with 20 or more participants receiving AHSCT for MS, infection was reported to occur in 31% to 58%.[26] Infection is the leading cause of TRM.[25] The most worrisome time for an infection to arise during AHSCT is during the pancytopenic period following conditioning before immune reconstitution. Increased incidence of urinary tract infections, herpes virus illnesses, gastroenteritis, and pneumonia has been reported.[6,27]

Epstein Barr virus (EBV) and Cytomegalovirus (CMV) may reactivate after AHSCT and could be life threatening. Therefore, routine monitoring for both viruses is recommended.[11] In one study of MS participants undergoing AHSCT,[28] all were found to have increasing EBV levels after transplant, with 28% of these individuals experiencing symptoms including fever, lymphadenopathy, and/or EBV-related B cell proliferative disorders. This usually occurred about 1 month after transplant and the majority required treated with rituximab, which decreased viral load and symptoms. Symptomatic EBV reactivation and high levels of paraproteinemia are associated with EDSS worsening after AHSCT.[23] ASHCT protocols typically include EBV antiviral prophylactic therapy until there is immune reconstitution.

CMV reactivation has been reported to occur on a similar timeline as EBV[27] and may be more common in those who received anti-CD20 treatment before AHSCT.[29] In one cohort study of 120 MS participants undergoing AHSCT,[23] CMV reactivation occurred in 22% but with the use of valganciclovir or ganciclovir, no cases progressed to symptomatic CMV disease.

### *Impact on Fertility and Pregnancy*

With the use of chemotherapeutic agents in mobilization and conditioning regimens, risk of infertility is substantial, 70% to 90%, in both women and men undergoing AHSCT.[30] The risk of infertility seems less in patients undergoing AHSCT for autoimmune disease compared with oncologic indications. There are limited data in this area to date but in 1 multicenter study of AHSCT for MS,[31] 70% of women of childbearing age had recovered their menses by about 7 months. Among those aged 32 years and younger, 92% recovered or maintained their menses. There was no association with the conditioning regimen used. Successful pregnancies have been reported after AHSCT for both male and female MS patients, both naturally and with use of reproductive assistive technology and treatments. The births occurred without maternal or neonatal complications. However, spontaneous abortions have also been reported.[30–32] Given that AHSCT is typically considered in young adults with MS, they should receive counseling on the potential for infertility and consideration of fertility preservation procedures before initiating the AHSCT procedure.

### *Neurological Sequelae*

There is the possibility of MS disease flare during the transplant procedure especially during mobilization. Notably there has been a fatality reported related to one such disease flare, which involved a new cervical cord lesion.[6] The risk for disease flare is now often mitigated using cyclophosphamide in combination with G-CSF. In one large study of AHSCT for a variety of autoimmune diseases, including MS, there were no disease flares reported in mobilization for those participants who received concomitant cyclophosphamide.[33]

The AHSCT procedure itself involves some neurotoxicity. Increases in serum neurofilament light chain and glial fibrillary acidic protein, markers of neuronal damage, along with MRI gray matter volume loss have been demonstrated following AHSCT in MS patients.[34] Clinically, in one study, 17% of participants had "neurological toxicity" occurring within 60 days of AHSCT.[27] More recently, significant worsening in EDSS was noted at 6 months but by 12 months most participants remained clinically stable if not slightly improved compared with pre-AHSCT baseline.[34]

### *Secondary Autoimmunity*

MS patients undergoing AHSCT may develop a secondary autoimmune disease months to years later.[11] This was reported to occur in 8% of MS patients receiving AHSCT in the European Blood and Marrow Transplantation (EBMT) database.[35] Secondary autoimmune disorders included hemophilia, idiopathic thrombocytopenic purpura, autoimmune hemolytic anemia, and thyroiditis. Younger individuals and those undergoing AHSCT earlier in their disease course seem at greater risk. In some cases, secondary autoimmunity may be related to use of alemtuzumab and/or ATG during the transplant.[11]

### *Other Complications*

Other complications that may occur during or shortly after AHSCT include neutropenia, neutropenic fever, failure of mobilization (ie, inadequate quantities of stem cells collected), hemorrhagic cystitis, ATG-related fever, engraftment syndrome, deep vein thrombosis, and falls.[11,27,33] Other late sequelae, which may occur after the immediate transplant period, include endocrinopathies[36] as well as cancers.[37]

## IMMUNOLOGIC EFFECTS

The mechanisms of action in AHSCT for MS is thought to be elimination or reduction of pathogenic immune cells followed by immune reconstitution with reset T and B cells, normalized immunoregulation, and a decreased inflammatory environment.

### *Cell Elimination and Lymphopenia*

Conditioning regimens given in AHSCT deplete mature lymphocytic and myelocytic cells dependent to a degree on the chemotherapeutics and antibody treatments used. There is a decrease in the total lymphocyte count for a year following AHSCT, and CD4 T cells may be decreased for 2 years even when nonmyeloablative regimens are used.[24] Similarly, mucosal-associated invariant T cells, a type of CD8+ T cell found in MS plaques in postmortem studies, were demonstrated to be almost undetectable in blood for 2 years following AHSCT even with nonmyeloablative regimens.[24] Specifically, the ablation of circulating T cells seems to be important, as higher levels of T cells in the peripheral blood at baseline is associated with achieving a long duration of relapse freedom after AHSCT.[24] As such, there have also been attempts to eliminate T cells from the graft via manipulation. However, to date graft manipulation has not been demonstrated to have added benefits to conditioning alone. It may be that the use of cyclophosphamide, which destroys mature lymphocytes but not CD34+ cells and ATG, which depletes T cells, already ensures that those unwanted cells do not engraft.[38]

Following cell elimination there is lymphopenia-induced proliferation where surviving and engrafted cells receive strong signals to proliferate. The replicative drive may be exhaustive for these cells and ultimately lead to senescence and clonal attrition. This may help rid the patient of remaining pathogenic cells that survived conditioning or were present in the graft as well, as make way for a more diversified immune cell repertoire post-AHSCT.[38]

### *Resetting of T and B Cell Populations*

Various B and T cell populations recover with different kinetics. Naïve B cells initially dominate the posttransplant circulating B cell population with mature CD19+ B cells increasing at 18 to 24 months after transplant.[39] CD4+ T cells recover slower than CD8+ T cells,[39] and naïve T cells predominate over memory T cells for a few years.[38] CD8+ T cells expand first as part of the lymphopenia-induced proliferation. These cells are mostly those that survive conditioning and expand as cytotoxic cells. However, they may then undergo phenotypic switching and acquire an anergic or regulatory phenotype because they have been demonstrated to have weakened response on T cell receptor (TCR) activation with less cytokine release.[38] CD4+ T cells, however, are more often generated de novo from the thymus after AHSCT. Studies of CD4+ TCR clones show disappearance of pre-AHSCT dominant clones and replacement with new clonotypes in the blood and cerebrospinal fluid after AHSCT.[24]

Despite the turnover and cell changes, returning or residual T cells responsive to myelin epitopes have been identified even after high-intensity conditioning.[24] Moreover, as noted above, there are usually increasing levels of EBV following AHSCT. This observation is of interest with the accumulating evidence supporting EBV infection as a risk factor for the development of MS[40] and, early expanding T cells likely respond to EBV.[38] Yet, breakthrough inflammatory disease after AHSCT is uncommon. One possible explanation is that these possibly pathogenic T cells are part of the early T cell expansion and then undergo replicative senescence.[38]

### *Increased Immunoregulation*

There is an increase in regulatory immune cells in the immune reconstitution after AHSCT.[24] Immunoregulatory CD56hi natural killer cells are elevated at 3 and 12 months after AHSCT. Memory CD4+ T regulatory cells are significantly increased 6 months after AHSCT and return to baseline levels at 2 years. CD8+/CD57+ T cells, which have demonstrated an ability to suppress CD4+ T cell proliferation, are a greater proportion of the CD8+ T cell pool after AHSCT. Moreover, an increased presence of immunoregulatory receptors on immune cells has been associated with better clinical outcomes.[39] Higher expression levels of cytotoxic T-lymphocyte antigen 4 on CD4+ regulatory

T cells and programmed death 1 on both CD19+ B cells and CD8+/CD57+ T cells was associated with a long duration of relapse freedom after AHSCT.

***Decreased Inflammatory Environment***

The inflammatory environment also seems to be altered after AHSCT.[38] There is reduced function of proinflammatory TH17 and Th1/17 cells and decreased IL-17a levels following transplant. Moreover, the returned or persistence of myelin epitope autoreactive T cells have been demonstrated to elicit a reduced inflammatory response on stimulation assays following AHSCT. There are also changes in gene expression with the upregulation of genes associated with maintaining a tolerant cytokine environment and normalization of genes regulating intrinsic and extrinsic proapoptotic process.

## CURRENT STATUS AND TARGET POPULATION

Initially, AHSCT was pursued in people with progressive MS, severe disability, and lack of response to approved DMTs.[1] However, in a retrospective multicenter cohort of MS patients who had undergone AHSCT, it was found that neurological progression after transplant was associated with older age, progressive disease course, and previous use of more than 2 DMTs.[17] Moreover, a higher baseline level of disability was associated with worse survival. Recently, the American Society for Blood and Marrow Transplantation, International Advisory Committee on Clinical Trials in MS, National Multiple Sclerosis Society, and others proposed similar recommendations for appropriate candidates for AHSCT.[3–5] Based on these and other recent studies, characteristics of patients likely to benefit versus those likely to experience harm are summarized in **Box 1**.

## UNANSWERED QUESTIONS

Several questions remain surrounding ASHCT in MS including optimal protocol for the procedure, indications for use, and fit within the current treatment spectrum (**Box 2**).

**Box 1**
**Characteristics of current most appropriate patient for autologous hematopoietic stem cell transplantation**

Increased likelihood of benefit

- Younger age (eg, ≤50 y)
- Recent disease onset (eg, disease duration ≤15 y)
- Mild-to-moderate disability (ie, ambulatory with unilateral assistance or better)
- A relapsing form of MS with recent clinical or MRI lesion activity (ie, within the previous several years)
- Continued disease activity despite disease modifying therapy

Increased likelihood of harm

- Older age (≥60 y)
- Severe disability (ie, nonambulatory)
- Presence of medically significant comorbidities (including but not limited to chronic infection; cardiopulmonary, liver, kidney, hematologic disorders; poorly controlled diabetes, or malignancy)

Note: there are patients who do not fulfill these criteria for whom AHSCT might be considered.

*Data from* Refs.[2,3,5,46]

**Box 2**
**Key unanswered questions regarding autologous hematopoietic stem cell transplantation in multiple sclerosis**

Technical questions that affect benefit/risk profile
- What level of intensity of the conditioning regimen provides the optimal tradeoff between level and durability of efficacy versus safety and tolerability?
- Is there a way to personalize the choice of the conditioning regimen?
- Do the intensity or components of the conditioning regimen provide differential beneficial and deleterious effects on the varied pathophysiologic mechanisms of MS (eg, is central nervous system penetration advantageous, disadvantageous, or mixed)?
- Is CD34+ selection necessary?
- Is inclusion of ATG in the conditioning regimen necessary?

Patient selection to maximize the likelihood of benefit and minimize the risk of harm:
- What is the appropriate level of clinical activity (ie, number of relapses)?
- Is MRI lesion activity sufficient or is clinical activity required?
- How recent must the clinical or radiologic activity have been?
- Does the activity need to have been on DMT?
- How many prior DMTs need to have failed?
- What are the maximum age and level of disability?
- Are there other patients likely to benefit?
  - Early RRMS on high efficacy DMT with worsening disability but no activity (ie, does AHSCT treat PIRA?)
  - Treatment naïve RRMS considered at high risk?
  - Neuromyelitis optica spectrum disorders, myelin-oligodendrocyte antibody associated disease, autoimmune encephalitis, anti-GAD65 disease, and so forth?

Appropriate place in the sequence of treatment options
- Where to place AHSCT in the overall relapsing MS algorithm relative to high-efficacy DMTs?
- Is AHSCT an appropriate alternative for a sizable proportion of patients for whom a high-efficacy DMT is being considered?

*Abbreviations:* AHSCT, autologous hematopoietic stem cell transplantation, ATG, antithymocyte globulin, DMT, disease modifying therapy, MRI, magnetic resonance imaging, MS, multiple sclerosis, PIRA, progression independent of relapse activity, RRMS, relapsing-remitting MS.

### *Procedure*

Several elements of the AHSCT procedure remain areas of debate. First, there is no agreement on the optimal conditioning regimen.[41] Arguments for higher-intensity regimens include more consistent and durable efficacy with better suppression of MS disease activity but with higher risk of complications including possibly more TRM as noted above. Those in favor of lower intensity conditioning argue that disease activity can still be controlled with lower risks of complication.[22] However, the heterogeneity of studies to date in terms of patient enrollment, outcome measures, and conditioning agents used even within a given intensity level limit ability to effectively compare.[2] Beyond intensity level, the use of ATG has also been debated. The relative importance of its depletion of T cells versus the possible risks including allergic reactions, more delayed immune reconstitution, and increased risk of secondary autoimmunity is unclear. Moreover, there may be patient demographic and disease factors that determine which conditioning regimen is optimal.

The need for graft manipulation also is unresolved. In studies of AHSCT for MS both manipulated and unmanipulated grafts have been used, and manipulation strategies have varied.[4] A retrospective analysis from the EBMT group failed to demonstrate improved outcomes with graft manipulation and suggested possible increased risk of infection.[27] However, this study included less than 100 patients who had graft manipulation and reviewed data only up to the year 2000 when a substantial proportion of patients received high-intensity conditioning. Moreover, graft manipulation adds to the practical complexity of the protocol. EBMT now recommends that graft manipulation not be done except in clinical trial settings.[4] Finally, there are also variations in CD34+ cell dosing used and graft storage practices.[4]

### *Indication and Patient Selection*

The optimal indication for AHSCT is not yet fully determined. It seems sufficiently established that AHSCT is effective at reducing relapses and preventing new MRI lesions as discussed in the section on efficacy above. Yet in these studies, magnitude of clinical and/or radiographic disease activity varied as did the timing relative to transplant. Moreover, prior DMT use and definitions of DMT failure also varied. Finally, older age and higher levels of disability have been associated with an increased risk. The point at which potential harm outweighs potential benefit is yet to be established.

The impact of AHSCT in treating progression independent of relapse activity (PIRA) is less clear. NEDA status is more often lost after AHSCT due to continued disability progression as opposed to new relapse or inflammatory MRI.[1] Similarly the effectiveness of AHSCT at treating disability progression in SPMS and PPMS is unclear. In a retrospective analysis of patients with SPMS undergoing AHSCT, there was minimal impact on disability progression.[42] In a long-term follow-up of predominantly progressive patients with MS undergoing AHSCT, 5-year progression free survival was 46%.[17] However, treatments addressing progressive disease are presently limited and related ASHCT outcomes must be interpreted considering the current therapeutic landscape.

AHSCT also has appeal for pediatric onset MS as a potential one-time treatment option. Data from the EBMT registry on 21 pediatric onset MS patients undergoing AHSCT has been published with findings that progression free survival at 3 years was 100% with no TRM.[43] However, one patient required intensive care. Although these results are encouraging for AHSCT in pediatric onset MS, the numbers to date are small and data on long-term outcomes are lacking.

### *Role in the Spectrum of Multiple Sclerosis Treatment Options*

High efficacy for AHSCT in MS has been demonstrated in the studies detailed above. However, with the exception of a case series of 20 patients with aggressive MS and considered to be at high risk of disability,[44] AHSCT is not typically being used as first-line therapy to date. Thus, where to place AHSCT in the current spectrum of MS treatment options is uncertain.

When considering safety and tolerability, AHSCT has substantial upfront safety issues compared with DMTs, including need for multiple procedures, an inpatient hospital stay, risk of TRM, and others. Yet, much of this burden surrounds the early procedure period whereas burden and risk of treatment with approved DMTs is cumulative over time. As such, it remains to be seen where AHSCT fits into the safety and tolerability spectrum for patients, caregivers, and clinicians.

Finally, cost is an important consideration. AHSCT has high upfront costs but many patients have long-term stability without the need to restart DMT and, thus, avoid expensive drug costs. A study using the Polish National Health Fund database found that AHSCT became cost-efficient after 3.9 years.[45] Moreover, this study considered only direct medical costs. A more comprehensive look at cost considering lost wages for patients and caregivers, need for adaptive equipment, treatment-related travel expenses, and others may find that AHSCT reaches cost-effectiveness sooner.

## DISCUSSION

Ultimately, ongoing head-to-head comparison in randomized trials will provide the most robust assessment of the efficacy and safety of AHSCT (**Table 2**). BEAT-MS (NCT04047628) is a rater-masked phase 3 trial sponsored by the National Institute of Allergy and Infectious Diseases and conducted in collaboration with the Immune Tolerance Network in the United States and United Kingdom. The trial plans to enroll 156 participants with RR or SPMS and 2 episodes of disease activity in the prior 3 years, at least one occurring despite treatment with a moderate-efficacy or high-efficacy DMT. Eligible participants are randomized to AHSCT utilizing a BEAM-ATG conditioning regimen compared with best available therapy chosen from alemtuzumab, cladribine, natalizumab, ocrelizumab, ofatumumab, or rituximab by the treating neurologist. The primary endpoint is relapse-free survival at 3 years. Secondary outcomes include ARR, NEDA, confirmed EDSS worsening, confirmed EDSS improvement, brain volume change, serum neurofilament light chain, and safety. Exploratory outcomes include additional relapse analyses, disability measured by the MS Functional Composite, MRI lesion and regional volume analyses, patient reported quality of life, health economics, and blood and cerebrospinal fluid mechanistic studies. Results from BEAT-MS will be critical for the comparison of AHSCT to anti-CD20 monoclonal antibodies and other high efficacy DMTs but will not be expected until late 2026 or after.

Similar trials, although with some differences in the details of eligibility criteria, AHSCT regimen, duration of follow-up, and primary outcomes are underway in other countries. RAM-MS (NCT03477500) is a phase 3 trial conducted in Scandinavia that seeks to enroll 100 participants age 18 to 50 years with RRMS and EDSS 0 to 5.5. Participants are randomized to AHSCT with a cyclophosphamide + ATG conditioning regiment versus high-efficacy DMT (alemtuzumab, cladribine, or ocrelizumab). The primary endpoint is proportion with NEDA-3 at 2 years. StarMS (ISRCTN88667898) is a phase 3 trial conducted in the United Kingdom that seeks to enroll 198 participants age 16 to 55 years with RRMS and EDSS 0 to 6.0. Participants are randomized to AHSCT with a cyclophosphamide + ATG conditioning regiment versus high efficacy DMT (alemtuzumab, cladribine, ocrelizumab, or ofatumumab). The primary endpoint is proportion with NEDA-3 at 2 years. Results of RAMS-MS and StarMS are expected in 2026. The NET-MS phase 2 trial has also been in planning stages for a number of years in Italy and is expected to open enrollment later in 2023. The COAST (NCT04971005) phase 2 trial in Germany was terminated because of difficulty with start-up and enrollment due to the COVID-19 pandemic. It is anticipated that following the completion of these trials, results will provide more definitive information concerning the efficacy, safety, and cost effectiveness of AHSCT compared with currently relevant high-efficacy DMTs as an aggregate.

People with MS being considered for AHSCT should be referred to one of the ongoing trials. In situations where AHSCT is indicated but participation in a trial is not feasible, the procedure should be performed only in centers with experience and expertise not only with AHSCT but also with the diagnosis and management of MS. The transplant and neurology teams should work collaboratively to select candidates and coordinate care before, during, and after the procedure. Comprehensive safety and efficacy data should be collected and submitted to one of the existing registries, such as the Autoimmune Disease Working Party of the European Society for Blood and Marrow Transplant (EBMT) or the Autoimmune Diseases and Cellular Therapies Working Committee of the Center for International Blood and Marrow Transplant Research. When appropriate, the case results should be published. In this way, the role of ASHCT as MS therapy will be better defined.

**Table 2**
**Summary of ongoing randomized controlled trials of autologous hematopoietic stem cell transplantation in multiple sclerosis**

| Trial | Study Design | Sample Size | Age Range (y) | MS Type | EDSS | Conditioning Regimen | Comparator | Primary Outcome |
|---|---|---|---|---|---|---|---|---|
| BEAT-MS NCT04047628 | Phase 3 US, UK | 156 | 18–55 | RR, aSP | 0–6.0 | BEAM + ATG | Alem, Clad, NTZ, Ocr, Ofa, RTX | Relapse-free survival at 3y |
| COAST[a] NCT04971005 | Phase 2 Germany | 50 | 18–55 | RR | 0–6.0 | Cy + ATG | Alem, Ocr | Proportion with NEDA-3 at 2y |
| NET-MS[b] | Phase 2b Italy | 90 | 18–50 | RR, aSP | 2.0–6.0 | BEAM + ATG | Alem, Clad, NTZ, Ocr, Ofa | Proportion with NEDA-3 at 3y |
| RAM-MS NCT03477500 | Phase 3 Scandinavia | 100 | 18–50 | RR | 0–5.5 | Cy + ATG | Alem, Clad, Ocr, | Proportion with NEDA-3 at 2y |
| StarMS ISRCTN88667898 | Phase 3 UK | 198 | 16–55 | RR | 0–6.0 | Cy + ATG | Alem, Clad, Ocr, Ofa | Proportion with NEDA-3 at 2y |

*Abbreviations:* AHSCT, autologous hematopoietic stem cell transplantation; Alem, alemtuzumab; aSP, active secondary progressive; ATG, antithymocyte globulin; BEAM, carmustine/etoposide/cytarabine/melphalan; Clad, cladribine; Cy, cyclophosphamide; EDSS, expanded disability status scale; MS, multiple sclerosis; NTZ, natalizumab; Ocr, ocrelizumab; Ofa, ofatumumab; RR, relapsing-remitting; RTX, rituximab; UK, United Kingdom; US, United States.

[a] Terminated.

[b] Under development.

## CLINICS CARE POINTS

- Patient selection is key to increase the likelihood of benefit and lessen the risk of harm.
- Characteristics of people with MS who were more likely to benefit from AHSCT include younger age, relatively recent disease onset, mild-to-moderate disability, recent clinical relapse or MRI lesion activity, and continued disease activity despite disease therapy.
- Characteristics of people with MS less likely to experience harm from AHSCT include younger age, lack of severe disability, and absence of comorbidities that increase the risk of complications.
- AHSCT should be performed only in centers with experience and expertise not only with AHSCT but also with the diagnosis and management of MS, and the transplant and neurology teams should collaboratively select candidates and coordinate care.

## DISCLOSURE

Dr L.A. Ross reports grant funding from the National Multiple Sclerosis Society (Sylvia Lawry Physician Fellowship FP-1906–34,172). Dr L.M. Stropp reports grant funding from the National Multiple Sclerosis Society, United States (Clinical Care Physician Fellowship CF-2106–37,856). Dr J.A. Cohen reports personal compensation for consulting for Biogen, Convelo, EMD Serono, Gossamer Bio, Mylan, and PSI; and serving as an Editor of *Multiple Sclerosis Journal*.

## REFERENCES

1. Muraro PA, Martin R, Mancardi GL, et al. Autologous haematopoietic stem cell transplantation for treatment of multiple sclerosis. Nat Rev Neurol 2017;13:391–405.
2. Sormani MP, Muraro PA, Schiavetti I, et al. Autologous hematopoietic stem cell transplantation in multiple sclerosis: a meta-analysis. Neurology 2017;88:2115–22.
3. Cohen JA, Baldassari LE, Atkins HL, et al. Autologous hematopoietic cell transplantation for treatment-refractory relapsing multiple sclerosis: position statement from the American Society for Blood and Marrow Transplantation. Biol Blood Marrow Transplant 2019;25:845–54.
4. Sharrack B, Saccardi R, Alexander T, et al. Autologous haematopoietic stem cell transplantation and other cellular therapy in multiple sclerosis and immune-mediated neurological diseases: updated guidelines and recommendations from the EBMT Autoimmune Diseases Working Party (ADWP) and the Joint Accreditation Committee of EBMT and ISCT (JACIE). Bone Marrow Transplant 2020;55:283–306.
5. Miller AE, Chitnis T, Cohen BA, et al. Autologous hematopoietic stem cell transplant in multiple sclerosis: recommendations of the National Multiple Sclerosis Society. JAMA Neurol 2021;78:241–6.
6. Atkins H. Hematopoietic SCT for the treatment of multiple sclerosis. Bone Marrow Transplant 2010;45:1671–81.
7. Atkins HL, Bowman M, Allan D, et al. Immunoablation and autologous haematopoietic stem-cell transplanatation for aggressive multiple sclerosis: a multicentre single-group phase 2 trial. Lancet 2016;388:576–85.
8. Burt RK, Balabanov R, Han X, et al. Association of nonmyeloablative hematopoietic stem cell transplantation with neurologic disability in patients with relapsing-remitting multiple sclerosis. JAMA 2015;313:275–84.

9. Nash RA, Hutton GJ, Racke MK, et al. High-dose immunosuppressive therpay and autologous hematopoietic cell transplantation for relapsing-remitting multiple sclerosis (HALT-MS). A 3-year interim report. JAMA Neurol 2015;72:159–69.
10. Nash RA, Hutton GJ, Racke MK, et al. High-dose immunosuppressive therapy and autologus HCT for relapsing-remitting MS. Neurology 2017;88:842–52.
11. Ismail A, Sharrack B, Saccardi R, et al. Autologous haematopoietic stem cell therapy for multiple sclerosis: a review for supportive care clinicians on behalf of the Autoimmune Diseases Working Party of the European Society for Blood and Marrow Transplantation. Curr Opin Support Palliat Care 2019;13:394–401.
12. Burt RK, Loh Y, Cohen B, et al. Autologous non-myeloablative haemopoietic stem cell transplanatation in relapsing-remitting multiple sclerosis: a phase I/II study. Lancet Neurol 2009;8:244–53.
13. Shevchenko JL, Kuznetsov AN, Ionova TI, et al. Autologous hematopoietic stem cell transplantation with reduced-intensity conditioning in multiple sclerosis. Exp Hematol 2012;40:892–8.
14. Moore JJ, Massey JC, Ford CD, et al. Prospective phase II clinical trial of autologous haematopoietic stem cell transplant for treatment refractory multiple sclerosis. J Neurol Neurosurg Psychiatry 2019;90:514–21.
15. Mancardi GL, Sormani MP, Di Gioia M, et al. Autologous haematopoietic stem cell transplantation with an intermediate intensity conditioning regimen in multiple sclerosis: the Italian multi-centre experience. Mult Scler 2012;18:835–42.
16. Burman J, Iacobaeus E, Svenningsson A, et al. Autologous haematopoietic stem cell transplantation for aggressive multiple sclerosis: the Swedish experience. J Neurol Neurosurg Psychiatry 2014;85:1116–21.
17. Muraro PA, Pasquini M, Atkins HL, et al. Long-term outcomes after autologous hematopoietic stem cell transplantation for multiple sclerosis. JAMA Neurol 2017; 74:459–69.
18. Häußler V, Ufer F, Pöttgen J, et al. aHSCT is superior to alemtuzumab in maintaining NEDA and improving cognition in multiple sclerosis. Ann Clin Transl Neurol 2021;8:1269–78.
19. Sormani MP, Muraro PA, Saccardi R, et al. NEDA status in highly active MS can be more easily obtained with autologous hematopoietic stem cell transplantation than other drugs. Mult Scler J 2017;23:201–4.
20. Kalincik T, Sharmin S, Roos I, et al. Effectiveness of autologous haematopoietic stem cell transplantation versus fingolimod, natalizumab and ocrelizumab in highly active relapsing-remitting multiple sclerosis. JAMA Neurol.
21. Mancardi G, Sormani MP, Gualandi F, et al. Autologous hematopoietic stem cell transplantation in multiple sclerosis. A phase II trial. Neurology 2015;84:981–8.
22. Burt RK, Balabanov R, Burman J, et al. Effect of nonmyeloablative hematopoietic stem cell transplantation vs continued disease-modifying therapy on disease progression in patients with relapsing-remitting multiple sclerosis: a randomized clinical trial. JAMA 2019;321:165–74.
23. Nicholas RS, Rhone EE, Mariottini A, et al. Autologous hematopoietic stem cell transplantation in active multiple sclerosis: a real-world case series. Neurology 2021;97:e890–901.
24. Cencioni MT, Genchi A, Brittain G, et al. Immune reconstitution following autologous hematopoietic stem cell transplantation for multiple sclerosis: a review on behalf of the EBMT Autoimmune Diseases Working Party. Front Immunol 2022; 12:813957.

25. Ge F, Lin H, Li Z, et al. Efficacy and safety of autologous hematopoietic stem-cell transplantation in multiple sclerosis: a systematic review and meta-analysis. Neurol Sci 2019;40:479–87.
26. Bose G, Freedman MS. Recent advances and remaining questions of autologous hematopoietic stem cell transplantation in multiple sclerosis. J Neurol Sci 2021; 421:117324.
27. Saccardi R, Kozak T, Bocelli-Tyndall C, et al. Autologous stem cell transplantation for progressive multiple sclerosis: update of the European Group for Blood and Marrow Transplantation autoimmune diseases working party database. Mult Scler J 2006;12:814–23.
28. Mehra V, Rhone E, Widya S, et al. Epstein-Barr virus and monoclonal gammopathy of clinical significance in autologous stem cell transplantation for multiple sclerosis. Clin Infect Dis 2019;69:1757–63.
29. Ruder J, Dinner G, Maceski A, et al. Dynamics of inflammatory and neurodegenerative biomarkers after autologous hematopoietic stem cell transplantation in multiple sclerosis. Int J Mol Sci 2022;23:10946.
30. Snarski E, Snowden JA, Oliveira MC, et al. Onset and outcome of pregnancy after autologous haematopoietic SCT (AHSCT) for autoimmune diseases: a retrospective study of the EBMT autoimmune diseases working party (ADWP). Bone Marrow Transplant 2015;50:216–20.
31. Massarotti C, Sbragia E, Boffa G, et al. Menstrual cycle resumption and female fertility after autologous hematopoietic stem cell transplantation for multiple sclerosis. Mult Scler J 2021;27:2103–7.
32. Chatterton S, Withers B, Sutton IJ, et al. Pregnancy post autologous stem cell transplant with BEAM conditioning for multiple sclerosis. Mult Scler J 2021;27: 2112–5.
33. Burt RK, Fassas A, Snowden J, et al. Collection of hematopoietic stem cells from patients with autoimmune diseases. Bone Marrow Transplant 2001;28:1–12.
34. Thebault S, Lee H, Bose G, et al. Neurotoxicity after hematopoietic stem cell transplant in multiple sclerosis. Ann Clin Transl Neurol 2020;7:767–75.
35. Daikeler T, Labopin M, Di Gioia M, et al. Secondary autoimmune disease occurring after HSCT for an autoimmune disease: a retrospective study of the EBMT Autoimmune Disease Working Party. Blood 2011;118:1693–8.
36. DeFilipp Z, Duarte RF, Snowden JA, et al. Metabolic syndrome and cardiovascular disease following hematopoietic cell transplantation: screening and preventive practice recommendations from CIBMTR and EBMT. Bone Marrow Transplant 2017;52:173–82.
37. Majhail NS, Rizzo JD, Lee SJ, et al. Recommended screening and preventive practices for long-term survivors after hematopoietic cell transplantation. Biol Blood Marrow Transplant 2012;18:348–71.
38. Massey JC, Sutton IJ, Ma DDF, et al. Regenerating immunotolerance in multiple sclerosis with autologous hematopoietic stem cell transplant. Front Immunol 2018;9:410.
39. Arruda LCM, de Azevedo JTC, de Oliveira GLV, et al. Immunological correlates of favorable long-term clinical outcome in multiple sclerosis patients after autologous hematopoietic stem cell transplantation. Clin Immunol 2016;169:47–57.
40. Bjornevik K, Cortese M, Healy BC, et al. Longitudinal analysis reveals high prevalence of Epstein-Barr virus associated with multiple sclerosis. Science 2022; 375:296–301.

41. Willison A, Ruck T, Lenz G, et al. The current standing of autologous haemato-poietic stem cell transplantation for the treatment of multiple sclerosis. J Neurol 2022;269:3937–58.
42. Mariottini A, Filippini S, Innocenti C, et al. Impact of autologous haematopoietic stem cell transplantation on disability and brain atrophy in secondary progressive multiple sclerosis. Mult Scler J 2021;27:61–70.
43. Burman J, Kirgizov K, Carlson K, et al. Autologous hematopoietic stem cell trans-plantation for pediatric multiple sclerosis: a registry-based study of the Autoim-mune Diseases Working Party (ADWP) and Pediatric Diseases Working Party (PDWP) of the European Society for Blood and Marrow Transplantation (EBMT). Bone Marrow Transplant 2017;52:1133–7.
44. Das J, Snowden JA, Burman J, et al. Autologous haematopoietic stem cell trans-plantation as a first-line disease-modifying therapy in patients with 'aggressive' multiple sclerosis. Mult Scler J 2021;27:1198–204.
45. Orlewska K, Bogusz K, Podlecka-Piętowska A, et al. Impact of immunoablation and autologous hematopoietic stem cell transplantation on treatment cost of mul-tiple sclerosis: real-world nationwide study. Value Health Reg Issues 2021;25: 104–7.
46. Saccardi R, Freedman MS, Sormani MP, et al. A prospective, randomized, controlled, trial of autologous haematopoietic stem cell transplanatation for aggressive multiple sclerosis: a position paper. Mult Scler J 2012;18:825–34.

# Highly Effective Therapy Versus Escalation Approaches in Early Multiple Sclerosis

## What Is the Future of Multiple Sclerosis Treatment?

Nicole Bou Rjeily, MD[a], Ellen M. Mowry, MD, MCR[a,b], Daniel Ontaneda, MD, PhD[c], Alise K. Carlson, MD[c,*]

**KEYWORDS**

- Multiple sclerosis • Relapsing-remitting multiple sclerosis
- Disease-modifying therapy • Escalation therapy • Eary highly effective therapy

**KEY POINTS**

- There is no formal consensus on the optimal initial treatment approach to patients with newly diagnosed relapsing multiple sclerosis. Escalation and early highly effective therapy approaches are the 2 most widely recognized treatment paradigms.
- As experience and safety data with newer, highly effective therapies accumulates over time, neurologists are becoming more comfortable using these medications, managing the associated risks, and monitoring for adverse events.
- Initial disease-modifying treatment choice should be based on considerations for effectiveness, safety risks, cost, and patient preferences including administration and monitoring schedule and family planning.
- Two randomized clinical trials comparing escalation versus highly effective therapy in patients with newly diagnosed relapsing multiple sclerosis will provide valuable insights into the optimal treatment approach.

[a] Department of Neurology, Johns Hopkins University School of Medicine, 600 North Wolfe Street, Pathology 627, Baltimore, MD 21287, USA; [b] Department of Epidemiology, Johns Hopkins University School of Medicine, 600 North Wolfe Street, Pathology 627, Baltimore, MD 21287, USA; [c] Cleveland Clinic Mellen Center, 9500 Euclid Avenue U10, Cleveland, OH 44195, USA
* Corresponding author.
*E-mail address:* carlsoa4@ccf.org

Neurol Clin 42 (2024) 185–201
https://doi.org/10.1016/j.ncl.2023.06.004

neurologic.theclinics.com

## INTRODUCTION

Multiple sclerosis (MS) is a chronic disease of the central nervous system with a global prevalence of more than 2 million cases worldwide[1] and nearly one million cases in the US alone.[2] MS most commonly presents in young adults with an initial relapsing-remitting course (RRMS), characterized by focal immune-mediated, inflammatory, and demyelinating clinical or radiological disease activity interspersed with periods of relapse freedom. Up to 15% of individuals have gradual accrual of disability in the absence of relapses from the time of symptom onset (primary progressive MS (PPMS)),[3] and many individuals develop progression of disease-related disability following an initial relapsing-remitting course (secondary progressive MS (SPMS)) within 25 years of initial diagnosis.[4] Progressive MS is thought to be caused by neurodegeneration, and some evidence suggests it may start early in the disease course.

Over the past 2 decades, a diverse array of disease-modifying therapies (DMTs) has been developed and approved for the treatment of relapsing forms of MS. These therapies act on various targets involved in the inflammation of the central nervous system through unique mechanisms of action and have varying modes of delivery, efficacy, safety, and side-effect profiles (including associated adverse effects, toxicities, and pregnancy-related risks).

Currently, there are no formal consensus guidelines regarding a recommended initial treatment approach to people newly diagnosed with MS. The 2 most recognized therapeutic paradigms are an escalation (ESC) approach and an early highly effective treatment (EHT) approach. The ESC approach is characterized by the initiation of a lower- or moderate-efficacy DMT with a more favorable safety profile following diagnosis, with escalation to higher-efficacy therapy considered in the setting of breakthrough disease activity and/or medication intolerance. The EHT approach is characterized by the initiation of a higher-efficacy DMT, which may be associated with a less favorable safety profile (with regard to side effects or risk of serious adverse events), early in the course of the disease.[5] To date, evidence favoring either approach is based primarily on long-term follow-up of patient cohorts from phase 3 clinical trials and observational real-world data (often obtained through patient registries or collaborative efforts). As favorable long-term efficacy and safety data emerge on the more recently approved highly effective therapies, there has been mounting support for the EHT approach. However, concern about methodological limitations in these prior studies continues to make certainty in the benefits of this approach unclear. Herein we compare and summarize available evidence for these 2 treatments approaches and discuss ongoing research and future directions.

## DISEASE-MODIFYING THERAPY PROFILES

To develop a safe and effective treatment plan for an individual patient, an in-depth understanding of the risk-benefit profiles of each DMT is necessary. DMTs have historically been divided into efficacy categories based on their performance with regards to the reduction of clinical relapses, reduction of clinical and subclinical radiological activity, and sometimes prevention/slowing of disability progression. DMT efficacy figures are often derived from pivotal phase 3 clinical trial results, which typically compare the reduction of annualized relapse rates (ARR) either to placebo or a comparator DMT. Other secondary outcomes may also include measurements such as whole-brain atrophy and cognitive function. Composite clinical endpoints are intended to better capture the spectrum of disability, but questions remain particularly when DMTs are thought to have direct effects primarily on inflammatory outcomes rather than neurodegeneration. Comparing DMT efficacy across trials can also be challenging due to changes in the diagnostic criteria over time (eg, updated diagnostic criteria allowing for earlier diagnosis, such that people with "milder" MS become eligible), secular effects on ARR, and changes in the accuracy of outcome ascertainment over time. For purposes of this review, we arbitrarily consider the first-generation injectable therapies lower-efficacy, oral medications moderate-efficacy, and monoclonal antibodies higher-efficacy therapies, recognizing that many therapies could be considered to span two categories (**Fig. 1**).

### *First-Generation Injectable Therapies*

Interferon beta (IFN β) formulations (IFN β-1a, IFN β-1b, and PEGylated IFN β-1b) and glatiramer acetate (GA) are injectable immunomodulatory therapies approved for treatment of relapsing forms of MS. These medications are also referred to as first-generation or platform therapies and are considered lower-efficacy DMTs.

IFN β is a cytokine which suppresses T-cell activation by the downregulation of antigen-presenting cells, shifting of T-cell differentiation toward anti-inflammatory T2 helper cells (by inducing interleukin 10 production), and interfering with T-cell migration by blocking adhesion molecules and metalloproteases.[6] High-dose IFN β-1a reduced ARR by 32%, new gadolinium-enhancing (GdE) lesions by 67%, new T2 lesions by 78%, and disability progression by 29% (based on the Expanded Disability Status Scale (EDSS)) compared to placebo in a phase 3 clinical trial.[7] Similarly, IFN β-1b reduced ARR by 34%, GdE lesions by 83%, new T2 lesions by 75%, and disability progression by 29%,[8] and PEGylated IFN β-1b reduced ARR by 27%, GdE lesions by 86%, new T2 lesions by 67%, and disability progression by 38%.[9] Interferons are associated with common side effects including flu-like symptoms, headache, depression, and transaminitis. More serious complications including hepatic injury, congestive heart failure, and worsening of other autoimmune/rheumatologic conditions may occur but are rare.[10–13]

GA exerts its immunomodulatory effect by promoting an anti-inflammatory T-cell phenotype and reducing autoreactivity to myelin.[14] Compared to placebo, GA was shown to reduce ARR by 29% in a phase 3 clinical trial, but has not been shown to have a significant effect on disability progression.[15] GA is also well tolerated, with the most reported side effect being injection-site reactions. Other potential side-effects include lipoatrophy and skin necrosis at injection sites as well as vasodilatory reactions.[16,17] GA is also considered safe for use throughout pregnancy and the postpartum period.[16,17]

### *Oral Therapies*

Oral DMTs include teriflunomide, fumarates, sphingosine 1-phosphate receptor modulators (S1PRmodulators), and cladribine. Oral DMTs can be considered moderate efficacy medications, however based on ARR some differences can be noted, particularly for cladribine which some consider a high efficacy therapy and teriflunomide which some consider a lower efficacy DMT.

Teriflunomide acts via the inhibition of de novo pyrimidine synthesis. It selectively inhibits the dihydro-orotate dehydrogenase enzyme, which inhibits cell division and proliferation of activated T and B lymphocytes.[18] A phase 3 clinical trial of teriflunomide demonstrated a 32% reduction in ARR, 80% reduction in GdE lesions, 77% reduction in new T2 lesions, and 26% reduction in disability progression compared to placebo.[19] Common side effects include gastrointestinal upset (nausea) and hair thinning.[20] Teriflunomide is highly teratogenic (in both women and men). Other

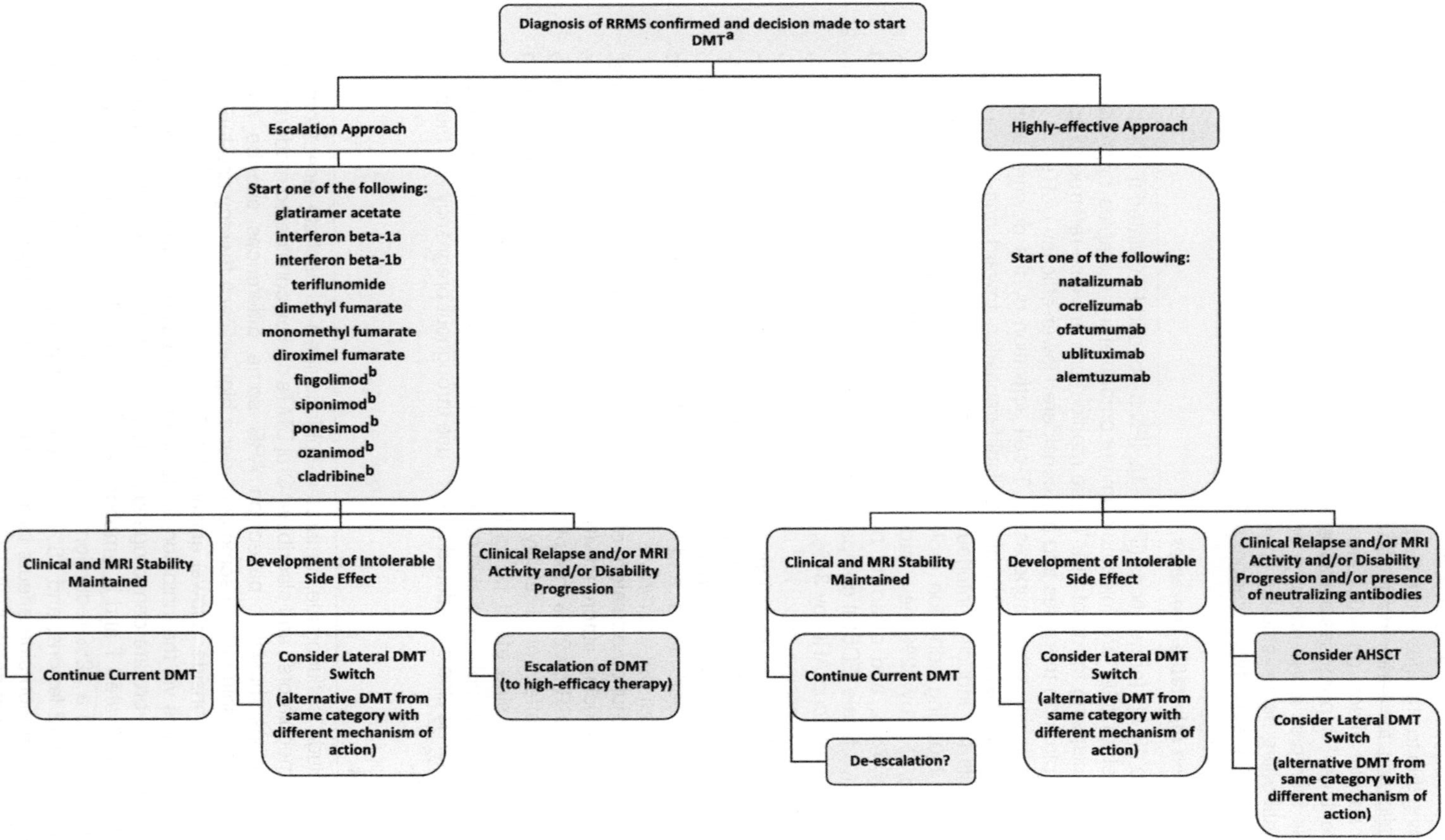


**Fig. 1.** Treatment approach to newly diagnosed relapsing-remitting multiple sclerosis. [a]Choice of therapy MUST consider DMT-specific risk-benefit profiles, preferred route/frequency of administration, cost and insurance coverage, family planning, disease burden and prognostic factors, and medical comorbidities; [b]Controversy among experts as to whether these medications belong in the escalation or early highly effective approach.

potentially serious side effects include hypertension, neuropathy, and reactivation of latent tuberculosis.[20]

The fumarates (dimethyl fumarate, diroximel fumarate, and monomethyl fumarate) are immunomodulating agents that are thought to act through the activation of nuclear factor-like 2.[21] Two phase 3 trials of dimethyl fumarate compared to placebo revealed a reduction of ARR by 44/53%, GdE lesions by 74/90%, new T2 lesions by 71/85%, and disability progression by 38%.[22,23] Common class effects of fumarate medications include flushing and gastrointestinal symptoms, the latter which tend to dissipate after 4 to 6 weeks of treatment. Lymphopenia, transaminitis, and increased risk of infection (including progressive multifocal leukoencephalopathy (PML)) may also occur.[24–26] Fumarates are not considered safe for use in pregnancy.[24–26]

The S1PRmodulators (fingolimod, siponimod, ozanimod, and ponesimod) cause lymphocyte sequestration in lymph nodes through the inhibition of the S1P gradient which leads to decreased lymphocytes in the blood and reduced migration of inflammatory cells into the central nervous system.[27] Compared to placebo, fingolimod reduces ARR by 54%, GdE lesions by 82%, new T2 lesions by 75%, and disability progression by 32%.[28] Siponimod was shown to have a 55% reduction in ARR, 82% reduction in GdE lesions, 80% reduction in new T2 lesions, and 80% reduction in disability progression compared to placebo.[29] Two phase 3 studies of ozanimod demonstrated a 48/38% reduction in ARR, 63/53% reduction in GdE lesions, 48/42% reduction in new T2 lesions, and 10.8/8.6% reduction (based on 3- and 6-month confirmed disability progression respectively) compared to IFN- β1a.[30,31] When compared to teriflunomide, ponesimod reduced ARR by 31%, MRI activity (combined and unique active lesions) by 56%, and disability progression by 17%.[32] Class effects of S1PRmodulators include lymphopenia, transaminitis, increased risk of infection (including the reactivation of varicella zoster virus (VZV) and PML), and headache. All S1PRmodulators have also been associated with cardiac arrhythmias (including heart block, symptomatic bradycardia), hypertension, macular edema, skin cancer, and worsening of reactive airway disease.[33–36] S1PRmodulators are not considered safe for use during pregnancy.[33–36]

Cladribine impairs DNA synthesis and leads to the preferential destruction of B and T cells.[37] In a phase 3 trial of cladribine (compared to placebo), ARR was reduced by 58%, GdE lesions by 86%, new T2 lesions by 73%, and disability progression by 47%.[37] Minor side effects include headache, fatigue, and increased risk of upper respiratory infections. Cladribine is also associated with several more serious potential side effects and adverse events including lymphopenia, liver and hematological toxicity, risk of serious infection (including VZV reactivation), graft-versus-host disease, and malignancy.[38] There is also a risk for teratogenicity, and therefore use is strictly avoided during pregnancy.[38]

### *High-efficacy Monoclonal Antibody Therapies*

Natalizumab is a monoclonal antibody, administered via once monthly infusion, which targets the alpha chain of the integrin VLA-4, effectively inhibiting the adhesion of lymphocytes to the endothelium of the blood–brain barrier and therefore blocking entry into the central nervous system.[39] Compared to placebo, natalizumab reduced ARR by 68%, GdE lesions by 92%, new T2 lesions by 83%, and disability progression by 42%.[40] Side effects include infusion reactions and systemic symptoms including fatigue, joint pain, and headaches. The primary concern with natalizumab is a strong association with PML, for which patients require close monitoring and testing for the presence of JC virus before and during treatment. Other rare but serious infections including respiratory, urinary tract, and herpes zoster infections, and liver failure may also occur.[41] Use of natalizumab during pregnancy is generally not advised, though may be considered in exceptional circumstances (ie, severe relapse during pregnancy) and should be used with caution during the third trimester.[42]

Ocrelizumab, ofatumumab, ublituximab, and rituximab are all anti-CD20 monoclonal antibodies which lead to B-cell depletion.[43–46] Ocrelizumab, rituximab, and ublituximab are all administered via infusion once every 6 months following treatment initiation, while ofatumumab is administered via subcutaneous injection once every month following initial loading doses. Phase 3 clinical trials of ocrelizumab versus IFN- β1a showed a 46/47% reduction in ARR, 94/95% reduction in GdE lesions, 77/83% reduction in new T2 lesions, and 40% reduction in disability progression (pooled result).[47] Ofatumumab was shown to be similarly efficacious, showing a 51/52% reduction in ARR, 97/94% reduction in GdE lesions, 82/85% reduction in new T2 lesions, and 34% reduction in disability progression (pooled) compared to teriflunomide.[48] Phase 3 clinical trials comparing ublituximab to teriflunomide showed a 58/50% reduction in ARR, 97/96% reduction in GdE lesions, and 92/90% reduction in new T2 lesions.[49]

In general, B-cell depleting therapies are considered to be similar with regard to efficacy and safety. Effects common to all these medications include infusion/injection-related reactions, reduction in immunoglobulins (which may be associated with severe or recurrent infections), and reactivation of hepatitis B virus.[43–46] There is also a concern for increased risk of malignancy, though some longer term data suggest that the risk of malignancy is not significantly different from that of the general population.[50,51] Although none of these medications are recommended to be continued throughout pregnancy, some have advocated they can be dosed 2 to 3 months prior to attempting to conceive.[42–46]

Alemtuzumab is an anti-CD52 monoclonal antibody that leads to the depletion of B- and T-cells.[52] In phase 3 clinical trials comparing alemtuzumab to IFN- β1a, ARR was reduced by 55/49%, GdE lesions by 63/62%, new T2 lesions by 17/32%, and disability progression by 27/42%.[53,54] Although effective in achieving the reduction of disease activity, alemtuzumab is associated with a multitude of adverse effects, many of which must be monitored for long after the course of treatment has been completed. These include, but are not limited to, novel autoimmune disease (thyroid disease, immune thrombocytopenic purpura, Goodpasture syndrome, hepatitis), increased infection risk (including PML, listeria meningitis, HSV, and VZV), hemophagocytic lymphohistiocytosis, stroke, and malignancy.[55] Alemtuzumab is not safe for use in pregnancy.[55]

## THE ESCALATION APPROACH

The ESC (or stepwise) approach to treatment initiation consists of starting a low- or moderate-efficacy DMT with a more favorable risk profile at disease outset. Patients are then monitored for evidence of disease activity, which may manifest as either clinical relapses or subclinical MRI activity. In the presence of new or ongoing disease activity, a different, most commonly higher-efficacy, therapy is considered. See **Fig. 1**. Because clinical trial outcomes represent averages of carefully selected subjects, patients in real-world scenarios (especially those who do not match the inclusion criteria used in the trials) may have either more or less favorable outcomes than the cohorts described in registration trials. Many patients do well on first-line or moderate-efficacy therapies and never require escalation to a higher-efficacy DMT to attain disease control. However, it is difficult to predict which patients might fall into this category, and which may experience suboptimal response early in the disease course.

A switch in therapy may also be considered in the event of treatment intolerance, where a higher-efficacy DMT may be selected as the next therapy choice.

For the escalation approach to be effective, the detection of non- or sub-optimal response to treatment is critical, as ongoing disease activity can set a course for sustained disability accumulation. Unfortunately, there are no clear guidelines regarding the approach and frequency of monitoring disease activity. Several composite outcome measures have been suggested to detect breakthrough disease activity warranting a change in treatment.[56–58] The Rio score and the modified Rio score are examples which were developed to assess response during the first year of treatment. Both scores include a combination of clinical and MRI criteria, which were developed in European cohorts and based on data from patients with RRMS treated with interferon β.[56,57] The concept of "no evidence of disease activity," or NEDA, with its several iterations also combines clinical relapses, MRI findings, and disability progression.[58] All of the aforementioned composite outcome measures have certain shortcomings that lead to challenges in their application and generalizability.[59] Moreover, it may be difficult to discriminate between a true clinical relapse and other possible etiologies in certain situations, leading to relapses being under-reported or under-documented. This is especially true for symptoms related to cognitive and sexual dysfunction.[60] As such, disease monitoring with outcome measures and biomarkers that are more sensitive for the detection of subclinical disease activity will be necessary to more effectively identify those not optimally responding to treatment.[61] Such tools may include the use of automated MRI measures, serum neurofilament light chain (sNfL) and optical coherence tomography.[62–64] One study suggested that sNfL can be used as a measure of disease activity and may be a useful tool to detect subclinical disease not otherwise detected by imaging or clinical evaluation,[63] though prior studies have shown mixed results, and further validation is needed. Although sNfL is associated with inflammatory disease activity, interpretation of sNfL levels is further complicated by its wide inter-subject variability and association with patient characteristics and comorbidities.[65]

The lack of a sensitive monitoring strategy to assess treatment response also contributes to difficulty in defining a threshold of disease activity that determines therapy failure. Moreover, monitoring with serial MRI is not widely integrated in clinical practice around the world, in which cases practitioners rely on clinical measures to identify evidence of ongoing disease activity. One risk associated with ESC is the potential delay in switching to a higher-efficacy therapy if the initial DMT fails. In one study this delay was found to be 2.4 (95% CI [2.1, 3.5]) years, associated with a time to sustained accumulation of disability which was much shorter in the ESC cohort (3.3 [1.8, 5.6] years) compared to the EHT cohort (6.0 [3.4, 8.2] years), although notably, a very small fraction of the people in the ESC cohort switched, leaving open the possibility that the non-switchers with incomplete treatment response drove this difference in disability.[66] The goal of treatment is to prevent the accumulation of new inflammatory disease activity, with the hope that this will decrease the risk of progressive neurologic decline and disability. Without a sufficiently sensitive monitoring strategy, ESC may be associated with undetected/subclinical disease activity. One argument against this proposed risk is that having a low threshold for the escalation of treatment at the earliest sign of disease activity would prevent such disability accrual. In other words, it is unclear whether the failure of an initial moderate-efficacy DMT due to subclinical disease activity would significantly alter the course of disability progression or redefine the disease course that was set in motion before treatment was initiated. Therapeutic inertia, a term used to describe when treatment is not escalated despite the presence of breakthrough disease activity, is also a concern as it could lead to failure of a prompt and successful escalation of therapy. This is a common phenomenon which has been observed in MS cohorts around the world and should be considered when selecting an initial therapy.[67–69]

Another challenge with ESC is the choice of the next DMT once the decision to change treatment has been made. Switching to either a higher-efficacy DMT or another moderate-efficacy DMT with a different mechanism of action (a so-called "lateral switch") are 2 plausible options. One study comparing both strategies showed that there was no difference in time to the first clinical relapse after switching, and that the proportion of patients who reached NEDA-3 after 24 months was similar.[70] Another study, however, showed that escalation to a higher-efficacy DMT delayed risk and time to clinical relapse compared to lateral switching.[71] A discussion weighing the risks and benefits of both strategies with the individual patient, addressing goals of treatment, risk profile, and patient preference regarding administration schedule and safety monitoring are often helpful in the shared decision making process.

## THE EARLY HIGHLY EFFECTIVE TREATMENT APPROACH

The EHT approach consists of initiating a higher-efficacy DMT promptly after the diagnosis of MS has been made. See **Fig. 1**. With the availability of several higher-efficacy DMTs (with variable mechanisms of action and side effects profiles), many neurologists are starting to favor this approach. Because most inflammatory activity occurs early in the disease course (and tends to decrease with age), proponents of this approach argue that the optimal time for the use of these medications is at the onset of treatment, leading to greater control of disease activity when inflammatory mechanisms are most prominent (and subsequently reducing long-term risk of disability accumulation).

One meta-analysis demonstrated that higher-efficacy DMTs were more effective compared to moderate-efficacy therapies in controlling disease activity in patients younger than 40.5 years of age, though the same effect was not demonstrated in older individuals.[72] Immuno-senescence associated with aging not only makes highly effective DMTs less necessary, but may also increase the risk of adverse events associated with treament.[73] Therefore, higher-efficacy DMTs may have a more favorable risk-benefit ratio earlier in the disease course.[73]

The primary concern for use of higher-efficacy DMTs is related to the less favorable safety profiles associated with those medications in comparison to lower- or moderate-efficacy DMTs. The adverse events most often associated with these medications include increased risk of serious infections and malignancy (as described above).

One proposed challenge associated with the EHT approach is the decision regarding the de-escalation of treatment. Given inflammatory disease activity decreases and the associated risks of higher-efficacy therapies increase with age, de-escalation of therapy is often considered once patients reach the seventh or eighth decade.[74,75] De-escalation may be accomplished in several ways including the discontinuation of treatment all together, switching to a moderate-efficacy DMT, using an extended interval dosing schedule, or implementing a reduced dosing regimen. Future development of more accurate biomarkers of disease activity may be useful in informing such decisions.[76] Regardless of when de-escalation is considered, there remains some degree of risk for return of disease activity once the highly effective therapy is withdrawn. The Discontinuation of DMTs in MS (DISCOMS; NCT03073603) trial and its extension study (NCT04754542) are evaluating the risk of developing new inflammatory disease activity with DMT discontinuation. Moreover, some DMTs (particularly natalizumab and fingolimod) may be associated with an increased risk of rebound disease activity, which may further complicate this process.[77,78]

## COMPARING ESCALATION AND EARLY HIGHLY EFFECTIVE TREATMENT

Although data from clinical trials demonstrate superior results for high-efficacy DMTs compared to lower- and moderate-efficacy DMTs, care must be taken when extrapolating these findings to clinical practice. As discussed previously, comparing the efficacy of DMTs across trials is challenging. Such trials also did not require a prompt escalation approach when breakthrough disease is detected, and thus did not address the clinical question about whether ESC or EHT is more effective.

Most observational studies that have attempted to compare ESC and EHT treatment strategies have favored the initial use of higher-efficacy DMTs due to the association with more favorable outcomes related to disease control (including decreased risk of relapses, slowing time to confirmed disability progression, or conversion to SPMS).[66,79–81] Other studies have shown that use of higher-efficacy DMTs immediately following disease onset is associated with lower risk of disability progression over time.[79,82] As data mount, more physicians are favoring EHT, especially in patients with poor prognostic features at the time of onset,[83] though many argue that higher-efficacy DMT should be initiated early irrespective of prognostic features.[73] However, these small observational studies must be interpreted with caution. Because these studies lack control over treatment allocation, confounding by indication cannot be eliminated. Moreover, some of these studies compare cohorts from different epochs, when different diagnostic criteria for MS were employed and different DMTs were clinically available, while others compared cohorts from different countries with different demographic profiles. The absence of a unified and rigorous monitoring approach to identify breakthrough disease activity, the prolonged time for second-line/escalation therapies to be initiated, and the lack of availability of certain therapies at the time that some of these studies were conducted may have resulted in suboptimal execution of escalation. Reporting bias, especially in EHT groups where disease activity may have been overlooked or under-reported due to a lack of available alternative treatment options with better efficacy, may have also led to the EHT approach appearing more effective. Randomized clinical trials are needed to better address the shortcomings seen in these studies.

### *Current Evidence*

When comparing treatment paradigms of EHT and ESC, there is currently little evidence to suggest that one approach is superior to the other with regards to long-term outcomes from well powered randomized controlled trials. As previously discussed, several studies have demonstrated the benefits of initiating higher-efficacy DMTs at the time of disease onset,[66,79–82] but these studies have consisted of mostly observational studies with limitations due to small sample sizes and confounding by indication. More importantly, the lack of standardized MRI outcomes and long-term follow-up of patients limit the conclusions that may be drawn about disease outcomes and rates of adverse events in real-world populations.

One widely accepted standard in the treatment of MS is the importance of starting treatment early, no matter which approach is selected. Natural history studies have shown how up to 50% to 60% of patients who initially have a relapsing-remitting course eventually progress to a secondarily progressive form with the accumulation of disability.[84,85] With the introduction of DMTs and several revisions of the MS diagnostic criteria which have allowed for earlier diagnosis and treatment initiation, the natural course of MS has been altered, with a much smaller proportion of patients with RRMS progressing to SPMS.[86] The American Academy of Neurology and the European Committee for Treatment and Research in Multiple Sclerosis both support early treatment after diagnosis to improve long-term disease outcomes.[87,88]

### Considerations

An important aspect of patient care is the inclusion of patients in the decision-making process for DMT selection. In addition to non-modifiable patient characteristics, non-neurological comorbidities, and exposures which may preclude use of certain DMTs, patients often also have their own treatment goals, preferred mode of delivery and monitoring schedule, safety concerns, and pregnancy plans.[59] Cost, which may be influenced by type or lack of insurance coverage, is also a potential contributing factor affecting DMT choice. Lastly, in some regions of the world, certain DMTs are not available, or insurance coverage of higher-efficacy medications may only be obtained following failure of one or more first-line therapies.[59] All of these factors must be considered when developing an individualized treatment plan once a diagnosis of MS has been made. See **Table 1**.

**Table 1**
**Comparison of treatment approaches for newly diagnosed relapsing-remitting multiple sclerosis**

| | Escalation Approach | Early Highly Effective Approach |
|---|---|---|
| Benefits | • More favorable safety profile<br>• Fewer concerns with long-term use<br>• Often more affordable/covered by most insurance plans<br>• May be required as initial therapy in certain countries | • Lower risk of breakthrough disease (clinical relapses and subclinical MRI activity)<br>• Lower risk of medication intolerance<br>• Lower risk of patient non-compliance |
| Risks | • Increased risk of breakthrough disease (clinical relapses and subclinical MRI activity) in some patients<br>• Increased risk of patient non-compliance due to more complex/frequent administration schedules | • Less favorable safety profile (higher risk of adverse events including infections and malignancy) |
| Challenges | • Detection of subclinical disease activity is challenging<br>• No defined threshold of disease activity that would warrant treatment escalation<br>• No definitive methods to predict which patients may have suboptimal response to low- or moderate-efficacy therapies<br>• Risk of rebound disease activity with the discontinuation of select therapies (eg, fingolimod) | • May be cost prohibitive/may not be covered by all insurance plans<br>• Risk of rebound disease activity with the discontinuation of select therapies (eg, natalizumab)<br>• No clear guidelines on best time to de-escalate treatment |
| Common goals | • Prompt treatment initiation<br>• Maximization of treatment adherence<br>• Patient engagement in shared decision making | |

Participation of patients in their care, along with a clear understanding of their disease and the risks and benefits associated with different treatment options, has been shown to improve satisfaction with the care provided as well as adherence to their treatment regimen.[89] Irrespective of DMT, poor adherence increases the risk of uncontrolled disease activity and subsequent clinical deterioration.[90] Therefore, interventions to improve compliance with DMT are essential to decrease the burden of MS-related disability.[90]

Some physicians rely on prognostic factors to guide their decision regarding treatment approach. However, predicting disease course is not an easy task due to the lack of well-characterized prognostic biomarkers. Efforts have been made to estimate MS prognosis and disability progression from disease onset. Some markers associated with aggressive MS include male sex, older age at onset, frequent relapses at onset, short inter-relapse interval, high T2 lesion burden, early discernible atrophy, and infratentorial lesions.[91] These prognostic factors were deduced from observational studies with limitations, specifically pertaining to generalizability. A study using prospective data from a large clinical cohort found that younger age, higher EDSS at baseline, more relapses in the previous year, and presence of GdE lesions at baseline were all associated with increased risk of relapse and new MRI lesions.[92] Nonetheless, further work is needed to better define and more effectively implement the use of these prognostic markers in clinical practice.

## FUTURE DIRECTIONS

Efforts to increase understanding of MS pathophysiology and develop mechanism-directed therapies are ongoing. New DMTs targeting novel pathologic mechanisms are expected to be developed in the coming years. Additionally, greater experience with therapies newer to the field, including autologous hematopoietic stem cell transplant (AHSCT), may further change the scope of treatment considered for patients with newly diagnosed MS. The question of how early to start treatment, including in patients with radiologically isolated syndrome before a formal diagnosis of MS is made, is also being investigated.[93,94]

Two pragmatic clinical trials which aim to directly compare the effectiveness of ESC and EHT approaches are currently being conducted. These studies, named TRaditional versus Early Aggressive Therapy for Multiple Sclerosis (TREAT-MS; NCT03500328) and Determining the Effectiveness of earLy Intensive versus Escalation approaches for the Treatment of Relapsing-remitting Multiple Sclerosis (DELIVER-MS; NCT03535298), are enrolling newly diagnosed patients with RRMS and randomizing to either ESC or EHT. The primary endpoint of TREAT-MS is time to sustained disability progression using EDSS-plus, while the primary endpoint of DELIVER-MS is whole brain volume loss at 36 months.[95] These randomized controlled studies will provide high-quality evidence and valuable insights as to which might be the optimal treatment approach.

## SUMMARY

Although the body of evidence has grown in recent years, the optimal approach to the treatment of those newly diagnosed with MS is unclear. Many DMTs with variable efficacy and safety profiles are now available, facilitating individualized decisions based upon efficacy, risk, cost, and personal preferences such as administration schedule and family planning. Although higher-efficacy therapies are associated with an increased risk of adverse events compared to lower- and moderate-efficacy therapies, the risk profiles of these medications are now better understood and more manageable with risk stratification tools developed in recent years. Results of pivotal pragmatic clinical trials will provide valuable insights regarding the optimal approach to the management of this population.

## CLINICS CARE POINTS

- Early treatment initiation after diagnosis, irrespective of DMT choice and treatment strategy, is important to improve long-term disease outcomes in patients with MS.
- Shared decision-making and patient satisfaction with the plan of care are important aspects of management that improve adherence to treatment and disease control.
- Caution must be exercised when interpreting results from observational studies due to inherent limitations in design that may lead to confounding by indication and other biases which may hinder generalizability.

## DISCLOSURE

N. Bou Rjeily has no disclosures. E.M. Mowry discloses research for Biogen, Genentech, and Teva, consulting for Be Care Link, LLC, and royalties for editorial duties for UpToDate. D. Ontaneda has received funding from the National Institutes of Health, National Multiple Sclerosis Society, Patient Centered Outcomes Research Institute, Race to Erase MS Foundation, Genentech, Genzyme, and Novartis. Consulting fees from Biogen Idec, Bristol Myers Squibb, Genentech/Roche, Genzyme, Janssen, Novartis, and Merck. A.K. Carlson has received fellowship funding (Grant 16696-P-FEL) from Biogen and institutional clinical training award (ICT-1805-31154) from National MS Society and has served as a consultant for Vigil Neuro.

## REFERENCES

1. Wallin MT, Culpepper WJ, Nichols E, et al. Global, regional, and national burden of multiple sclerosis 1990–2016: a systematic analysis for the Global Burden of Disease Study 2016. Lancet Neurol 2019;18(3):269–85.
2. Wallin MT, Culpepper WJ, Campbell JD, et al. The prevalence of MS in the United States. Neurology 2019;92(10):e1029–40.
3. Confavreux C, Vukusic S. Natural history of multiple sclerosis: a unifying concept. Brain 2006;129(3):606–16.
4. Rovaris M, Confavreux C, Furlan R, et al. Secondary progressive multiple sclerosis: current knowledge and future challenges. Lancet Neurol 2006;5(4):343–54.
5. Amin M, Hersh CM. Updates and advances in multiple sclerosis neurotherapeutics. Neurodegener Dis Manag 2023;13(1):47–70.
6. Jakimovski D, Kolb C, Ramanathan M, et al. Interferon β for Multiple Sclerosis. Cold Spring Harb Perspect Med 2018;8(11):a032003.
7. Ebers GC, Rice G, Lesaux J, et al. Randomised double-blind placebo-controlled study of interferon β-1a in relapsing/remitting multiple sclerosis. Lancet 1998; 352(9139):1498–504.
8. Duquette P, Girard M, Despault L, et al. Interferon beta-1b is effective in relapsing-remitting multiple sclerosis. I. Clinical results of a multicenter, randomized, double-blind, placebo-controlled trial. The IFNB Multiple Sclerosis Study Group. Neurology 1993;43(4):655–61.

9. Calabresi PA, Kieseier BC, Arnold DL, et al. Pegylated interferon β-1a for relapsing-remitting multiple sclerosis (ADVANCE): a randomised, phase 3, double-blind study. Lancet Neurol 2014;13(7):657–65.
10. Avonex (interferon beta-1a) [package insert]. Cambridge, MA: Biogen; 2021.
11. Rebif (interferon beta-1a) [package insert]. Rockland, MA: EMD Serono; 2014.
12. Betaseron (interferon beta-1b) [package insert]. Whippany, NJ: Bayer HealthCare Pharmaceuticals; 2021.
13. Plegridy (peginterferon beta-1a) [package insert]. Cambridge, MA: Biogen; 2014.
14. Yang JH, Rempe T, Whitmire N, et al. Therapeutic Advances in Multiple Sclerosis. Front Neurol 2022;13:824926.
15. Johnson KP, Brooks BR, Cohen JA, et al. Copolymer 1 reduces relapse rate and improves disability in relapsing-remitting multiple sclerosis: results of a phase III multicenter, double-blind placebo-controlled trial. The Copolymer 1 Multiple Sclerosis Study Group. Neurology 1995;45(7):1268–76.
16. Copaxone (glatiramer acetate) [package insert]. Parsippany, NJ: Teva Pharmaceuticals Industries; 2023.
17. Glatopa (glatiramer acetate) [package insert]. Princeton, NJ: Novartis Pharmaceuticals; 2018.
18. Bar-Or A, Pachner A, Menguy-Vacheron F, et al. Teriflunomide and its mechanism of action in multiple sclerosis. Drugs 2014;74(6):659–74.
19. O'Connor P, Wolinsky JS, Confavreux C, et al. Randomized trial of oral teriflunomide for relapsing multiple sclerosis. N Engl J Med 2011;365(14):1293–303.
20. Aubagio (teriflunomide) [package insert]. Cambridge, MA: Genzyme Corporation; 2021.
21. Faissner S, Gold R. Oral Therapies for Multiple Sclerosis. Cold Spring Harb Perspect Med 2019;9(1):a032011.
22. Gold R, Kappos L, Arnold DL, et al. Placebo-controlled phase 3 study of oral BG-12 for relapsing multiple sclerosis. N Engl J Med 2012;367(12):1098–107.
23. Fox RJ, Miller DH, Phillips JT, et al. Placebo-controlled phase 3 study of oral BG-12 or glatiramer in multiple sclerosis. N Engl J Med 2012;367(12):1087–97.
24. Tecfidera (dimethyl fumarate) [package insert]. Cambridge, MA: Biogen; 2019.
25. Bafiertam (monomethyl fumarate) [package insert]. High Point, NC: Banner Life Sciences; 2021.
26. Vumerity (diroximel fumarate) [package insert]. Cambridge, MA: Biogen; 2020.
27. McGinley MP, Cohen JA. Sphingosine 1-phosphate receptor modulators in multiple sclerosis and other conditions. Lancet 2021;398(10306):1184–94.
28. Kappos L, Radue E-W, O'Connor P, et al. A placebo-controlled trial of oral fingolimod in relapsing multiple sclerosis. N Engl J Med 2010;362(5):387–401.
29. Kappos L, Bar-Or A, Cree BAC, et al. Siponimod versus placebo in secondary progressive multiple sclerosis (EXPAND): a double-blind, randomised, phase 3 study. Lancet 2018;391(10127):1263–73.
30. Comi G, Kappos L, Selmaj KW, et al. Safety and efficacy of ozanimod versus interferon beta-1a in relapsing multiple sclerosis (SUNBEAM): a multicentre, randomised, minimum 12-month, phase 3 trial. Lancet Neurol 2019;18(11):1009–20.
31. Cohen JA, Comi G, Selmaj KW, et al. Safety and efficacy of ozanimod versus interferon beta-1a in relapsing multiple sclerosis (RADIANCE): a multicentre, randomised, 24-month, phase 3 trial. Lancet Neurol 2019;18(11):1021–33.
32. Kappos L, Fox RJ, Burcklen M, et al. Ponesimod compared with teriflunomide in patients with relapsing multiple sclerosis in the active-comparator phase 3 OPTIMUM study: a randomized clinical trial. JAMA Neurol 2021;78(5):558–67.

33. Gilenya (fingolimod) [package insert]. East Hanover, NJ: Novartis Pharmaceuticals Corporation; 2022.
34. Mayzent (siponimod) [package insert]. East Hanover, NJ: Novartis Pharmaceuticals Corporation; 2023.
35. Zeposia (ozanimod) [package insert]. Princeton, NJ: Bristol Meyers Squibb; 2022.
36. Ponvory (ponesimod) [package insert]. Titusville, NJ: Janssen Pharmaceuticals; 2022.
37. Giovannoni G, Comi G, Cook S, et al. A placebo-controlled trial of oral cladribine for relapsing multiple sclerosis. N Engl J Med 2010;362(5):416–26.
38. Chen E. Mavenclad. www.fda.gov/medwatch. Accessed April 30, 2023.
39. Khoy K, Mariotte D, Defer G, et al. Natalizumab in Multiple Sclerosis Treatment: From Biological Effects to Immune Monitoring. Front Immunol 2020;11:549842.
40. Polman CH, O'Connor PW, Havrdova E, et al. A randomized, placebo-controlled trial of natalizumab for relapsing multiple sclerosis. N Engl J Med 2006;354(9): 899–910.
41. Tysabri (natalizumab) [package insert]. Cambridge, MA: Biogen; 2023.
42. Carlson AK, Ontaneda D, Rensel MR, et al. Reproductive issues and multiple sclerosis: 20 questions. Cleve Clin J Med 2023;90(4):235–43.
43. Ocrevus (ocrelizumab) [package insert]. South San Francisco, CA: Genentech; 2022.
44. Ruxience (rituximab-pvrr) [package insert]. Ireland: Pfizer Ireland Pharmaceuticals Cork; 2021.
45. Briumvi (ublituximab-xiiy) [package insert]. Morrisville, NC: TG Therapeutics; 2022.
46. Kesimpta (ofatumumab) [package insert]. East Hanover, NJ: Novartis Pharmaceuticals Corporation; 2022.
47. Hauser SL, Bar-Or A, Comi G, et al. Ocrelizumab versus Interferon Beta-1a in Relapsing Multiple Sclerosis. N Engl J Med 2017;376(3):221–34.
48. Hauser SL, Bar-Or A, Cohen JA, et al. Ofatumumab versus Teriflunomide in Multiple Sclerosis. N Engl J Med 2020;383(6):546–57.
49. Steinman L, Fox E, Hartung H-P, et al. Ublituximab versus Teriflunomide in Relapsing Multiple Sclerosis. N Engl J Med 2022;387(8):704–14.
50. Hauser SL, Kappos L, Montalban X, et al. Safety of Ocrelizumab in Patients With Relapsing and Primary Progressive Multiple Sclerosis. Neurology 2021;97(16): e1546–59.
51. Fleury I, Chevret S, Pfreundschuh M, et al. Rituximab and risk of second primary malignancies in patients with non-Hodgkin lymphoma: A systematic review and meta-analysis. Ann Oncol 2016;27(3):390–7.
52. Ruck T, Bittner S, Wiendl H, et al. Alemtuzumab in Multiple Sclerosis: Mechanism of Action and Beyond. Int J Mol Sci 2015;16(7):16414–39.
53. Cohen JA, Coles AJ, Arnold DL, et al. Alemtuzumab versus interferon beta 1a as first-line treatment for patients with relapsing-remitting multiple sclerosis: a randomised controlled phase 3 trial. Lancet 2012;380(9856):1819–28.
54. Coles AJ, Twyman CL, Arnold DL, et al. Alemtuzumab for patients with relapsing multiple sclerosis after disease-modifying therapy: a randomised controlled phase 3 trial. Lancet 2012;380(9856):1829–39.
55. Lemtrada (alemtuzumab) [package insert]. Cambridge, MA: Genzyme Corporation; 2022.
56. Río J, Castilló J, Rovira A, et al. Measures in the first year of therapy predict the response to interferon β in MS. Mult Scler 2009;15(7):848–53.

57. Sormani MP, Rio J, Tintorè M, et al. Scoring treatment response in patients with relapsing multiple sclerosis. Mult Scler 2013;19(5):605–12.
58. Rotstein D, Solomon JM, Sormani MP, et al. Association of NEDA-4 With No Long-term Disability Progression in Multiple Sclerosis and Comparison With NEDA-3. Neurol - Neuroimmunol Neuroinflammation 2022;9(6). https://doi.org/10.1212/NXI.0000000000200032.
59. Rotstein D, Montalban X. Reaching an evidence-based prognosis for personalized treatment of multiple sclerosis. Nat Rev Neurol 2019;15(5):287–300.
60. Tallantyre EC, Causon EG, Harding KE, et al. The aetiology of acute neurological decline in multiple sclerosis: Experience from an open-access clinic. Mult Scler J 2015;21(1):67–75.
61. Ontaneda D, Tallantyre E, Kalincik T, et al. Early highly effective versus escalation treatment approaches in relapsing multiple sclerosis. Lancet Neurol 2019;18(10): 973–80.
62. Wattjes MP, Ciccarelli O, Reich DS, et al. 2021 MAGNIMS–CMSC–NAIMS consensus recommendations on the use of MRI in patients with multiple sclerosis. Lancet Neurol 2021;20(8):653–70.
63. Benkert P, Meier S, Schaedelin S, et al. Serum neurofilament light chain for individual prognostication of disease activity in people with multiple sclerosis: a retrospective modelling and validation study. Lancet Neurol 2022;21(3):246–57.
64. Lambe J, Saidha S, Bermel RA. Optical coherence tomography and multiple sclerosis: Update on clinical application and role in clinical trials. Mult Scler J 2020;26(6):624–39.
65. Sotirchos ES, Fitzgerald KC, Singh CM, et al. Associations of sNfL with clinico-radiological measures in a large MS population. Ann Clin Transl Neurol 2023; 10(1):84–97.
66. Harding K, Williams O, Willis M, et al. Clinical Outcomes of Escalation vs Early Intensive Disease-Modifying Therapy in Patients With Multiple Sclerosis. JAMA Neurol 2019;76(5):536–41.
67. Saposnik G, Montalban X, Selchen D, et al. Therapeutic inertia in multiple sclerosis care: A study of canadian neurologists. Front Neurol 2018;9:781.
68. Almusalam N, Oh J, Terzaghi M, et al. Comparison of Physician Therapeutic Inertia for Management of Patients With Multiple Sclerosis in Canada, Argentina, Chile, and Spain. JAMA Netw Open 2019;2(7). https://doi.org/10.1001/JAMANETWORKOPEN.2019.7093.
69. Rodrigues R, Rocha R, Bonifácio G, et al. Therapeutic inertia in relapsing-remitting multiple sclerosis. Mult Scler Relat Disord 2021;55:103176.
70. D'Amico E, Leone C, Zanghì A, et al. Lateral and escalation therapy in relapsing-remitting multiple sclerosis: a comparative study. J Neurol 2016;263(9):1802–9.
71. Chalmer TA, Kalincik T, Laursen B, et al. Treatment escalation leads to fewer relapses compared with switching to another moderately effective therapy. J Neurol 2019;266(2):306–15.
72. Weideman AM, Tapia-Maltos MA, Johnson K, et al. Meta-analysis of the Age-Dependent Efficacy of Multiple Sclerosis Treatments. Front Neurol 2017;8:577.
73. Filippi M, Amato MP, Centonze D, et al. Early use of high-efficacy disease-modifying therapies makes the difference in people with multiple sclerosis: an expert opinion. J Neurol 2022;269(10):5382.
74. Hua LH, Fan TH, Conway D, et al. Discontinuation of disease-modifying therapy in patients with multiple sclerosis over age 60. Mult Scler J 2019;25(5):699–708.
75. Birnbaum G. Stopping Disease-Modifying Therapy in Nonrelapsing Multiple Sclerosis Experience from a Clinical Practice. Int J MS Care 2017;19(1):11–4.

76. Vollmer BL, Wolf AB, Sillau S, et al. Evolution of Disease Modifying Therapy Benefits and Risks: An Argument for De-escalation as a Treatment Paradigm for Patients With Multiple Sclerosis. Front Neurol 2022;12:2646.
77. Vidal-Jordana A, Tintoré M, Tur C, et al. Significant clinical worsening after natalizumab withdrawal: Predictive factors. Mult Scler 2015;21(6):780–5.
78. Barry B, Erwin AA, Stevens J, et al. Fingolimod Rebound: A Review of the Clinical Experience and Management Considerations. Neurol Ther 2019;8(2):241.
79. Brown JWL, Coles A, Horakova D, et al. Association of Initial Disease-Modifying Therapy with Later Conversion to Secondary Progressive Multiple Sclerosis. JAMA 2019;321(2):175–87.
80. Buron MD, Chalmer TA, Sellebjerg F, et al. Initial high-efficacy disease-modifying therapy in multiple sclerosis: A nationwide cohort study. Neurology 2020;95(8):e1041–51.
81. Iaffaldano P, Lucisano G, Caputo F, et al. Long-term disability trajectories in relapsing multiple sclerosis patients treated with early intensive or escalation treatment strategies. Ther Adv Neurol Disord 2021;14. https://doi.org/10.1177/17562864211019574.
82. He A, Merkel B, Brown JWL, et al. Timing of high-efficacy therapy for multiple sclerosis: a retrospective observational cohort study. Lancet Neurol 2020;19(4):307–16.
83. Amato MP, Tent M. Updated EAN-ECTRIMS guideline on pharmacological MS treatment. 2022;271(20):11761-11766. doi.
84. Tremlett H, Zhao Y, Devonshire V. Natural history of secondary-progressive multiple sclerosis. Mult Scler 2008;14(3):314–24.
85. Tedeholm H, Skoog B, Lisovskaja V, et al. The outcome spectrum of multiple sclerosis: disability, mortality, and a cluster of predictors from onset. J Neurol 2015;262(5):1148–63.
86. Cree BAC, Gourraud PA, Oksenberg JR, et al. Long-term evolution of multiple sclerosis disability in the treatment era. Ann Neurol 2016;80(4):499–510.
87. Rae-Grant A, Day GS, Marrie RA, et al. Practice guideline recommendations summary: Disease-modifying therapies for adults with multiple sclerosis: Report of the Guideline Development, Dissemination, and Implementation Subcommittee of the American Academy of Neurology. Neurology 2018;90(17):777–88.
88. Montalban X, Gold R, Thompson AJ, et al. ECTRIMS/EAN Guideline on the pharmacological treatment of people with multiple sclerosis. Mult Scler J 2018;24(2):96–120.
89. Tintoré M, Alexander M, Costello K, et al. The state of multiple sclerosis: Current insight into the patient/health care provider relationship, treatment challenges, and satisfaction. Patient Prefer Adherence 2016;11:33–45.
90. Washington F, Langdon D. Factors affecting adherence to disease-modifying therapies in multiple sclerosis: systematic review. J Neurol 2022;269(4):1861.
91. Rush CA, MacLean HJ, Freedman MS. Aggressive multiple sclerosis: proposed definition and treatment algorithm. Nat Rev Neurol 2015;11(7):379–89.
92. Zhang Y, Cofield S, Cutter G, et al. Predictors of Disease Activity and Worsening in Relapsing-Remitting Multiple Sclerosis. Neurol Clin Pract 2022;12(4):e58.
93. Okuda DT, Kantarci O, Lebrun-Frénay C, et al. Dimethyl Fumarate Delays Multiple Sclerosis in Radiologically Isolated Syndrome. Ann Neurol 2023;93(3):604–14.

94. Freedman MS, Comi G, De Stefano N, et al. Moving toward earlier treatment of multiple sclerosis: Findings from a decade of clinical trials and implications for clinical practice. Mult Scler Relat Disord 2014;3(2):147–55.
95. Ontaneda D, Tallantyre EC, Raza PC, et al. Determining the effectiveness of early intensive versus escalation approaches for the treatment of relapsing-remitting multiple sclerosis: The DELIVER-MS study protocol. Contemp Clin Trials 2020; 95. https://doi.org/10.1016/J.CCT.2020.106009.

# Leveraging Real-World Evidence and Observational Studies in Treating Multiple Sclerosis

Albert Aboseif, DO[a],
Izanne Roos, MBChB, MMed (Neurology), FRACP, PhD[b,c],
Stephen Krieger, MD[d], Tomas Kalincik, MD, PhD, PGCertBiostat, FRACP[c,e],
Carrie M. Hersh, DO, MSc[f,*]

**KEYWORDS**

- Multiple sclerosis • Real-world evidence • Observational studies
- Randomized controlled trials • Propensity score analysis
- Disease-modifying therapies

**KEY POINTS**

- Observational studies evaluate heterogenous real-world patient cohorts with multiple sclerosis (MS).
- Observational studies complement randomized controlled trials by harnessing population-specific treatment strategies.
- Analytical methods can be used to reduce the bias and confounding inherent to observational data.
- Leveraging real-world evidence enhances personalized MS care.

## INTRODUCTION

In a rapidly evolving treatment landscape for multiple sclerosis (MS), the utilization of real-world observational studies has become increasingly valuable for decision-making at the bedside. Real-world observational studies may be more generalizable

[a] Department of Neurology, Neurological Institute, Cleveland Clinic, 9500 Euclid Avenue S10, Cleveland, OH 44195, USA; [b] Department of Neurology, Neuroimmunology Centre, Royal Melbourne Hospital, L7 635 Elizabeth Street, Melbourne 3000, Australia; [c] Department of Medicine, CORe, University of Melbourne, Melbourne, Australia; [d] Corinne Goldsmith Dickinson Center for MS Icahn School of Medicine at Mount Sinai, 5 East 98th Street, Box 1138, New York, NY 10029, USA; [e] Department of Neurology, Neuroimmunology Centre, Royal Melbourne Hospital, L6 635 Elizabeth Street, Melbourne 3000, Australia; [f] Lou Ruvo Center for Brain Health, Cleveland Clinic, 888 West Bonneville Avenue, Las Vegas, NV 89106, USA
* Corresponding author. 888 West Bonneville Avenue, Las Vegas, NV 89106.
*E-mail address:* hershc@ccf.org

Neurol Clin 42 (2024) 203–227
https://doi.org/10.1016/j.ncl.2023.06.003
0733-8619/24/

to the broader population than randomized controlled trials (RCTs) and can offer realistic insights into the effectiveness and safety of disease-modifying therapies (DMTs). However, clear limitations and biases inherent to observational studies exist, many of which are addressed by RCTs featuring more regimented study conditions. This article reviews the benefits and challenges of real-world observational studies and how they can complement RCTs in providing guidance on the use of DMTs in clinical practice. The work also summarizes recent real-world data (RWD) that provide insights into more contemporary aspects of MS care and highlights some of the advanced statistical methods that may be used to mitigate challenges intrinsic to observational studies. Future opportunities and applications of these studies within the sphere of routine clinical practice are also reviewed. Finally, updates on various patient registries and learning health systems are discussed, including how their applications can further the understanding of present day DMT approaches and future perspectives.

## BENEFITS AND CHALLENGES OF RANDOMIZED CONTROLLED TRIALS

RCTs are considered the highest level of evidence. The process of randomization produces comparable groups minimizing indication bias and unmeasured confounders. Observed differences in outcomes can therefore be attributed to the intervention rather than between-group differences. RCTs are thus the gold standard for generating efficacy and safety data for investigational treatments and are often required for regulatory approval. RCTs have resulted in the approval of greater than 20 DMTs to date,[1,2] with a growing number of agents in the pipeline. RCTs evaluate the efficacy of an intervention under idealized study conditions with strict quality control measures. In addition to determining clinical efficacy and drug safety, RCTs also evaluate imaging and laboratory biomarkers, which are not collected in a standardized way during routine clinical care.[3] Furthermore, source data verification in RCTs for the purpose of quality control ensures a high degree of semantic validity of the data reported.[4]

Although one of the greatest strengths of RCTs is high internal validity, their rigor and constraints simultaneously reduce external validity, or generalizability to the "real world." RCTs are governed by carefully designed inclusion and exclusion criteria, chosen to select homogenous patient groups from the overall MS population. Although the details of these criteria differ among trials, patients at the extremes of age or with certain medical comorbidities are nearly uniformly excluded from RCT participation. Furthermore, RCTs are more often performed in large well-resourced urban centers. Trials may not enroll racial and ethnic minorities commensurate with their representation in the overall population. Lower participation in RCTs can influence risk patterns and treatment recommendations.[5] The use of ideal study conditions and frequent clinical monitoring in RCTs therefore limits the generalizability to patients managed as part of routine clinical care. Thus, external validity can often be challenged by study cohorts that are ultimately not representative of the general population.

RCTs are also costly and time-intensive, limiting the evaluation of long-term drug efficacy and adverse outcomes.[6–8] Open label extension studies, where patients continue unblinded follow-up after core study completion help to mitigate these limitations but, like observational studies, are subject to selection bias (described below).[9] More recently, extension of RCT follow-up duration using a method of trial population recapture has allowed for reevaluation of drug outcomes decades later.[10,11] Finally, RCTs are limited in their ability to compare multiple therapies simultaneously,[7,8] thus challenging personalized decision-making.

## BENEFITS AND CHALLENGES OF REAL-WORLD OBSERVATIONAL STUDIES

Because it is neither ethical, feasible, nor pragmatic to answer all clinical questions through an RCT, there has been increased interest in using longitudinal observational studies to guide MS care. In contrast to RCTs, which demonstrate treatment efficacy under idealized conditions, observational studies evaluate treatment effectiveness, that is, performance under "real world" conditions.[12] The inclusion of heterogeneous study cohorts that are more representative of the breadth of patients with MS allows observational studies to be more generalizable and clinically applicable.[13] In addition, the utilization of large-scale international MS databases allows for greater global representation of patients.[14] Guidance on the use of treatments during pregnancy and breastfeeding and in vulnerable patient populations can only be obtained from observational studies.[8] Given their capacity for long-term follow-up, which far exceeds the duration of the core phases of RCTs, observational studies improve the assessment of delayed risks and long-term benefits of various DMTs and differing treatment strategies.[7,8] Observational studies may offer a more primary focus on patient-centered and patient-reported outcomes, resulting in increased attention on functional status and quality of life.[15]

Responsible use of these data is however conditional on well-designed research questions, the recognition of various forms of bias and careful attention to data quality. In a treatable chronic condition such as MS, treatment indication (ie, nonrandom treatment exposure) is the most prominent source of bias. The choice of therapy is usually determined by patients' clinical status and prognosis, both of which ultimately determine future clinical outcomes. Other common sources of bias inherent to observational studies are summarized in **Table 1**. A detailed explanation of bias can be found elsewhere.[6] The benefits and challenges of RCTs and observational data are summarized in **Table 2**.

## METHODS FOR IMPROVING REAL-WORLD OBSERVATIONAL STUDIES

Although randomization is the key instrument to eliminating treatment-related indication bias at the time of treatment decisions and a standard feature of RCTs, nonrandomized cohorts rely on other techniques. Typically, these are statistical methods aimed at balancing recorded patient characteristics at the time of treatment decision. Many statistical methods are available and have been used in MS research over the past decade. Matching on a predefined set of patient characteristics is the most direct method, but when applied retrospectively in an existing cohort, it can lead to considerable patient exclusion and a reduction of generalizability of the study findings. Therefore, propensity score (PS)-based methods have become popular in MS research, inspired by cardiology, diabetes, and human immunodeficiency virus (HIV) research. These methods allow researchers to first identify the recorded patient characteristics associated with differential allocation of compared therapies, such as demographics (eg, age, biological sex, race, socioeconomic factors), baseline disease characteristics (eg, MS phenotype, disease duration, measures of inflammatory activity and disability, prior DMTs), and medical comorbidities and lifestyle factors (eg, tobacco smoking)- and then use only the salient characteristics to account for systematic differences in treatment allocation. This can be achieved through several approaches, including PS matching, weighting, stratification, or adjustment (**Fig. 1**).

PS matching and weighting are more efficient at minimizing imbalance between compared groups than adjustment and stratification.[16] One may view PS matching as an extreme of inverse probability of treatment weighting. For instance, a weighted comparison of disability outcomes showed that patients treated in Sweden (where six

**Table 1**
**Types of bias inherent to observational studies in multiple sclerosis**

| Types of Bias | Definition | Examples in MS Observational Studies |
|---|---|---|
| Indication bias | Treatment exposure is nonrandom, instead based on clinical characteristics | DMT choice is nonrandom, often based on demographics, disease characteristics, comorbidities, and patient preferences |
| Selection bias | Cohort selection is nonrandom, with preferential inclusion of specific subgroups | Inclusion criteria are often based on age, disease status and duration, absence of certain comorbidities/co-medications, and treatment status |
| Attrition bias | Follow-up duration is non-standardized and nonrandom with variable participant dropout | High nonrandom variability exists in the length of follow-up among patients |
| Detection bias | Systematic differences between groups in how outcomes are determined | Non-standardized follow-up frequency with variability based on clinical characteristics such as disease severity, treatment status, and compliance |
| Immortal time bias | Non-standardized entry protocols across cohorts, for which there is an interval during the observation period that the outcome cannot occur | Variability in the time of study inclusion, notably between treated and untreated patients, leading to incorrect handling of the period between cohort entry and first treatment exposure |
| Hidden bias | Unmeasured confounders or an incomplete understanding of causal mechanisms | Unaccounted characteristics important for DMT assignment may lead to unrecognized confounding |

**Table 2**
**Benefits and challenges of real-world evidence and randomized controlled trials**

| Study Type | Benefits | Challenges |
|---|---|---|
| Real-world evidence | Studies effectiveness<br>Cost-effective<br>Uses existing data<br>Generalizable, heterogenous patient groups<br>Longer follow-up | Variable data quality and completeness<br>Susceptible to various forms of bias warranting analytical consideration, including indication bias and unmeasured data |
| Randomized controlled trials | Studies efficacy<br>High-quality data<br>Randomization produces directly comparable patient groups | Expensive: money and time<br>Less generalizable cohorts<br>Rigorous monitoring not a reflection of real-world practice<br>Ethics of randomization<br>Short duration |

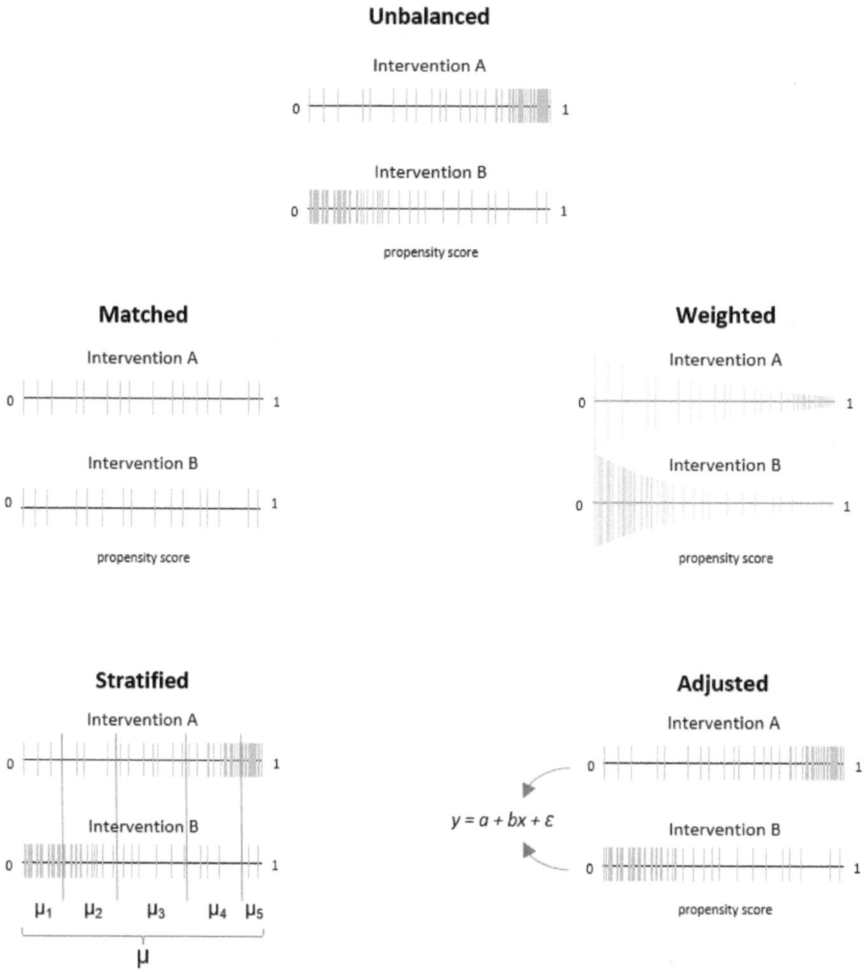


**Fig. 1.** Illustration of basic applications of PS in balancing comparisons of interventions in observational data. Although weighting assigns an inverse probability of treatment weight to each individual based on the probability of being exposed to the treatment of interest, matching only retains patients who are represented in both compared groups (which is equivalent to using weights 0 for cases only represented in one group). Stratification of analyses on PS uses a meta-analytical approach to combine treatment effects observed in several strata of the study sample. Occasionally, PS is used to parsimoniously adjust the model of outcome for relevant determinants of treatment allocation.

times more patients initiated natalizumab or rituximab as their first DMT) accumulated disability at a slower rate than patients treated in Denmark.[17] The weights allowed for use of all patient data in the analyses, but the contribution of each patient to the overall result was determined by the continuous weight representing the probability of being treated in Denmark or Sweden conditional on the patient's characteristics. Another study arrived at the same conclusion by matching patients from an international registry who initiated a high-efficacy therapy (HET) within 2 years versus between years 4 to 6 from MS onset.[18] This approach dictated that patients with characteristics that were not represented in both compared groups were excluded, whereas information from all of the matched patients contributed to the overall result to the same extent.

Matching also allows for pairwise censoring to reduce informed censoring and attrition bias.[6] Although PS matching tends to be more robust to model misspecification than weighting, it is only able to estimate average treatment effect among the treated (ATT[19]). In contrast, weighting provides the option of estimating average treatment effect (**Box 1**). Another advantage of PS matching, stratification, and, to some extent, weighting, is that they separate the balancing of compared groups from the estimation of the treatment effect on the outcome. In practice, this means that the study sample with balanced groups is established before analyzing the outcomes in the compared groups, similar to an RCT. The balance can be objectively assessed, using metrics independent on sample size—such as standardized mean differences. The use of statistical inference (*P*-values) to quantify balance between compared groups is a common error that should be avoided.[20]

The key limitation of PS-based methods is their ability to only account for measured determinants of treatment allocation. This is a result of its assumption of "absence of unmeasured confounding." Because in reality the full range of potential confounders of MS outcomes cannot be documented, a careful analyst would explore robustness of their conclusions to potential unmeasured bias. Rosenbaum bounds or Hodges–Lehmann $\Gamma$ are commonly used methods.[21] They quantify the amount of unmeasured bias that would be required before the conclusion of a study could be changed. For example, natalizumab was more effective in controlling relapses than fingolimod in an analysis that was robust to strong potential unmeasured confounding (up to 80% of the characteristics associated with treatment allocation, as indicated by $\Gamma = 0.8$).[22] This effect remained unchanged whether the analysis accounted for imputed missing MR imaging data or not. Although these methods do not eliminate unmeasured bias, they provide clinical readers with a quantification of the robustness of the study's findings.[23]

To meet another essential assumption of PS-based analyses, every patient must have a nonzero chance to receive either of the compared interventions (referred to as the positivity assumption).[24] In practice, treatment approaches should only be compared over a time period when, and in regions where, both interventions were available. Comparative analyses between nonoverlapping historical and contemporary cohorts may lead to erroneous conclusions.[25]

Both RCTs and observational studies balanced at study baseline remain vulnerable to imbalance that may be introduced during the post-baseline follow-up. This often neglected source of bias reflects the fact that treatment decisions are revised throughout the study follow-up. As an example, informed censoring may differentially affect treatments with substantially different tolerability profiles. To preserve the balance after baseline, an analyst may use pairwise censoring (in matched groups) or methods of causal inference that rebalance time-varying determinants of treatment allocation and censoring throughout the follow-up (**Box 2**).[26] Examples used in

**Box 1**
**Definition of average treatment effect**

Average treatment effect: Average difference between the effects of compared interventions on the outcome generalized to the entire study population.

Average treatment effect among the treated: Average difference between the effects of compared interventions among the sample of patients who received one of the treatments.

**Box 2**
**Definition of causal inference**

Causal inference: Methodological approach to establish causal relationship between intervention and outcome. This can be achieved through appropriately powered RCTs accounting for potential sources of bias, or observational studies with statistical methods emulating a target trial and accounting for measured bias.

comparisons of MS therapies include G-estimation, marginal structural modeling and doubly robust estimators.[27] The doubly robust estimators are also robust to misspecification of the underlying statistical models.

Additional important components of reliable and informative studies using observational data are rigorous study design, high-quality data, and clearly postulated and feasible research questions. Although clinical data present the most relevant information from the perspective of patients' long-term outcomes, a representative summary of the complexities of neurologic status is challenging. Among the available instruments, Expanded Disability Status Scale (EDSS) offers the advantage of quantifying a standard neurologic assessment and is therefore accessible to all specialists.[28] On the other hand, this complex instrument requires appropriate benchmarking.[29] As a key outcome and adjustment/balancing variable, it is important that quantitative disability data are recorded as part of standard clinical follow-up. The main criticism of EDSS includes the significant variability in the size of its ordinal steps and can be mitigated by derived outcomes, such as confirmed disability worsening or disability milestones.[30] Second, EDSS is insensitive to change in many neurologic domains once a patient develops a significant limitation of gait. Complementary assessments of neurologic systems with superior statistical properties—such as MS Functional Composite—help address some of these shortcomings.[31]

In routine clinical care, data missingness and inaccuracies are inevitable. Objective approaches to establishing and improving data quality are available. Such processes help establish data completeness, syntactic accuracy, consistency, and believability.[32] Semantic accuracy provides the highest level of data quality assurance. It is, however, reliant on primary source verification and therefore significant resources. Further, standardized data definitions should be used to improve data metric uniformity and reduce intra-rater and inter-rater variability in multisite cohorts. The research landscape in MS has benefitted from access to high-quality data sources, both at national (eg, Observatoire français de la sclérose en plaques [OFSEP], Danish MS Registry, Czech National MS Registry [ReMuS], Swiss MS Registry, Italian MS Registry) and international levels (eg, MSBase, BigMSData) and in focused cohorts (eg, North American Research Committee on Multiple Sclerosis [NARCOMS], MS Partners Advancing Technology and Health Solutions [MS PATHS]).

## CONTINUED CHALLENGES AND OPPORTUNITIES FOR IMPROVING REAL-WORLD EVIDENCE GENERATION

Despite the broader and more informed use of advanced statistical methods in the analyses of observational data in MS, certain limitations persist. Observational studies rely on retrospective data collection and thus depend heavily on accurate documentation of key variables such as DMT start and stop dates and reasons for initiation and discontinuation. Insufficient accounting for bias in observational studies is partially attributable to insufficient or inaccurate reporting on these data, some of which is self-reported by the patient.[33] Furthermore, the definition of various types of treatment discontinuation is not standardized across centers leading to additional inconsistencies. In this context, the integration of a standardized template into the electronic medical record (EMR) to allow for more accurate and consistent documentation of DMT start and stop reasons may allow observational studies to better account for treatment indication bias.[33] This approach is currently being explored in the learning health system MS PATHS,[34] using a standardized template known as the MS SmartForm, to document details on DMT initiation and discontinuation in addition to other clinician-reported disease characteristics.

In the above context, few observational studies on MS DMTs account for physician-reported reasons for which patients initiate a specific therapy, potentially biasing results. As such, Simpson and colleagues conducted a study to characterize reasons for DMT selection and assess whether including indications for DMT choice can improve overall covariate balance when developing PS models in comparative effectiveness studies.[33] The investigators concluded that PS models accounting for DMT start indication improved overall prediction models compared with those that only included standard confounding variables.

The advent of MS registries and learning health systems has offered major contributions to studying large heterogeneous patient populations, which are often infeasible or unavailable in RCTs. These advantages include the exploration of patient-reported outcome measures, imaging tools such as standardized MR imaging, and biological markers such as serum neurofilament light chain.[8,34–37] However, these databases are not without their own set of limitations. Data standardization is a pervasive issue in observational studies due to the reliance on retrospective data collection, which can be incomplete and variable.[38] The expansion of a data set across multiple centers serves only to further compound this issue due to differences across centers in data capture and quality control.[14] Finally, the reporting of DMT safety information as well as the collection of clinician-reported outcome measures is not pervasively available across all MS registries and large databases. In contrast, due to their prospective nature, RCTs are often less subject to the degree of data missingness encountered with observational studies.[6]

Large data registries can also have a high degree of variability in methods of data production, further yielding inconsistent data quality. There is often a lack of standardization across MR imaging machines and imaging protocols, resulting in image variability and compromising the ability to pool imaging data sets across centers.[39] One possible solution to this issue is the preprocessing of images using intensity normalization methods across centers.[39] Treatment-dependent follow-up protocols may also differ across centers as well as among various patients within a single center. For instance, patients with more active disease or those on higher efficacy DMTs may present more frequently to a provider than patients with stable or inactive disease or those on lower efficacy DMTs. These differences in follow-up time can result in detection and recall bias—potentially creating an opportunity where higher event rates are documented in patients following-up more frequently compared with those with less active disease who present to the clinic less frequently. In addition, the frequency of EDSS follow-up influences the probability of detecting confirmed EDSS change.[30]

## HARNESSING INSIGHTS FROM REAL-WORLD EVIDENCE: RECENT OBSERVATIONAL STUDIES IN MULTIPLE SCLEROSIS

An increase in observational studies over the last decade has altered the landscape of MS care globally, influencing diagnostics and management, and shifting focus to a patient-centered care model. Leveraging real-world evidence (RWE) has been especially crucial for identifying treatment strategies in clinical practice and improving MS care for underserved populations that have historically been poorly represented in large clinical trials. Further, the use of advanced statistical methods, including PS analyses as described above, has allowed for well-designed observational studies to inform on comparative effectiveness between individual DMTs and treatment approaches. A summary of select studies is described below and shown in **Table 3**.

### *Underrepresented Populations*

Observational studies allow for the study of older and underrepresented populations with MS on a larger scale in whom DMT response may differ compared with other cohorts. Such studies focusing on late-onset MS (≥50 years at symptom onset) revealed a poorer overall prognosis, increased disability progression over time despite initial course, and a lack of disability reduction despite interferon beta exposure.[40,41] On the other hand, older patients with long-standing MS discontinuing DMT in the setting of relatively stable disease have demonstrated low likelihood of clinical relapses and EDSS progression.[42–44]

Meanwhile, Black patients are more likely to have an aggressive disease course, higher overall disability level, and a shorter time to conversion to secondary progressive MS relative to other racial and ethnic groups.[45–47] A recent retrospective comparative study evaluating Black, Hispanic, and White patients with MS showed higher rates of disease progression in Black patients, despite similar sociodemographic profiles and DMT exposure relative to the other cohorts.[48] Meanwhile Hispanic patients often develop symptoms at a younger age, are more likely to develop relapsing MS, and tend to have worse disability if migrating to the United States after the age of 15 years-old.[49] The results of these studies are a call to action on an important unmet need in tailoring multifaceted approaches to DMT selection in racial and ethnic minority groups. These findings also highlight the utility of observational studies in identifying important sociodemographic, comorbidity, and clinical features of a population often excluded from RCTs, and emphasize the need for additional treatment-based studies specific to these underrepresented groups. The advent of multiregional and international databases has led to an increase in the diversity of patients when generating RWE and offers the potential for future patient-centered treatment strategies in these underrepresented populations.

### *Comparison of Oral Disease-Modifying Therapies*

The use of large-scale multicenter databases allows for simultaneous comparisons of multiple DMTs in diverse populations, resulting in greater real-world applicability.[8,50] Numerous observational studies comparing the effectiveness of oral DMTs—fingolimod, dimethyl fumarate (DMF), and teriflunomide—using PS methodologies have provided insights into the use of these drugs in clinical practice. For example, Ontaneda and colleagues and Buron and colleagues showed lower relapse rates among DMF- versus teriflunomide-treated patients.[51,52] The investigators also demonstrated comparable effectiveness between fingolimod- and DMF-treated patients after switching from first-line self-injectable therapies.[51] There were no significant differences in disability accrual across DMF and teriflunomide.[52] Of note, in patients who completed at least 3 months of therapy, those on fingolimod were less likely to discontinue treatment compared with teriflunomide and DMF.[53]

Other comparative effectiveness studies using data from the EMR, health claims insurance databases, and matching-adjusted indirect analyses from prior clinical trials[54–57] showed similar performance between fingolimod and DMF. Subgroup analyses from large heterogenous databases also demonstrated the ability to evaluate

**Table 3**
**Summary of observational studies exploring comparative effectiveness of disease-modifying therapies and treatment approaches**

| Comparisons of Interest | Reference | Exposure | Analysis and Data Source | Outcomes | Summary |
|---|---|---|---|---|---|
| Oral DMTs | Ontaneda et al,[51] 2019 | INJ switching to DMF ($n$ = 833) vs TFN ($n$ = 279)<br>INJ switching to DMF ($n$ = 1602) vs FTY ($n$ = 534)<br>Duration: ≥ 90 d | PS matching 3:1 DMF to TFN and 3:1 DMF to FTY<br>Source: health claims database | ARR: DMF < TFN (RR = 0.667, 95% CI 0.486, 0.914); DM = FTY (RR = 1.07, 95% CI 0.861, 1.328) | Comparable ARR between DMF and FTY and lower ARR in DMF vs TFN after switching from INJ |
| | Buron et al,[52] 2019 | DMF ($n$ = 767) vs TFN ($n$ = 1469)<br>Duration: average 2 y | IPTW<br>Source: nationwide registry | ARR: DMF < TFN (RR = 0.58, 95% CI 0.46, 0.73); 42% lower relapse rate in DMF vs TFN<br>EDSS worsening: DMF = TFN (−0.02; SD [0.98] vs 0.03; SD[1.06])<br>Discontinuations due to breakthrough disease: DMF < TFN (10.7%, 95% CI 8.7%, 12.6% vs.22.4%, 95% CI 20.1%, 24.7%)<br>Discontinuation due to AE: DMF = TFN (18.0%, 95% CI 15.9%, 20.2% vs 18.5%, 95% CI 16.7%, 20.2%) | Lower ARR and discontinuation due to disease breakthrough in DMF vs TFN<br>Comparable EDSS worsening and discontinuation due to AE between DMF and TFN |
| | Kalincik et al,[53] 2019 | DMF ($n$ = 782) vs TFN ($n$ = 614)<br>FTY ($n$ = 2332) vs TFN ($n$ = 614)<br>FTY ($n$ = 2332) vs DMF ($n$ = 782)<br>Duration: 2.5 y | PS matching without replacement 2:1 (DMF:TFN), 4:1 (FTY:TFN), or 5:1 (FTY:DMF) using nearest neighbor matching with a caliper of 0.15 SDs of PS<br>Source: international registry, MSBase | ARR: DMF = TFN (0.19 vs 0.22; $P = 0.55$); FTY < TFN (0.18 vs 0.24; $P = 0.05$); FTY < DMF (0.20 vs 0.26; $P = 0.01$)<br>Disability accumulation: DMF = FTY = TFN ($P \geq 0.59$)<br>Disability improvement: DMF = FTY = TFN ($P \geq 0.14$)<br>Discontinuation rate: FTY < TFN and DMF ($P < 0.001$); TFN = DMF ($P$ = 0.68) | Lower ARR and discontinuation in FTY vs TFN and DMF<br>Comparable disability outcomes with all three DMTs |
| | Vollmer et al,[55] 2019 | DMF ($n$ = 737) vs FTY ($n$ = 535)<br>Duration: 3 y | ATT PS weighting Source: EMR | Proportion with clinical relapses: DMF = FTY (OR = 1.27, 95% CI 0.90, 1.79)<br>Proportion with GdE lesions: DMF = FTY (OR = 1.25, 95% CI 0.85, 1.84)<br>Proportion with new T2 lesions: DMF = FTY (OR = 0.99, 95% CI 0.74, 1.32)<br>Discontinuation: DMF > FTY (58.3% vs 45.2%; OR = 1.81, 95% CI 1.41, 2.31) | Comparable effectiveness for DMF and FTY over 36 mo with increased discontinuation in DMF<br>Within 12 m of DMF and FTY discontinuation, switchers to HET vs other DMTs (INJ/orals) had fewer relapses |
| | Boster et al,[58] 2017 | DMF ($n$ = 3352) vs IFN beta ($n$ = 884), GA ($n$ = 1057), TFN ($n$ = 500) and FTY ($n$ = 579)<br>Duration: 1 y | Poisson and negative binomial regression<br>Source: health claims database | Relapses: DMF = FTY (IRR = 1.03, 95% CI 0.88, 1.21); DMF < IFN beta (IRR = 1.27, 95% CI, 1.10, 1.46), GA (IRR = 1.34, 95% CI 1.17, 1.53) and TNF (IRR = 1.23, 95% CI 1.05, 1.45) | Comparable effectiveness between DMF and FTY<br>DMF and FTY demonstrated superior effectiveness vs IFN beta, GA and TFN |

| | | | | | |
|---|---|---|---|---|---|
| Monoclonal antibodies | Vollmer et al,[56] 2018 | NTZ ($n$ = 451) vs FTY ($n$ = 271)<br>NTZ ($n$ = 451) vs DMF ($n$ = 342)<br>Duration: 2 y | PS matching with 1:1 nearest neighbor with replacement<br>ATT doubly robust weighting estimator<br>Source: EMR | Odds of new T2 lesion, GdE lesion, or clinical relapse: FTY > NTZ (OR = 2.0, 95% CI 1.41, 2.85); DMF > NTZ (OR = 2.38, 95% CI 1.68, 3.37)<br>Discontinuation: FTY = NTZ ($P$ = 0.634); DMF > NTZ ($P$ < 0.001)<br>Discontinuation reason: FTY: disease activity ($P$ < 0.001) and AE ($P$ < 0.001); DMF: disease activity ($P$ < 0.001) and AE ($P$ < 0.001); NTZ: JCV positivity ($P$ < 0.001) | NTZ had superior effectiveness and tolerability than FTY and DMF |
| | Granqvist et al,[58] 2018 | RTX ($n$ = 120) vs INJ ($n$ = 215)<br>RTX ($n$ = 120) vs. DMF ($n$ = 86)<br>RTX ($n$ = 120) vs FTY ($n$ = 17)<br>RTX ($n$ = 120) vs NTZ ($n$ = 50) | PS analysis stratified quintiles in the regression models<br>Source: national registry and EMR | ARR: INJ > RTX (HR = 7.0, 95% CI 2.5, 19.6); DMF vs RTX (HR = 3.4, 95% CI 1.0, 11.8); FTX vs RTX (HR = 3.8, 95% CI 0.6, 24.2); NTZ vs RTX (HR = 4.1, 95% CI 1.0, 17.2)<br>GdE Lesions: INJ > RTX (OR = 10.1, 95% CI 2.3, 73.0); DMF > RTX (OR = 8.4, 95% CI 1.7, 72.1); FTY = RTX (OR = 3.0, 95% CI 0.1, 85.0); NTZ = RTX (OR = 8.5, 95% CI 0.9, 109.1)<br>Discontinuation: INJ > RTX (HR = 11.4, 95% CI 4.7, 27.4); DMF > RTX (HR = 15.1, 95% CI 3.9, 58.0); FTY > RTX (HR = 5.9, 95% CI 1.5, 23.4); NTZ > RTX (HR 11.3, 95% CI 3.2, 39.4) | RTX demonstrated superior discontinuation rates vs all other compared DMTs and superior effectiveness compared with INJ and DMF, borderline significance vs NTZ and FTY (likely due to small sample sizes) |
| | Vollmer et al,[59] 2020 | FTY (n = 271) vs RTX (n = 182)<br>NTZ (n = 451) vs RTX (n = 182)<br>DMF (n = 342) vs RTX (n = 182)<br>Duration: 2 y | PS matching with replacement, 1:2 nearest neighbor<br>ATT doubly robust weighting estimator<br>Source: EMR | Clinical relapse, GdE, and/or T2 Lesion: FTY > RTX (OR = 3.17, 95% CI 1.81, 5.55); DMF > RTX (OR = 2.68, 95% CI 2.68, 4.29); NTZ = RTX (OR = 1.36, 95% CI 0.83, 2.23); NTZ > RTX (OR = 2.21, 95% CI 1.20, 4.06)<br>between 6 and 24 mo<br>Discontinuation: FTY > RTX (OR = 2.02, 95% CI 1.24, 3.30); DMF > RTX (OR = 3.27, 95% CI 2.15, 4.97); NTZ = RTX (OR = 1.39, 95% CI 0.88, 2.20), NTZ > RTX (OR = 2.36, 95% CI 1.44, 3.88) when excluding insurance | RTX showed superior effectiveness and discontinuation outcomes vs. FTY and DMF, superior effectiveness to NTZ between 6–24 mo<br>RTX demonstrated comparable discontinuation rates due to any reason with NTZ, superior discontinuation when excluding insurance as a reason for discontinuation |
| | Kalincik et al,[61] 2018 | Cladribine ($n$ = 37) vs NTZ ($n$ = 1410)<br>Cladribine ($n$ = 37) vs IFN beta ($n$ = 1940)<br>Cladribine ($n$ = 37) vs FTY ($n$ = 1893)<br>Duration: ≥ 1 y on-treatment | PS matching without replacement, 10:1 nearest neighbor with caliper 0.5 SD of PS<br>Source: international registry, MSBase | Clinical relapse: Cladribine < IFN beta (HR = 0.6, 95% CI 0.38, 0.95); Cladribine = FTY (HR = 1.2, 95% CI 0.83, 1.8); Cladribine > NTZ (HR = 1.8, 95% CI 1.08, 2.97) | Cladribine had relapse activity comparable to FTY, disability accrual comparable to FTY and IFN beta, and superior disability improvement vs FTY, IFN beta, and NTZ |

(*continued on next page*)

Table 3 (*continued*)

| Comparisons of Interest | Reference | Exposure | Analysis and Data Source | Outcomes | Summary |
|---|---|---|---|---|---|
| | | | | Disability accumulation: Cladribine = IFN beta (HR = 0.61, 95% CI 0.20, 1.82); cladribine = FTY (HR = 1.8, 95% CI 0.91, 3.7); cladribine > NTZ (HR=2.5, 95% CI 1.2, 5.6)<br>Disability improvement: Cladribine > IFN beta (HR = 15, 95% CI 3.6, 59); cladribine > FTY (HR: 3.9, 95% CI 1.6, 9.6); cladribine > NTZ (HR = 4, 95% CI 1.8, 9.2) | |
| | Kalincik et al,[62] 2017 | ATZ (*n* = 189) vs IFN beta (*n* = 2155)<br>ATZ (*n* = 189) vs FTY (*n* = 828)<br>ATZ (*n* = 189) vs NTZ (*n* = 1160)<br>Duration: up to 5 y on-treatment | PS matching without replacement in a variable (2:1 to 1:1) ratio, nearest neighbor with caliper 0.1 SD of PS<br>Source: international registry, MSBase | ARR: ATZ < IFN beta (0.19 vs 0.53; *P*<.0001); ATZ < FTY (0.15 vs 0.34, *P*<.0001); ATZ = NTZ (0.20 vs 0.19, *P* = .78)<br>Disability accumulation: ATZ = IFN beta (HR = 0.66, 95% CI 0.36, 1.22), ATZ = FTY (HR = 1.27, 95% CI 0.60, 2.70), ATZ = NTZ (HR 0.81, 95% CI 0.47, 1.39)<br>Disability improvement: ATZ = IFN beta (HR = 0.98, 95% CI 0.65, 1.49), ATZ = FTY (HR = 0.50, 95% CI 0.25, 1.01), ATZ < NTZ (HR = 0.35, 95% CI 0.20, 0.59) | ARR for ATZ superior to IFN beta and FTY and similar to NTZ, similar disability accumulation across all compared DMTs, and less disability improvement for ATZ vs NTZ |
| | Hersh et al,[63] 2021 | NTZ (n = 145) vs OCR (n = 520)<br>Duration: Mean follow-up 6 mo from NTZ/OCR start | IPTW with trimming of 2% PS outliers<br>Source: international learning health system, MSPATHS | Positive affect and well-being: NTZ > OCR (*P* = 0.02)<br>Sleep: NTZ > OCR (*P* =0.003)<br>Satisfaction with social roles and activities:<br>NTZ >OCR (*P* = 0.03) | NTZ was associated with greater improvements in positive affect and well-being, sleep, and social satisfaction compared with OCR |

| | | | | | |
|---|---|---|---|---|---|
| DMT Discontinuation and sequencing | Zhu et al,[64] 2022 | FTY ($n$ = 1045) switching to OCR ($n$ = 445) vs NTZ ($n$ = 524)<br>FTY ($n$ = 1045) switching to Cladribine ($n$ = 76) vs NTZ ($n$ = 524)<br>Duration: ≥6 mo after switching from FTY | IPTW<br>Source: international registry, MSBase | ARR: OCR < NTZ (RR = 0.67, 95% CI 0.47, 0.96); cladribine > NTZ (RR = 2.31, 95% CI 1.30, 4.10)<br>Time to relapse: OCR < NTZ (HR 0.57, 95% CI 0.40, 0.83); cladribine = NTZ (HR 1.18, 95% CI 0.47, 2.93)<br>Disability accumulation: OCR = NTZ (HR = 0.81, 95% CI 0.49, 1.35); comparison to cladribine not performed due to small sample size<br>Disability improvement: OCR < NTZ (HR = 0.49, 95% CI 0.32, 0.73); comparison to cladribine not performed due to small sample size<br>Discontinuation: NTZ = cladribine (HR = 0.74, 95% CI 0.26, 2.10); OCR < NTZ (HR = 0.11, 95% CI 0.07, 0.20) | Following FTY cession, cladribine had higher ARR compared with NTZ<br>Following FTY cessation, NTZ had higher ARR and shorter time to first relapse than OCR, yet NTZ had higher probability of sustained disability improvement<br>There were no significant differences in disability accumulation between OCR and NTZ<br>OCR had lower discontinuation rates than NTZ |
| | Hersh et al,[65] 2020 | NTZ (n = 556) switching to moderate DMT<br>(DMF: n = 130, FTY: n = 140) vs HET<br>(OCR: n = 106, RTX: n = 17, ATZ: n = 7)<br>Duration: 2 y | ATT PS weighting<br>Source: EMR | 24 mo (on-treatment):<br>ARR ratio: Moderate DMT = HET (OR=1.44, 95% CI 0.69, 1.59)<br>Time to first relapse: Moderate DMT = HET (HR = 2.12, 95% CI 0.87, 5.17)<br>GdE lesions: Moderate DMT > HET (OR = 3.62, 95% CI 1.56, 5.21)<br>T2 lesions: Moderate DMT > HET (OR = 2.23, 95% CI 1.17, 3.88)<br>Absence of disease activity: Moderate DMT < HET (OR = 0.41, 95% CI 0.21, 0.71) | Switching from NTZ to moderate efficacy therapy was associated with increased risk of disease activity compared with HET over 24 mo |
| | Alping et al,[66] 2016 | NTZ ($n$ = 256) switching to FTY ($n$ = 142) vs RTX ($n$ = 114)<br>Duration: within 1.5 y of NTZ discontinuation due to JCV antibody positivity | Logistic regression for categorical variables<br>Kaplan–Meier curves and Cox proportional hazards models for survival analysis<br>Source: national MS registry and EMR | Clinical relapse: RTX < FTY (HR = 0.10, 95% CI 0.02, 0.43)<br>GdE lesions: RTX < FTY (OR = 0.05, 95% CI 0.00, 0.22)<br>Adverse events: RTX < FTY (HR = 0.25, 95% CI 0.10. 0.59)<br>Discontinuation: RTX < FTY (HR = 0.07, 95% CI 0.02, 0.30) | Greater effectiveness and tolerability of RTX vs FTY after switching from NTZ over 1.5 y |
| | Iaffaldano et al,[68] 2015 | NTZ ($n$ = 613) switching to FTY ($n$ = 135) vs BRACE (IFN beta $n$ = 160, GA $n$ = 138)<br>Duration: 1 y on switched DMT | PS matching 1:1 and 5:1 greedy matching<br>Source: national MS registry | Relapse: FTY < BRACE (IRR = 0.52, 95% CI 0.37, 0.74)<br>Disability progression: FTY = BRACE (HR = 0.58, 95% CI 0.26, 1.31) | FTY was superior to BRACE in controlling relapses after NTZ discontinuation; there was no between-group differences in disability progression |

(continued on next page)

**Table 3 (continued)**

| Comparisons of Interest | Reference | Exposure | Analysis and Data Source | Outcomes | Summary |
|---|---|---|---|---|---|
| | Roos et al,[70] 2022 | 14,213 patients with RRMS on seven different DMTs (MTX $n = 214$, NTZ $n = 2,453$, FTY $n = 1,279$, DMF $n = 553$, TFN $n = 389$, IFN beta $n = 8,993$, GA $n = 2,891$) with 18,029 discontinuation epochs<br>Duration: 1 y since discontinuing DMT | IPTW<br>Source: two international MS registries: OFSEP and MSBase | Discontinuation ARR: post-NTZ (months 2–4 ARR = 0.47, 95% CI 0.43, 0.51); post-FTY (months 1–2 ARR = 0.80, 95% CI 0.70, 0.89)<br>New therapy ARR: post-NTZ (mean ARR difference = 0.15, 95% CI 0.08, 0.22); post-FTY (mean ARR difference = 0.14, 95% CI −0.01, 0.29)<br>Starting a subsequent DMT reduced both the risk of relapse (HR= 0.76, 95% CI 0.72, 0.81) and disability accumulation (HR = 0.73, 95% CI 0.65, 0.80) | Disease reactivation after DMT discontinuation varied between therapies, with peak relapse activity 1–10 mo in untreated cohorts<br>Untreated intervals should be minimized after discontinuing NTZ and FTY<br>Predictors of relapse were higher relapse rate in the year before DMT discontinuation, female sex, younger age, and higher EDSS score |
| | Vollmer et al,[70] 2022 | Oral DMTs: FTY ($n = 271$), DMF ($n = 342$) vs infusible<br>DMTs: RTX ($n = 182$), NTZ ($n = 451$)<br>Duration: 2 y | PS matching with 1:1 nearest neighbor with replacement<br>Source: EMR | Disease activity: Age < 45 years old: Oral DMT > Infusible DMT (OR = 2.18, 95% CI 1.34, 3.53); age ≥ 45 years old: Oral DMT = Infusible DMT (OR 1.16; 95% CI 0.59, 2.27)<br>Clinical relapse: Age < 45 years old: Oral DMT > Infusible DMT (OR = 2.93, 95% CI 1.71, 5.14); age ≥45 years old: Oral DMT = Infusible DMT (OR = 1.49, 95% CI 0.67, 3.32) | High-efficacy DMTs demonstrated less benefit in older patients |
| | Hillert et al,[71] 2021 | 184,013 observed DMT discontinuations<br>Observed treatments: IFN beta ($n = 116,551$), NTZ ($n = 33,974$), GA ($n = 32,324$), FTY ($n = 19,675$)<br>Duration: Study period between 1996 and 2017 | Descriptive statistics<br>Source: five national/international registries, Italian, OFSEP, Danish, Swedish, MSBase | DMT discontinuation: FTY: 19.7/100 PY (95% CI 19.2, 20.1) < NTZ: 22.6/100 PY (95% CI 22.2, 23.0) < IFN beta 23.3/100 PY (95% 23.2, 23.5) < GLA 25.8/100 PY (95% CI 25.4, 26.2)<br>DMT restart: 86.6% switched to an alternate DMT within 6 mo<br>Discontinuation reason: Lack of efficacy (23.3%) > AE (16.1%) > intolerance (13.8%) | DMT discontinuation reasons and rates were mostly stable over time, slightly increased in recent years likely driven by greater number of available DMTs<br>DMT discontinuation was most commonly due to DMT properties |

| | | | | | |
|---|---|---|---|---|---|
| DMT approaches | He et al,[18] 2020 | Early HET within 2 y of disease onset ($n$ = 213) vs late HET 4–6 y after disease onset ($n$ = 253)<br>HET: RTX, OCR, MTX, ATZ, NTZ<br>Duration (median follow-up): 7.8 y | PS matching without replacement, nearest neighbor, caliper 0.1, variable matching ratio 1:5<br>Source: national/international registries, Swedish and MSBase | Disability progression: Early HET < Late HET (HR = 0.34, 95% CI 0.23, 0.51)<br>Disability progression 6–10 y: Early HET < Late HET (HR = 0.38, 95% CI 0.17, 0.81)<br>Discontinuation: Early HET = Late HET (HR = 0.80, 95% CI 0.63, 1.03) | Early HET started within 2 y of disease onset was associated with less disability after 6–10 y than if started later in the disease course |
| | Kalincik et al,[72] 2021 | 14, 717 MS patients treated vs untreated | IPTW<br>Source: international registry, MSBase | Relapses: Treated < Untreated (HR = 0.60, 95% CI 0.43, 0.82)<br>Disability progression: Treated < Untreated (HR = 0.56, 95% CI 0.38, 0.82)<br>Disability progression to EDSS 6.0: Treated < Untreated (HR = 0.33, 95% CI 0.19, 0.59)<br>Relapses (≥15 year follow-up): Treated < Untreated (HR = 0.59, 95% CI 0.50, 0.70)<br>Disability progression (≥15 y follow-up): Treated < Untreated (HR = 0.81, 95% CI 0.67, 0.99) | DMT was effective in improving long-term disability outcomes in RRMS |
| | Harding et al,[73] 2019 | EIT ($n$ = 104) vs escalation ($n$ = 488)<br>EIT: ATZ and NTZ<br>Escalation: IFN beta, GA, DMF, FTY, TFN<br>Duration: 18 y | *t* test, Mann–Whitney *U* test, X2 test, linear regression, Cox proportional hazards regression models<br>Source: national database, southeast Wales, UK | ARR: EIT < Escalation (0.16 vs 0.0 ; $P$ = 0.02)<br>Δ EDSS over 5 y: EIT < Escalation (+0.3 vs +1.2, 95% CI −1.38, −0.32)<br>Sustained disability accumulation: EIT < Escalation(6.0 vs 3.1, $P$ = 0.05) | Patients starting EIT vs Escalation acquired less disability accumulation long term |
| | Brown et al,[74] 2019 | IFN beta/GA ($n$ = 407) vs untreated ($n$ = 213)*<br>FTY ($n$ = 85) vs untreated ($n$ = 174)*<br>NTZ ($n$ = 82) vs untreated ($n$ = 164)*<br>ATZ ($n$ = 44) vs untreated ($n$ = 92)*<br>*Initial treatments<br>Duration: median 13.4 y | PS matching 10:1 to 1:1 by nearest neighbor, caliper 0.1<br>Source: international database, MBase, Bristol, Cardiff, Swansea, Dublin, Dresden, Southeast Wales | Conversion to SPMS: IFN beta/GA < Untreated (HR = 0.71, 95% CI 0.61, 0.81), FTY < Untreated (HR = 0.37, 95% CI 0.22, 0.62), NTZ < Untreated (HR =0.61, 95% CI 0.43, 0.86), ATZ < Untreated (HR = 0.52, 95% CI 0.32, 0.85)<br>Conversion to SPMS: FTY, ATZ, NTZ < IFN beta/GA (HR = 0.66, 95% CI 0.44, 0.99)<br>Conversion to SPMS: IFN beta/GA within 5 y of disease onset < IFN beta/GA > 5 y of disease onset (HR = 0.77, 95% CI 0.61, 0.98)<br>Conversion to SPMS: IFN beta/GA escalation to FTY, ATZ, NTZ within 5 y of disease onset < IFN beta/GA escalation to FTY, ATZ, NTZ > 5 y of disease onset (HR = 0.76, 95% CI 0.66, 0.88) | Initial treatment with FTY, NTZ, or ATZ resulted in a lower risk of conversion to SPMS compared with starting IFN beta/GA |

(*continued on next page*)

**Table 3 (continued)**

| Comparisons of Interest | Reference | Exposure | Analysis and Data Source | Outcomes | Summary |
|---|---|---|---|---|---|
| | Spelman et al,[17] 2021 | Danish Cohort: Low–moderate efficacy DMT ($n$ = 1966) (92%) vs high-efficacy DMT ($n$ = 165) (7.6%)<br>Low–moderate: TFN ($n$ = 907) (42.0%); IFN beta-1a ($n$ = 643) (29.8%)<br>Swedish Cohort: Low–moderate DMT ($n$ = 1769) (65.5%) vs high-efficacy DMT ($n$ = 931) (34.5%)<br>Low–moderate: DMF ($n$ = 615 )(22.8%); IFN beta-1a ($n$ = 616) (22.8%)<br>High-efficacy: RTX ($n$ = 484) (17.9%); NTZ ($n$ = 299) (11.1%),<br>FTY ($n$ = 148) (5.5%)<br>Duration: maximum follow-up 7 y | IPTW<br>Source: national registries, Swedish and Danish | 24 week disability worsening:<br>Swedish < Danish (HR = 0.76, 95% CI 0.57, 0.90); Swedish strategy associated with 29% reduction in post-baseline 24-week confirmed disability worsening vs Danish strategy<br>Time to Milestone EDSS 3.0: Swedish < Danish (HR = 0.76, 95% CI 0.60, 0.97); Swedish strategy associated with 24% reduction in rate of reaching EDSS 3.0 vs. Danish strategy<br>Time to milestone EDSS 4.0: Swedish < Danish (HR = 0.75, 95% CI 0.61, 0.96); Swedish strategy associated with 25% reduction in rate of reaching EDSS 4.0 vs Danish strategy | Efficacy of DMT escalation in terms of disease progression was inferior to HET as initial DMT |

*Abbreviations:* AE, adverse effects; ARR, annualized relapse rate; ATT, average treatment effect on treated; ATZ, alemtuzumab; BRACE, betaseron, rebif, avonex, copaxone, or extavia; DMF, dimethyl fumarate; DMT, disease-modifying therapy; EDSS, expanded disability status scale; EIT, early intensive therapy; EMR, electronic medical record; FTY, fingolimod; GA, glatiramer acetate; GdE, gadolinium-enhancing; HET, highly effective therapy; IFN, interferon; INJ, platform self-injectable DMT; IPTW, inverse probability of treatment weights; IRR, incidence rate ratio; MS PATHS, Multiple Sclerosis Partners Advancing Technology and Health Solutions; MTX, mitoxantrone; NTZ, natalizumab; OCR, ocrelizumab; PS, propensity score; PY, person-years; RR, rate ratio; RRMS, relapsing-remitting multiple sclerosis; RTX, rituximab; SD, standard deviation; SPMS, secondary progressive MS; TFN, teriflunomide.

Notation of "=" refers to equal or comparable, ">" refers to greater than probability of the specified endpoint, and "<" refers to less than probability of the specified endpoint.

populations of interest (eg, male/female, older/younger, DMT naive/experienced, contrast-enhancing lesions/no contrast-enhancing lesions at baseline) and DMT sequencing practices following fingolimod and DMF discontinuation.[54,55] Taken together from different data repositories, these observational studies substantiated comparable effectiveness of fingolimod and DMF in real-world practice (see **Table 3**).

### *Comparison of Monoclonal Antibodies*

The use of monoclonal antibodies—natalizumab, rituximab, ocrelizumab, ofatumumab, and alemtuzumab—in clinical practice has steadily increased given their robust ability to suppress active inflammatory disease, along with improvements in safety mitigation strategies. There has not been a single RCT comparing their efficacy. Here, observational studies have the advantage of providing real-world insights into their use, specifically demonstrating how monoclonal antibodies compare within and outside their own broad efficacy group. For example, studies comparing monoclonal antibodies with alternative DMTs showed fewer clinical relapses, MR imaging lesions, and discontinuations with rituximab versus DMF, fingolimod, and first-line self-injectable therapies.[58,59] Reassuringly, findings from these RWD were similar to those of the RIFUND trial of rituximab versus DMF,[60] highlighting consistent results from two different study designs. In another study, relapses on cladribine were less frequent than on interferon-beta, similar to fingolimod, and more frequent than on natalizumab, although the probability of disability improvement on cladribine was higher than all three comparators.[61]

Several studies also reported on comparisons between monoclonal antibodies. For example, although rituximab showed overall similar clinical and radiographic effectiveness and discontinuation rates compared with natalizumab, rituximab resulted in less disease activity between 6 and 24 months and fewer discontinuations when excluding those due to cost coverage issues.[59] In another study, alemtuzumab demonstrated similar annualized relapse rate to natalizumab, although natalizumab was associated with a higher probability of overall disability improvement.[62] From a quality-of-life perspective, natalizumab showed significant improvements in positive affect and well-being, sleep, and satisfaction with social roles and activities compared with ocrelizumab.[63] Comparing the performance of natalizumab versus another HET on patient-reported outcomes (PROs) allowed the investigators to surmise that expectation bias was an unlikely potential confounder.

### *Disease-Modifying Therapy Discontinuation and Sequencing*

The lack of formal guidance on DMT sequencing approaches has led to variable use of therapies in clinical practice. DMTs may be discontinued due to disease inactivity over several years or due to safety risks. Observational studies can be useful for offering insights on switching strategies, a common and often challenging clinical dilemma at the bedside. Recent studies revealed that patients who discontinued DMF or fingolimod and switched to a monoclonal antibody versus another therapy experienced fewer clinical relapses.[54,64] Similarly, patients who switched from natalizumab to another monoclonal antibody (eg, rituximab, ocrelizumab, or alemtuzumab) versus an oral DMT (eg, fingolimod, DMF) had lower risk of new MR imaging lesions and disability progression and a higher proportion of absence of disease activity.[65] Alping and colleagues showed similar findings in a different study cohort evaluating relapsing-remitting MS (RRMS) patients who switched from natalizumab to rituximab versus fingolimod.[66]

Washout periods should be considered when balancing safety versus the need for prompt DMT switching while accounting for time to full drug effect. Observational studies are well positioned to evaluate such practices and provide guidance for health care providers. For example, several studies investigating relapses after natalizumab discontinuation showed that rebound disease was largely prevented with timely DMT switch, notably within 2 months, with HET providing somewhat better protection than moderate-efficacy therapies.[65,67–69] However, there are a few caveats when collectively interpreting de-escalation data: (1) all patients regardless of age are typically included; (2) disease freedom before de-escalation are not always controlled for; and (3) natalizumab—a therapy that can demonstrate a prompt resumption of inflammatory activity on drug interruption—has largely been the HET examined to date. Therefore, evaluating long-term effectiveness of other de-escalation strategies using RWD, such as switching from anti-CD20 therapies—where the efficacy of DMT discontinuation is associated with a relatively slow re-population of CD20 cells that allow a greater window for the next therapy to become active—will have high clinical utility. This is especially important when evaluating de-escalation in a patient population of increasing age and time on therapy where the difference in efficacy between DMTs becomes less pronounced.[70]

Frequent DMT interruptions, switching, and discontinuations remain a major challenge for replicating treatment efficacy observed in RCTs in real-world clinical practice. Therefore, understanding DMT switching patterns derived from RWD is important for informing health care providers when educating their patients on therapeutic options. For example, a large study investigating greater than 110,000 patients on various DMTs from five international MS registries over the course of 20 years showed that discontinuation rates were lowest for fingolimod, followed by natalizumab and interferon beta. Of the observed who discontinued DMT, 86% of patients switched to an alternative DMT within 6 months.[71] Among all DMTs, lack of efficacy was the most common overall reason for DMT discontinuation, likely driven by early market domination of first-line injectable therapies over the observed period and later availability of alternative DMTs, followed by adverse effects and intolerance.[71]

### *Early Initiation of Highly Effective Therapies Versus Disease-Modifying Therapy Escalation*

Observational studies investigating longitudinal outcomes have shed light on treatment initiation strategies. However, it is important to note that definitions of HET and escalation DMTs are quite variable across practices and national and international databases that challenge comparisons across studies. This affects the ability to establish practice guidelines and therefore requires large pragmatic prospective studies with similar definitions to garner evidence-based data.

Despite limitations, we can use earlier works to lay the foundation for different early initiation treatment approaches. For example, early initiation of HET within the first 2 years of disease onset was found to be associated with lower disability compared with late initiation (>4–6 years) at 6 to 10-year follow-up.[18] Further, treated versus untreated patients yielded superior long-term clinical outcomes.[72] Clinical equipoise remains as to whether early initiation of HET yields better long-term outcomes compared with traditional escalation approaches. Various observational studies to date have offered insights on this important clinical question,[17,73,74] suggesting better long-term outcomes in early intensive therapy versus lower efficacy DMT. A population-based study using the Swedish and Danish registries showed a 29% reduction in the rate of post-baseline 24-week confirmed disability worsening and a 24% rate reduction in reaching an EDSS score of 3.0 in patients starting HET versus escalation approach.[17] However, some important caveats to consider are non-standardized assessment frequencies and switching practices and an inability to account for relevant comorbidities and environmental exposures (eg, tobacco smoking).

Owing to such limitations comparing initial DMT approaches from retrospective observational cohorts, two large pragmatic clinical trials were designed and are currently underway to offer robust evidence regarding these two treatment philosophies (clinicaltrials.gov, NCT03535298; clinicaltrials.gov, NCT03500328). Often, observational studies build on a foundation from prior RCTs; in this case, a set of RCTs will build on prior RWE.

## DISCUSSION AND FUTURE PERSPECTIVES

Despite their limitations, well-designed observational studies continue to inform clinical decision-making in MS treatment, and in combination with RCT data, may allow more nuanced and personalized MS care. RWE can help identify patterns and trends in the use of specific DMTs or treatment strategies, ultimately directing the development of guidelines and clinical practice recommendations. Advancing our understanding of various DMT approaches across populations of interest, in addition to finessing the use of advanced statistical methods when forming conclusions on treatment effects, will continue to drive RWE forward.

An emerging area and next frontier using RWD is the concept of heterogeneous treatment effects (HTEs). Personalized predictions of treatment effects are crucial for clinical decision-making, especially given the varying safety profiles of DMTs, and are poorly understood and implemented at the bedside. Patients often experience different outcomes under the same treatment. The baseline risk of patients is often a determinant of HTE, and in turn, patient characteristics affect baseline risk. Published two-stage models of HTE in MS were derived from clinical trials,[75–77] but although they showed potential for improving personalized medicine, they have limited generalizability. Generating models from real-world MS data can have additional complexities due to their intrinsic limitations. However, RWD-based HTE studies have the advantage of external validity relative to RCTs, providing an excellent substrate for risk prediction. In this context, using the MS PATHS real-world research network, investigators are conducting a proof-of-concept study for two-stage HTE models for various outcomes of interest (eg, relapses, brain atrophy), inclusive of all DMTs—categorized into low, moderate, and high efficacy—and pertinent disease characteristics using RWD and PS analyses.[78,79] If successful, these early developed models could potentially enhance personalized treatment of patients with different disease characteristics by better predicting response to a certain DMT based on their baseline risks.

Quality and semantic validity of routinely recorded data represent other areas for ongoing improvement for generating RWE. Outside of the original research question, RCTs represent sources of high-quality data, which can be repurposed to answer new questions using statistical approaches in the analyses of observational data. Causal inference, with more complex methods that allow adjustment for various sources of bias that change over time, represents the next frontier in the exploration of causal associations inherent in clinical data sets. Causal inference from large observational databases can also attempt to emulate RCTs that would target a specific research question,[80] especially valuable when evaluating comparative effectiveness across multiple DMTs. As the complexity of analytical methodology in clinical research evolves, the demands on investigators and readers increase. Therefore, standardization of reporting of concepts, methods, and results of analyses of observational data has become a necessity, allowing clinical readership to appreciate the strengths and limitations of the individual studies, which over time are advancing the evidence-based management of MS.

## SUMMARY

The application of observational studies in daily clinical practice has enabled or facilitated informed decision-making in several important clinical situations. Such topics include an individualized approach to underrepresented MS populations, guidance on comparative effectiveness between DMTs, DMT discontinuation and switching in the longitudinal setting, and insight into strategies for early DMT initiation. Observational studies provide direction on complex treatment decisions and may inform practices in populations of interest. They have ultimately transformed MS care and demonstrate the continued need for these types of studies, in combination with RCTs, to enhance evidence-generation in treating MS.

## CLINICS CARE POINTS

- Randomized controlled trials (RCTs) are prospective studies that evaluate the *efficacy* of disease-modifying therapies (DMTs) in multiple sclerosis (MS) and are necessary for drug regulatory approval, but their results may not be directly applicable to all real-world clinical decisions.
- Observational studies, often retrospective in nature, are more generalizable and can offer insights into the *effectiveness* and safety of MS DMTs.
- Propensity score-based methods can mitigate biases that are inherent to observational studies.
- Observational studies allow for deep investigation of large heterogeneous patient populations in a real-world setting, allowing longer term patient follow-up and evaluation of DMTs in populations of interest not always studied in RCTs (eg, underserved/underrepresented populations and older patients).
- Observational studies can provide comparisons of interventions when RCTs are unavailable or infeasible and allow real-world insights into initial DMT choice, sequencing, and discontinuation.

## DISCLOSURES

A. Aboseif has no disclosures. I. Roos has served on scientific advisory boards, received conference travel support and/or speaker honoraria from Roche, Novartis, Merck and Biogen. She is supported by MS Australia and the Trish Multiple Sclerosis Research Foundation. S. Krieger reports consulting or advisory work with Baim Institute, Biogen, Cycle, EMD Serono, Genentech, Novartis, Octave, Genzyme/Sanofi, and TG Therapeutics, and non-promotional speaking with Biogen, EMD Serono, and Genentech. Grant and research support from Biogen, BMS, Novartis and Sanofi. T. Kalincik served on scientific advisory boards for MS International Federation and World Health Organization, BMS, United States, Roche, Janssen, Sanofi Genzyme, Novartis, Merck and Biogen, steering committee for Brain Atrophy Initiative by Sanofi Genzyme, received conference travel support and/or speaker honoraria from WebMD Global, Eisai, Novartis, Biogen, Roche, Sanofi-Genzyme, Teva, BioCSL and Merck and received research or educational event support from Biogen, United States, Novartis, Genzyme, United States, Roche, Switzerland, Celgene and Merck. C.M. Hersh has received speaking, consulting, and advisory board fees from Genentech, United States, Genzyme, Biogen, Novartis, EMD-Serono, Bristol Myers Squibb, TG

Therapeutics, and Alexion. She has received research support paid to her institution by Biogen, Novartis, Switzerland, Genentech, Patient-Centered Outcomes Research Institute, United States (PCORI) and NIH, United States - NINDS 1U01NS111678 to 01A1 sub-award.

## REFERENCES

1. McGinley MP, Goldschmidt CH, Rae-Grant AD. Diagnosis and Treatment of Multiple Sclerosis: A Review [published correction appears in JAMA. 2021 Jun 1;325(21):2211. JAMA 2021;325(8):765–79.
2. Amin M, Hersh CM. Updates and advances in multiple sclerosis neurotherapeutics. Neurodegener Dis Manag 2022. https://doi.org/10.2217/nmt-2021-0058 [published online ahead of print, 2022 Oct 31].
3. Spieth PM, Kubasch AS, Penzlin AI, et al. Randomized controlled trials - a matter of design. Neuropsychiatr Dis Treat 2016;12:1341–9.
4. Tudur Smith C, Stocken DD, Dunn J, et al. The value of source data verification in a cancer clinical trial. PLoS One 2012;7(12):e51623.
5. Avasarala J. Inadequacy of clinical trial designs and data to control for the confounding impact of race/ethnicity in response to treatment in multiple sclerosis. JAMA Neurol 2014;71(8):943–4.
6. Kalincik T, Butzkueven H. Observational data: Understanding the real MS world. Mult Scler 2016;22(13):1642–8.
7. Sormani MP, Bruzzi P. Can we measure long-term treatment effects in multiple sclerosis? Nat Rev Neurol 2015;11(3):176–82.
8. Trojano M, Tintore M, Montalban X, et al. Treatment decisions in multiple sclerosis - insights from real-world observational studies. Nat Rev Neurol 2017;13(2): 105–18.
9. Taylor GJ, Wainwright P. Open label extension studies: research or marketing? BMJ 2005;331(7516):572–4.
10. Goodin DS, Reder AT, Ebers GC, et al. Survival in MS: a randomized cohort study 21 years after the start of the pivotal IFNβ-1b trial. Neurology 2012;78(17): 1315–22.
11. Davies G, Jordan S, Brooks CJ, et al. Long term extension of a randomised controlled trial of probiotics using electronic health records. Sci Rep 2018;8(1): 7668.
12. Singal AG, Higgins PD, Waljee AK. A primer on effectiveness and efficacy trials. Clin Transl Gastroenterol 2014;5(1):e45.
13. Concato J, Shah N, Horwitz RI. Randomized, controlled trials, observational studies, and the hierarchy of research designs. N Engl J Med 2000;342(25): 1887–92.
14. Cook JA, Collins GS. The rise of big clinical databases. Br J Surg 2015;102(2): e93–101.
15. Porter ME, Larsson S, Lee TH. Standardizing Patient Outcomes Measurement. N Engl J Med 2016;374(6):504–6.
16. Austin PC. An Introduction to Propensity Score Methods for Reducing the Effects of Confounding in Observational Studies. Multivariate Behav Res 2011;46(3): 399–424.
17. Spelman T, Magyari M, Piehl F, et al. Treatment Escalation vs Immediate Initiation of Highly Effective Treatment for Patients With Relapsing-Remitting Multiple Sclerosis: Data From 2 Different National Strategies. JAMA Neurol 2021;78(10): 1197–204.

18. He A, Merkel B, Brown JWL, et al. Timing of high-efficacy therapy for multiple sclerosis: a retrospective observational cohort study. Lancet Neurol 2020;19(4): 307–16.
19. Austin PC, Stuart EA. The performance of inverse probability of treatment weighting and full matching on the propensity score in the presence of model misspecification when estimating the effect of treatment on survival outcomes. Stat Methods Med Res 2017;26(4):1654–70.
20. Greenland S, Senn SJ, Rothman KJ, et al. Statistical tests, P values, confidence intervals, and power: a guide to misinterpretations. Eur J Epidemiol 2016;31(4): 337–50.
21. Rosenbaum PR. Overt bias in observational studies. New York, NY: Springer; 2002.
22. Kalincik T, Horakova D, Spelman T, et al. Switch to natalizumab versus fingolimod in active relapsing-remitting multiple sclerosis. Ann Neurol 2015;77(3):425–35.
23. Rosenbaum PR. Sensitivity analysis in observational studies. In: Everitt BS, Howell DC, editors. Encyclopedia of Statistics in Behavioral ScienceVol. 4. Chichester: John Wiley & Sons, Ltd; 2005. p. 1809–14.
24. Westreich D, Cole SR. Invited commentary: positivity in practice. Am J Epidemiol 2010;171(6):674–81.
25. Signori A, Pellegrini F, Bovis F, et al. Comparison of Placebos and Propensity Score Adjustment in Multiple Sclerosis Nonrandomized Studies. JAMA Neurol 2020;77(7):902–3.
26. Hernán MA. Methods of Public Health Research - Strengthening Causal Inference from Observational Data. N Engl J Med 2021;385(15):1345–8.
27. Funk MJ, Westreich D, Wiesen C, et al. Doubly robust estimation of causal effects. Am J Epidemiol 2011;173(7):761–7.
28. Amato MP, Fratiglioni L, Groppi C, et al. Interrater reliability in assessing functional systems and disability on the Kurtzke scale in multiple sclerosis. Arch Neurol 1988;45(7):746–8.
29. D'Souza M, Ö Yaldizli, John R, et al. Neurostatus e-Scoring improves consistency of Expanded Disability Status Scale assessments: A proof of concept study. Mult Scler 2017;23(4):597–603.
30. Kalincik T, Cutter G, Spelman T, et al. Defining reliable disability outcomes in multiple sclerosis. Brain 2015;138(Pt 11):3287–98.
31. Meyer-Moock S, Feng YS, Maeurer M, et al. Systematic literature review and validity evaluation of the Expanded Disability Status Scale (EDSS) and the Multiple Sclerosis Functional Composite (MSFC) in patients with multiple sclerosis. BMC Neurol 2014;14:58.
32. Batini C, Cappiello C, Francalanci C, et al. Methodologies for data quality assessment and improvement. ACM Comput Surv 2009;41(3):1–52.
33. Simpson A, Hu C, Hersh C, Mowry E, Fitzgerald K. Inclusion of indications for start of disease-modifying therapies can improve predictive models used in comparative effectiveness studies in multiple sclerosis. In: Vol 27. SAGE PUBLICATIONS LTD 1 OLIVERS YARD, 55 CITY ROAD, LONDON EC1Y 1SP, ENGLAND; 2021:686-686.
34. Mowry EM, Bermel RA, Williams JR, et al. Harnessing Real-World Data to Inform Decision-Making: Multiple Sclerosis Partners Advancing Technology and Health Solutions (MS PATHS). Front Neurol 2020;11:632.
35. Issa NT, Byers SW, Dakshanamurthy S. Big data: the next frontier for innovation in therapeutics and healthcare. Expert Rev Clin Pharmacol 2014;7(3):293–8.

36. Benkert P, Meier S, Schaedelin S, et al. Serum neurofilament light chain for individual prognostication of disease activity in people with multiple sclerosis: a retrospective modeling and validation study. Lancet Neurol 2022;21(3):246–57.
37. Boesen MS, Blinkenberg M, Thygesen LC, et al. Magnetic resonance imaging criteria at onset to differentiate pediatric multiple sclerosis from acute disseminated encephalomyelitis: A nationwide cohort study. Mult Scler Relat Disord 2022;62:103738.
38. Kahn MG, Brown JS, Chun AT, et al. Transparent reporting of data quality in distributed data networks. EGEMS (Wash DC) 2015;3(1):1052.
39. Carré A, Klausner G, Edjlali M, et al. Standardization of brain MR images across machines and protocols: bridging the gap for MRI-based radiomics. Sci Rep 2020;10(1):12340.
40. Shirani A, Zhao Y, Petkau J, et al. Multiple sclerosis in older adults: the clinical profile and impact of interferon Beta treatment. BioMed Res Int 2015;2015: 451912.
41. Guillemin F, Baumann C, Epstein J, et al. Older Age at Multiple Sclerosis Onset Is an Independent Factor of Poor Prognosis: A Population-Based Cohort Study. Neuroepidemiology 2017;48(3–4):179–87.
42. Kister I, Spelman T, Patti F, et al. Predictors of relapse and disability progression in MS patients who discontinue disease-modifying therapy. J Neurol Sci 2018; 391:72–6.
43. Hua LH, Fan TH, Conway D, et al. Discontinuation of disease-modifying therapy in patients with multiple sclerosis over age 60. Mult Scler 2019;25(5):699–708.
44. Kaminsky AL, Omorou AY, Soudant M, et al. Discontinuation of disease-modifying treatments for multiple sclerosis in patients aged over 50 with disease Inactivity. J Neurol 2020;267(12):3518–27.
45. Cree BA, Khan O, Bourdette D, et al. Clinical characteristics of African Americans vs Caucasian Americans with multiple sclerosis. Neurology 2004;63(11): 2039–45.
46. Klineova S, Nicholas J, Walker A. Response to disease modifying therapies in African Americans with multiple sclerosis. Ethn Dis 2012;22(2):221–5.
47. Amezcua L, Rivas E, Joseph S, et al. Multiple Sclerosis Mortality by Race/ Ethnicity, Age, Sex, and Time Period in the United States, 1999-2015. Neuroepidemiology 2018;50(1–2):35–40.
48. Pérez CA, Lincoln JA. Racial and ethnic disparities in treatment response and tolerability in multiple sclerosis: A comparative study. Mult Scler Relat Disord 2021;56:103248.
49. Amezcua L, Lund BT, Weiner LP, et al. Multiple sclerosis in Hispanics: a study of clinical disease expression. Mult Scler 2011;17(8):1010–6.
50. Hersh CM, Marrie RA. Harnessing real-world data to inform treatment decisions in multiple sclerosis. Neurology 2019;93(7):285–6.
51. Ontaneda D, Nicholas J, Carraro M, et al. Comparative effectiveness of dimethyl fumarate versus fingolimod and teriflunomide among MS patients switching from first-generation platform therapies in the US. Mult Scler Relat Disord 2019;27: 101–11.
52. Buron MD, Chalmer TA, Sellebjerg F, et al. Comparative effectiveness of teriflunomide and dimethyl fumarate: A nationwide cohort study. Neurology 2019;92(16): e1811–20.
53. Kalincik T, Kubala Havrdova E, Horakova D, et al. Comparison of fingolimod, dimethyl fumarate and teriflunomide for multiple sclerosis. J Neurol Neurosurg Psychiatry 2019;90(4):458–68.

54. Vollmer B, Ontaneda D, Harris H, et al. Comparative discontinuation, effectiveness, and switching practices of dimethyl fumarate and fingolimod at 36-month follow-up. J Neurol Sci 2019;407:116498.
55. Vollmer BL, Nair KV, Sillau S, et al. Natalizumab versus fingolimod and dimethyl fumarate in multiple sclerosis treatment. Ann Clin Transl Neurol 2018;6(2):252–62.
56. Fox RJ, Chataway J. Advancing trial design in progressive multiple sclerosis. Mult Scler 2017;23(12):1573–8.
57. Boster A, Nicholas J, Wu N, et al. Comparative Effectiveness Research of Disease-Modifying Therapies for the Management of Multiple Sclerosis: Analysis of a Large Health Insurance Claims Database. Neurol Ther 2017;6(1):91–102.
58. Granqvist M, Boremalm M, Poorghobad A, et al. Comparative Effectiveness of Rituximab and Other Initial Treatment Choices for Multiple Sclerosis. JAMA Neurol 2018;75(3):320–7.
59. Vollmer BL, Nair K, Sillau S, et al. Rituximab versus natalizumab, fingolimod, and dimethyl fumarate in multiple sclerosis treatment. Ann Clin Transl Neurol 2020; 7(9):1466–76.
60. Svenningsson A, Frisell T, Burman J, et al. Safety and efficacy of rituximab versus dimethyl fumarate in patients with relapsing-remitting multiple sclerosis or clinically isolated syndrome in Sweden: a rater-blinded, phase 3, randomised controlled trial. Lancet Neurol 2022;21(8):693–703.
61. Kalincik T, Jokubaitis V, Spelman T, et al. Cladribine versus fingolimod, natalizumab and interferon β for multiple sclerosis. Mult Scler 2018;24(12):1617–26 [published correction appears in Mult Scler. 2017 Dec;23(14):NP1].
62. Kalincik T, Brown JWL, Robertson N, et al. Treatment effectiveness of alemtuzumab compared with natalizumab, fingolimod, and interferon beta in relapsing-remitting multiple sclerosis: a cohort study. Lancet Neurol 2017;16(4):271–81.
63. Hersh CM, Kieseier B, de Moor C, et al. Impact of natalizumab on quality of life in a real-world cohort of patients with multiple sclerosis: Results from MS PATHS. Mult Scler J Exp Transl Clin 2021;7(2). 20552173211004634.
64. Zhu C, Zhou Z, Roos I, et al. Comparing switch to ocrelizumab, cladribine or natalizumab after fingolimod treatment cessation in multiple sclerosis. J Neurol Neurosurg Psychiatry 2022;93(12):1330–7.
65. Hersh CM, Harris H, Conway D, et al. Effect of switching from natalizumab to moderate- vs high-efficacy DMT in clinical practice. Neurol Clin Pract 2020; 10(6):e53–65.
66. Alping P, Frisell T, Novakova L, et al. Rituximab versus fingolimod after natalizumab in multiple sclerosis patients. Ann Neurol 2016;79(6):950–8.
67. Iaffaldano P, Lucisano G, Pozzilli C, et al. Fingolimod versus interferon beta/glatiramer acetate after natalizumab suspension in multiple sclerosis. Brain 2015; 138(Pt 11):3275–86.
68. Naegelin Y, Rasenack M, Andelova M, et al. Shortening the washout to 4 weeks when switching from natalizumab to fingolimod and risk of disease reactivation in multiple sclerosis. Mult Scler Relat Disord 2018;25:14–20.
69. Roos I, Malpas C, Leray E, et al. Disease Reactivation After Cessation of Disease-Modifying Therapy in Patients With Relapsing-Remitting Multiple Sclerosis. Neurology 2022;99(17):e1926–44.
70. Vollmer BL, Wolf AB, Sillau S, et al. Evolution of Disease Modifying Therapy Benefits and Risks: An Argument for De-escalation as a Treatment Paradigm for Patients With Multiple Sclerosis. Front Neurol 2022;12:799138.

71. Hillert J, Magyari M, Soelberg Sørensen P, et al. Treatment Switching and Discontinuation Over 20 Years in the Big Multiple Sclerosis Data Network. Front Neurol 2021;12:647811.
72. Kalincik T, Diouf I, Sharmin S, et al. Effect of Disease-Modifying Therapy on Disability in Relapsing-Remitting Multiple Sclerosis Over 15 Years. Neurology 2021;96(5):e783–97.
73. Harding K, Williams O, Willis M, et al. Clinical Outcomes of Escalation vs Early Intensive Disease-Modifying Therapy in Patients With Multiple Sclerosis. JAMA Neurol 2019;76(5):536–41.
74. Brown JWL, Coles A, Horakova D, et al. Association of Initial Disease-Modifying Therapy With Later Conversion to Secondary Progressive Multiple Sclerosis [published correction appears in JAMA. 2020 Apr 7;323(13):1318]. JAMA 2019; 321(2):175–87.
75. Varadhan R, Seeger JD. *Estimation and Reporting of Heterogeneity of Treatment Effects*. Agency for Healthcare Research and Quality (US); 2013 https://www.ncbi.nlm.nih.gov/books/NBK126188/. Accessed January 29, 2023.
76. Gong X, Hu M, Basu M, et al. Heterogeneous treatment effect analysis based on machine-learning methodology. CPT Pharmacometrics Syst Pharmacol 2021; 10(11):1433–43.
77. Chalkou K, Steyerberg E, Egger M, et al. A two-stage prediction model for heterogeneous effects of treatments. Stat Med 2021;40(20):4362–75.
78. Hersh C, Sun Z, Grossman C, et al. A 2-Stage Model of Heterogenous Treatment Effects for Brain Atrophy in MS Utilizing the MS PATHS Research Network (S27. 001). 2023. 100(7, Suppl_2), Wolters Kluwer Health, Inc.
79. Hersh C, Sun Z, Grossman C, Shen C, Pellegrini F, Campbell N. Proof of concept for 2-stage models of heterogeneous treatment effects derived from the real-world MS PATHS research network. In: Vol 28. SAGE PUBLICATIONS LTD 1 OLIVERS YARD, 55 CITY ROAD, LONDON EC1Y 1SP, ENGLAND; 2022:389-390.
80. Hernán MA, Robins JM. Using Big Data to Emulate a Target Trial When a Randomized Trial Is Not Available. Am J Epidemiol 2016;183(8):758–64.

# Health, Wellness, and the Effect of Comorbidities on the Multiple Sclerosis Disease Course: Tackling the Modifiable

Devon S. Conway, MD*, Amy B. Sullivan, PsyD, Mary Rensel, MD

**KEYWORDS**

• Multiple sclerosis • Wellness • Mental health • Comorbidities • Brain reserve

**KEY POINTS**

- There is a high burden of mood disorders in patients with multiple sclerosis. Numerous approaches are available for addressing mood disturbances and doing so represents an important aspect of multiple sclerosis care.
- Comorbidities are known to impact multiple sclerosis patients in a number of ways, including diagnostic delays and selection of treatment strategies. Cardiovascular comorbidities, in particular, have been tied to more rapid disability accumulation in patients with multiple sclerosis. Aggressive management of comorbidities may have a positive influence on the multiple sclerosis disease course.
- Wellness is a state of emotional, physical, and social well-being. Comprehensive strategies addressing behavioral factors such as nutrition, exercise, and social engagement are key to optimizing wellness in patients with multiple sclerosis.
- A multidisciplinary team approach is needed for multiple sclerosis care with contributions from the neurology team, psychologists, psychiatrists, rehabilitation specialists, and primary care, among others.

## INTRODUCTION

Multiple sclerosis (MS) is a complex disorder of the central nervous system that causes a combination of inflammatory demyelination and neurodegeneration, resulting in accumulation of physical, emotional, and cognitive disability. Numerous disease-modifying therapies (DMTs) are available for MS, but these treatments have several limitations including that they primarily impact the inflammatory component of the disease and are only partially effective.[1] The lack of a definitive treatment of MS means that not

Mellen Center for Multiple Sclerosis, Neurological Institute, Cleveland Clinic, Cleveland, OH, USA
* Corresponding author. 9500 Euclid Avenue /U10, Cleveland, OH 44195.
*E-mail address:* conwayd2@ccf.org

Neurol Clin 42 (2024) 229–253
https://doi.org/10.1016/j.ncl.2023.06.007 neurologic.theclinics.com

only should MS care teams emphasize effective DMT use, but that overall optimization of MS patient health is essential. Significant opportunities exist to address modifiable patient health behaviors, many of which may positively impact the MS disease course.

This review focuses on 3 aspects of MS care that fall outside of DMT management: mental health, physical comorbidities, and wellness. Increasing evidence suggests that these domains can significantly impact outcomes in patients with MS and deserve careful attention. For instance, depression can impact adherence to DMT,[2] quality of life,[3] and MS symptoms such as pain and fatigue.[4,5] Physical comorbidities have been well documented as complicating the timing of the diagnosis of MS[6] and the MS disease course, including highly prevalent conditions such as hypertension,[7] obesity,[8] and hyperlipidemia.[9] An emphasis on wellness can also benefit patients with MS,[10] with data accumulating on the positive impact of interventions targeting exercise,[11] mindfulness,[12] and diet.[13]

Although the traditional focus of MS care is on DMT management, the evidence described below accentuates the importance of a comprehensive approach to the care of patients with MS (**Fig. 1**). Such an approach needs to be team-based with participation from neurologists, primary care physicians, relevant specialists, psychiatrists and psychologists, physical, occupational, and speech and language therapists, social workers, and dietitians, among others. The collective contributions of such a care team can be expected to improve outcomes for patients with MS in a variety of ways, as will be reviewed.

## MENTAL HEALTH COMORBIDITIES

Mental health challenges are common before and after the diagnosis of MS. Depression and anxiety have been identified as frequently predating the onset of MS, making

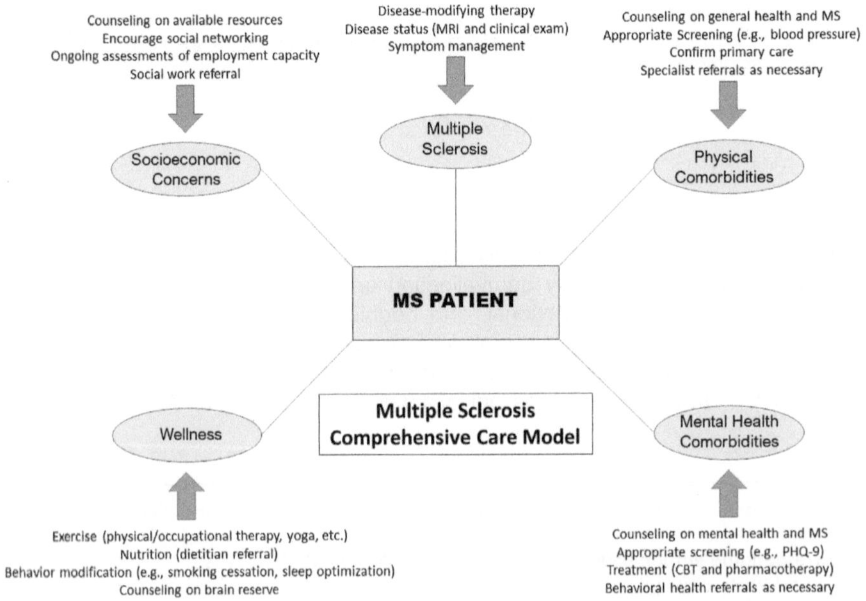


**Fig. 1.** Multiple sclerosis comprehensive care model. MS, multiple sclerosis; MRI, magnetic resonance imaging; PHQ-9, Patient Health Questionnaire 9; CBT, cognitive behavioral therapy.

them prominent components of the MS prodrome.[14] Major challenges face patients with MS including unpredictable relapses and the risk of disability progression, which can be significant stressors. Anxiety and depression are among the most common complaints in patients with MS and are seen at higher rates in patients with MS than in the general population. It is important to recognize that although MS often presents with an adjustment reaction, there are other reasons why patients with MS may have neuropsychiatric symptoms, including a reaction to DMT, or a biologically mediated reaction that may be influenced by lesion location.[15]

Reports on the prevalence of depression, bipolar disorder (BPD), and anxiety disorders in the MS population have varied widely. In a well-known systematic review, reports of the prevalence of psychiatric disorders ranged from 4.98% to 58.9% for depression, 0% to 16.2% for BPD, and 1.2% to 44.6% for anxiety disorders.[16] People with MS also have an increased prevalence of adjustment disorder (20%) and pseudobulbar affect (6%–46%).[17]

### *Depression*

Depression occurs 4 times more frequently in MS than in other neurologic conditions, including potentially more disabling ones such as Parkinson's disease and amyotrophic lateral sclerosis.[18] Increasing evidence suggests that depression deserves careful attention in patients with MS because it may impact adherence to DMT,[2] quality of life,[3] and also co-occurs frequently with MS symptoms such as pain and fatigue,[4] perhaps amplifying them.[5]

Mood disorders in MS are linked to higher rates of suicidal ideation and completed suicide. People with MS are nearly twice as likely to commit suicide compared with the general population and, strikingly, the completed suicide rate is 7.5 times higher in patients with MS than in age-matched controls.[19] In a 2012 systematic review investigating the relationship between MS and suicidal behavior, the majority of included studies found rates of completed suicide 1.6 to 14 times higher than in the general population.[20] A study of veterans showed risk factors for suicide in MS include male sex, depression, and alcohol abuse (**Table 1**).[21] Suicidal ideation has been associated

**Table 1**
**Suicide and suicidal ideation risk factors in people with multiple sclerosis**

| | |
|---|---|
| Suicide[a] | Male<br>Younger age<br>Earlier disease course<br>Loss of independence and/or functioning<br>Nonfuture oriented |
| Suicidal ideation[b,c] | Progressive disease subtype<br>Lifetime history of depression, anxiety, or alcohol abuse<br>Depression severity<br>Family history of mental illness<br>Social isolation<br>Greater disability<br>Lower income<br>Not driving |

[a] Stenager EN, Stenager E, Koch-Henriksen D, et al. Suicide and multiple sclerosis: an epidemiological investigation. *J Neurol Neurosurg Psychiatry.* 1992;55(7):542-545.
[b] Feinstein A. An examination of suicidal intent in patients with multiple sclerosis. *Neurology.* 2002;59(5):674-678.
[c] Turner AP, Williams RM, Bowen JD, et al. Suicidal ideation in multiple sclerosis. *Arch Phys Med Rehabil.* 2006;87(8):1073-1078.

with fatigue, poor social support, and poor sleep quality, which need to be preemptively addressed in the routine clinical care of the patient with MS.[22] It is imperative that mental health and suicide risk in patients with MS are assessed and managed by trained mental health professionals.

Depression and anxiety, if left undetected and untreated, can affect multiple functional domains including energy, cognition, perception of health, healthy aging, and sexual function and thereby affect the quality of life and risk of suicidal ideation in persons living with MS.[23] Moreover, patients with MS who have depression may have worse long-term disease-related outcomes as a result of decreased adherence to DMTs and other treatment recommendations such as physical therapy, occupational therapy, and behavioral medicine.[24] Routine mood disorder screening is essential with consultation to mental health professionals when appropriate.[17]

### *Stress*

Stress has been defined as "a state in which homeostasis is threatened or perceived to be so."[25] Acute stressful events and chronic stress can influence and impact MS in the short and long term. Considerable evidence supports a reciprocal relationship between stressful life events, MS symptoms, and MS exacerbations, possibly mediated by immune function and autonomic imbalance.[26–31] There is also a reciprocal relationship between disease progression and emotional distress such that disease progression can result in increased emotional distress, while greater emotional distress can increase the risk for further disease progression.[32] The link between emotional distress and its impact and influence on disease activity and outcomes dates back to the earliest research in MS.

Jean Martin Charcot, who first recognized MS as a unique disease entity in the 19th century, acknowledged the implications of stress on the MS disease process. Charcot wrote that grief, vexation, and adverse events in one's life were closely related to MS onset. In the 1930s, Hans Selye presented his initial concept of stress, which continues to guide our conceptualization today.[33] Briefly, from a physiologic perspective, he described the role of the hypothalamic–pituitary–adrenal (HPA) axis as the major stress-mediating signaling system. Upregulation of the HPA axis is conceptualized as a protective mechanism resulting in increased resistance to a given stressor. In the setting of sudden stress onset, sympathetic activation triggers increases in norepinephrine and epinephrine, which prompts activation of the HPA axis. Chronic stress can lead to dysfunction of the HPA axis, resulting in dysregulated levels of circulating cortisol.[34]

From a psychological perspective, Selye[35] recognized that the stress response can be mobilized not only in response to a stressor, but also in anticipation of a stressor, underscoring the important relationship between thoughts and physical disease processes, or the mind and the body. Rigorous study of the mind–body interaction and stress physiology began in the 21st century. It is now appreciated that many chronic diseases are preceded by lifestyle practices and perceptions but that it may take years for the disease to manifest itself through symptoms and signs.

The relationship between MS relapses, immune dysfunction, and depression suggests interventions that improve depression or other aspects of mental health could benefit long-term outcomes of patients with MS.[36] Patients newly diagnosed with MS or who experience acute disease activity may be particularly at risk for emotional distress, including adjustment reaction and mood disorders, which may contribute to impaired physical functioning.[37] The cognitive, emotional, and behavioral response to MS diagnosis and disease activity (eg, preoccupation with disability status, reductions in social interactions) can also be predictive of illness-related functional impairment.[38]

Evidence also shows that disease severity and time since diagnosis are strongly correlated with mood symptoms in patients with MS and that older individuals and those with more severe mood disorders are more likely to be referred to and seen by a behavioral medicine specialist.[39,40]

Several mind–body interventions have been reported to be helpful in managing mood symptoms and the occurrence of new brain lesions.[41] Nonpharmacologic interventions such as cognitive behavioral therapy (CBT)[38,42] and stress reduction[41] were shown to be beneficial to those living with MS. These psychological interventions provide patients with treatment-related improvements in emotional distress,[27] quality of life,[43] fatigue,[42] and the occurrence of new brain lesions.[41] Behavioral medicine includes a range of interventions and outcome measures to help manage mood. It is important for clinicians to recognize the high prevalence of mood disorders in the MS population and to facilitate referral of affected individuals to a behavioral medicine specialist.

### *Treatment of Mood Disorders*

The reciprocal relationship between MS and emotional distress as well as evidence that psychological interventions can improve both emotional and physical outcomes in patients with MS suggests the importance of treating mood disorders. Patients who are newly diagnosed with MS or are experiencing worsening levels of impairment may particularly benefit from psychological intervention.

Depression is often under-recognized and undertreated in patients with MS. Depression at the time of MS diagnosis is high in all ages and in both sexes and several large groups have suggested screening at each appointment.[44] Many mood disorder screening tests have been validated in MS and can be used for regular screenings in clinical practice. Both the Patient Health Questionnaire-9 (PHQ-9)[45] and the Generalized Anxiety Disorder-7 (GAD-7)[46] are free and widely used tools to screen for depression and anxiety, respectively, and each of these measures has been found to be both reliable and valid in the MS population.[47,48] Technology enabled distribution of the PHQ-9, GAD-7, or other questionnaires can even be used to assess mood status in advance of an appointment to facilitate efficient, comprehensive care.[49] Psychology and psychiatry teams can be involved as indicated.

Pharmacotherapy is commonly used for the treatment of depression in MS, and recent evidence suggests the proportion of patients with MS with depression receiving antidepressant treatment is increasing.[50] Studies specifically evaluating antidepressant therapy in patients with MS are limited, and there are no specific guidelines for antidepressant use in patients with MS.[51] However, the American Psychiatric Association recommends antidepressant therapy as an initial treatment choice in patients with major depressive disorder.[52] Extrapolating this to the MS population is reasonable and our practice is to offer antidepressant therapy as one treatment option to patients with MS with depression. **Table 2** shows commonly used antidepressants and their potential side effects. Many antidepressant therapies may have added benefits by addressing other symptoms commonly seen in MS such as paresthesias, headaches, and insomnia.

CBT techniques can be used to enhance coping strategies. In a 2006 Cochrane review, Thomas and colleagues[53] concluded there is evidence that CBT aspects enhance coping strategies in MS. In 2011, Plow and colleagues[54] reviewed 27 studies on self-management and health promotion concepts such as coping, depression, and stress management and found these beneficial in the treatment of anxiety and depression. There are also substantial effects from emotion-focused or acceptance oriented concepts such as mindfulness going back to the neurobiologist Kabat-Zinn.[55] Thus,

**Table 2**
**Antidepressant medications commonly used in patients with multiple sclerosis**

| Mechanism of Action | Drug Names | Common Side Effects |
|---|---|---|
| Selective serotonin reuptake inhibitor (SSRIs) | Citalopram<br>Escitalopram<br>Fluoxetine<br>Fluvoxamine<br>Paroxetine<br>Sertraline<br>Vortioxetine | Agitation/anxiety<br>Dizziness<br>Dry mouth<br>Gastrointestinal upset<br>Sexual dysfunction |
| Serotonin norepinephrine reuptake inhibitor (SNRI) | Desvenlafaxine<br>Duloxetine<br>Levomilnacipran<br>Venlafaxine | Agitation/anxiety<br>Dizziness<br>Dry mouth<br>Excessive sweating<br>Gastrointestinal upset<br>Sexual dysfunction |
| Norepinephrine-dopamine reuptake inhibitor (NDRI) | Buproprion | Dry mouth<br>Gastrointestinal upset<br>Insomnia<br>Weight loss |
| Tricyclic andtidepressants (TCA) | Amitriptyline<br>Amoxapine<br>Desipramine<br>Doxepin<br>Imipramine<br>Nortriptyline<br>Protriptyline<br>Trimipramine | Arrhythmia<br>Dizziness<br>Drowsiness<br>Dry mouth<br>Excessive sweating<br>Gastrointestinal upset<br>Weight gain |

by providing coping skills, stress management, and management of mood disorders such and anxiety and depression, improvement of outcomes in patient with MS is expected.[41] Feinstein and colleagues[56] reviewed evidence that supporting the use of CBT in patients with MS and found that pharmacologic treatment and CBT were equally effective. There is no one best treatment option for addressing depression in patients with MS and an individualized approach is recommended.

## PHYSICAL COMORBIDITIES

Most patients with MS have or will develop other health problems coexistent with MS, which are termed comorbidities. Comorbidities have special implications for patients with MS, including that they can lead to diagnostic delays,[57] more rapid disability accumulation,[58] and increased mortality risk.[59] Many comorbidities are preventable or manageable, which raises important questions such as which comorbidities patients with MS are most at risk for, which are most deleterious with respect to disability progression, and whether proper management can diminish or negate the harmful impact of comorbidities on the MS disease course.

### *Cardiovascular Comorbidities*

Cardiovascular disease, which is known to have detrimental effects on the brain structure even in the general population,[60,61] is increasing in incidence among patients with MS.[62] A number of autoimmune diseases have been associated with an increased burden of cardiovascular disease, including MS, in which patients were recently found to have an 85% increased hazard of cardiovascular disease relative to healthy controls.[63] Cardiovascular comorbidities of interest in patients with MS include hypertension, with an estimated prevalence of 16% to 20.8%, hyperlipidemia, with an estimated prevalence of 10.9%, and diabetes, with an estimated prevalence of 0% to 27.1%.[64]

Cardiovascular disease has a detrimental impact on the MS disease course. Presence of one vascular comorbidity at MS diagnosis is associated with a 51% increased risk of gait disability, while having 2 confers a 228% increased risk.[65] Diabetes and hypertension have been linked to worsened scores on neuroperformance testing and increased depression in patients with MS.[58] A recent post-hoc analysis of data from the CombiRx clinical trial revealed a 31.6% increased hazard of disease activity among patients with dyslipidemia,[66] supporting findings from a Canadian prospective study in which individuals with hyperlipidemia had a 67% increased relapse rate.[67] Smoking leads to a dose-dependent increase in the risk of MS,[68–71] and passive smokers also experience increased risk.[72] The impact of smoking on disease course is still being elucidated, but several studies suggest smokers experience increased disease activity,[73] and accelerated evolution to secondary progressive MS.[74,75]

Hypertension is of special interest in MS because several DMTs, including sphingosine-1-phosphate receptor modulators, teriflunomide, and alemtuzumab, may lead to increases in blood pressure.[76–78] Hypertension is more prevalent in patients with MS than the general population,[79] although patients with MS do not have an earlier age of onset.[80] A Canadian study suggests that patients with MS are as likely as controls to meet blood pressure targets,[81] although these findings need to be replicated in other countries. There is also evidence of racial and ethnic disparities in the diagnosis and management of hypertension in patients with MS,[82,83] indicating a need for increased attention to how this condition is handled in minority populations.[84]

Why cardiovascular comorbidities are associated with accelerated disability progression in patients with MS is unclear. It is possible that cardiovascular disease promotes a proinflammatory state but the overall explanation is probably complex and multifold. The impact of vascular disease on white matter integrity is a likely contributor as well. In fact, a recent post-mortem study of 85 patients with MS and 68 controls suggested that an increased burden of cerebral small vessel disease may account for differences in disability progression between MS patients with and without vascular disease.[85]

### *Cancer*

The chronic inflammation underlying MS may be protective against cancer due to increased immune surveillance for malignancy. However, there is concern that the immunomodulatory and immunosuppressive medications used to treat MS may heighten risk of cancer by impairing the anti-neoplastic activities of the immune system.[86] Notably, lifestyle risk factors that are associated with cancer[87] are known to increase MS risk as well, including smoking[88] and obesity.[89]

Investigations into the incidence and outcomes of cancer in patients with MS have produced varying results. A recent population-based matched cohort study from Canada investigated the incidence of 15 cancer types in patients with and without MS.[90] Bladder, central nervous system, and hematologic cancers had a significantly higher incidence rate in patients with MS than controls, but only for bladder cancer did patients with MS have an increased mortality rate. A systematic review from 2015 found that among population based studies, breast, cervical, and digestive cancers had the highest incidence.[91] Among women with breast cancer, those with MS have higher all-cause mortality than women without MS.[92] A Mendelian randomization analysis, which can help to reduce confounding and reverse causality bias, was recently used to analyze the relationship between lung cancer and MS.[93] In a cohort of patients with lung cancer and controls, the investigators uncovered a higher risk of lung cancer among those with genetic evidence of MS, suggesting a causal impact of MS on lung cancer. On the other hand, a Danish nationwide cohort study found no increased cancer incidence or cancer-specific mortality among patients with MS compared with the general population.[94] Thus, uncertainty continues to exist around the relationship between having MS and developing cancer and additional studies are needed.

The risk of malignancy with MS DMTs is a topic of ongoing research. Increased cancer risk with particular treatments may only become apparent with prolonged exposure in large populations, making this an important subject for continuous monitoring. Among approved DMTs, cladribine was initially rejected by the Food and Drug Administration (FDA) in 2011 after multiple types of malignancy were observed in the active treatment arm of the CLARITY study.[95] In 2018, after the CLARITY extension study and other analyses suggested no increased risk of malignancy with cladribine, the medication received FDA approval, although it still carries a black box warning pertaining to malignancy.[96,97] In the OPERA and ORATORIO studies of ocrelizumab,[98,99] there were 15 neoplasms noted in the ocrelizumab groups as compared with 4 in the group receiving placebo. These findings sparked concerns about an increased risk of cancer with ocrelizumab, but analyses of long-term data from extension studies and the post-marketing experience found that malignancies occurred at rates consistent with epidemiologic references.[100] Patients taking sphingosine-1 phosphate receptor modulators are known to have a higher incidence of basal cell carcinoma.[101] Whether there is also an increased risk of melanoma with this DMT class is debated.[102,103]

### *Other Comorbidities*

Numerous other comorbidities afflict patients with MS, often at rates higher than are experienced in the general population.[104] A recent population based study of asthma found an age and gender adjusted prevalence ratio of asthma in patients with MS to be 2.97 compared with the general population. MS patients with asthma are more likely to be female, obese, hypertensive, and living in medium or low-income neighborhoods.[105] Migraine has an estimated prevalence of 55% in patients with MS, whereas the prevalence of tension type headaches is 20%.[106] Headache deserves special attention in MS due to the proclivity of certain DMTs, such as fingolimod and interferons, to worsen headache disorders.[107,108] Other autoimmune diseases that have increased rates in patients with MS include thyroid disease, psoriasis, and inflammatory bowel disease.[109]

Having multiple comorbidities is common in MS. Of the 77.1% of patients with a physical comorbidity in the North American Registry for Care and Research in Multiple Sclerosis, 25.6% have 2 comorbidities and 44.1% have 3.[110] Age, obesity, higher disability, and being a woman were identified as risk factors for a higher comorbidity burden in a study of Australian MS patients.[111] Some data suggest a cumulative impact of comorbidities on the MS disease course. For instance, a study of MS patients with hypertension, hyperlipidemia, diabetes, and obstructive lung disease found that both measures of disability and depression incrementally worsened with each additional comorbidity.[58]

### *Physical Comorbidity Management Considerations*

The widespread impact of comorbidities on patients with MS suggests that addressing coexisting health conditions should be a key component of MS care. Careful comorbidity management is likely to negate at least some of the negative consequences of comorbidities on patients with MS, though additional research is needed to confirm this. Improvements in a patient's general health are also expected with comorbidity optimization, suggesting wide ranging benefits for patients.

Addressing comorbidities can be challenging as most fall outside the normal purview of neurologists. As such, a team-based approach involving the patient's primary care physician and relevant specialists is indicated. Numerous barriers to collaborative care exist including patients' lack of access to primary care and specialty providers, poor communication between specialties, complicated medication regimens, and incompatible electronic medical record systems that do not allow for easy sharing of notes and test results. Research is needed to facilitate development of appropriate care models for MS patients with comorbidities that can help to overcome such barriers.

Notably, many patients with MS see their neurology team more frequently than their primary care physician, which creates a unique opportunity for intervention. As discussed above, cardiovascular comorbidities have some of the most impactful consequences for patients with MS, and risk factors for these conditions such as obesity and smoking can be easily recognized. Attention to blood pressure trends, especially in patients on DMTs that can raise blood pressure, is another straightforward opportunity for intervention. Patients with concerning features should be educated about the risks of comorbidities to their general health as well as the recognized interactions between comorbidities and MS. Counseling about the benefits of exercise, healthy nutrition, and smoking cessation as well as the availability of treatment options that may mitigate the impact of many comorbidities is also an essential aspect of MS care. Finally, it is also important to recognize that minorities, many of whom tend to have a more aggressive course of MS, often bear a disproportionate burden of comorbidities and are also more likely to be receiving substandard care.[82–84]

### *Wellness and Multiple Sclerosis*

Comprehensive medical care for patients with MS should emphasize wellness and a comprehensive healthy lifestyle due to the modifiable nature and the associated risks of comorbidities in MS. Wellness is defined by the World Health Organization (WHO) as a state of complete physical, mental, and social well-being and not merely the absence of disease or infirmity. All 3 of these wellness components should be considered when caring for patients with MS (**Table 3**). In 2010, the WHO devised an action plan as part of a global strategy to prevent and control the noncommunicable diseases that account for 60% of deaths worldwide: cardiovascular disease, cancer, diabetes, and respiratory diseases.[112] Several risk factors associated with these 4 diseases are preventable and modifiable and include tobacco, harmful alcohol use, unhealthy diets, physical inactivity, and obesity. Notably, these risk factors can also contribute to worsening disability levels in MS and other neurologic conditions, such as vascular dementia.[65,113]

Preservation and enhancement of brain reserve through support and education about modifiable behaviors may lessen the risk of disability progression and improve quality of life in patients with MS. Hence, addressing wellness presents a unique opportunity to modify long-term risks.[114] An "urgent" call to educate patients with MS on

**Table 3**
**Physical, mental, and social approaches to wellness in patients with multiple sclerosis**

| MS Wellness | Physical | Mental | Social |
| --- | --- | --- | --- |
| Wellness actions at each MS visit | Discuss brain reserve<br>Confirm primary care<br>Wellness education<br>Resource management<br>Vitals<br>Nicotine use<br>Physical activity<br>Sleep efficacy<br>Nutritional plans<br>Vitamin D<br>Vascular risk factor education<br>Wellness goals and outcomes<br>Address barriers to wellness goals | Mood disorder screen (eg, PHQ-9 or GAD-7)<br>QOL measures<br>Wellness goals and outcomes<br>Address barriers to wellness goals | Social connections<br>Safety<br>Wellness goals and outcomes<br>Address barriers to wellness goals<br>QOL measures |
| Preventable factors related to MS wellness | Confirm primary care<br>Education and goal setting<br>Resource management<br>Nicotine use<br>Physical activity<br>Immunizations<br>Sleep efficacy<br>Nutritional plans<br>Vitamin D<br>Vascular risk factor education<br>Shared decision making | Education and goal setting<br>Resource management<br>Shared decision making | Social connections<br>Safety<br>Education and goal setting<br>Resource management<br>Shared decision making |
| Modifiable factors | Smoking/vaping<br>Excessive alcohol<br>Nutritional plans<br>Physical activity<br>Manage comorbidities | Stress level<br>Wellness practices | Social connection<br>Safety<br>Resource allocation |
| Resources to address wellness goals | Primary care<br>Physical therapy<br>Occupational therapy<br>Social work<br>Speech therapy<br>Nutritionist<br>Patient advocacy groups | Behavioral medicine<br>Psychology<br>Psychiatry<br>Social work<br>Patient advocacy groups | Social work<br>Patient advocacy groups |

PHQ-9, Patient Health Questionnaire-9; GAD-7, Generalized Anxiety Disorder-7; MS, multiple sclerosis; QOL, quality of life measures.

how to live a "brain healthy lifestyle" was published in 2016 due to emerging evidence that "brain reserve" is an important concept for optimal physical, mental, and social living with MS.[115] Because of increasing knowledge about the importance of modifiable well-being factors, the National MS Society also created a framework of wellness education aimed at well-being optimization in 2016.[116] This section will concentrate on preventable and modifiable behavioral activities with the goal of preserving and enhancing brain reserve to achieve the best possible long-term outcomes. Monitoring of MS well-being related data points, employing shared decision making, and goal setting will help patients realize this target. Efficacious DMT and regular monitoring of disease activity is essential for comprehensive treatment of MS and optimization of overall well-being, but will not be the focus of this section.

### *Brain Reserve*

The brain reserve theory posits that optimizing the treatment of medical comorbidities and behavioral risk factors is protective against structural and functional brain decline in those living with MS.[117] Brain volume appears to be primarily genetically determined, but the preservation or enrichment of brain volume is modifiable for optimal functionality.[118,119] To maximize brain reserve and overall well-being in those living with MS, patient data point need to be regularly monitored so that the health care team can provide education and address modifiable risk factors related to long-term neurologic functioning.[120] Primary care or preventive care is needed for age-appropriate health screening, staying up-to-date with immunizations, and management of medical comorbidities. Routine education on factors like body mass index (BMI), blood pressure, lipids, blood sugar, and smoking status is important because health-related quality of life is linked to the ability to access information on preventive lifestyle behaviors.[121] Further, a growing body of research suggesting that MS and cardiovascular risk factors may compound upon one another further emphasizes the need to urgently address modifiable behaviors.[122–124]

Education and engagement with patients and their families is key to promoting wellness in the MS population. This can be achieved through strategies such as clarifying patient priorities, motivational interviewing, and shared decision making. Motivational interviewing is a technique that can be used to clarify a patient's goals, listen, support, motivate, self-regulate, and identify barriers to goal achievement.[125] Motivational interviewing has been shown to improve outcomes in patients with MS when combined with counseling or rehabilitation, when used individually or in a group setting.[126] The duration of positive outcomes from motivational interviewing may be limited, suggesting a need for repetition and close monitoring.

Shared decision making is a collaborative process between the patient, their family, and health care professionals to clarify the patient's priorities as well as their current and past experiences. Shared decision making has shown a positive effect on patient adherence to MS therapies, thereby promoting optimal disease management and outcomes.[127] Improved long-term outcomes can be seen with a focus on the patient's preferences and involving them in focused discussions. Clarifying the priorities of the patient and their family may broadly enhance well-being with physical, psychological, and social benefits for those living with MS. Setting goals with measurable outcomes and continuously assessing the achievement of those goals can further help to bolster wellness and improve brain reserve.

### *Lifestyle*

Lifestyle wellness management is complex and requires a comprehensive team approach. General health, nutrition, exercise, sleep, vitamin D, mood disorder screening, and social connection assessment are the mainstay of a well-being program while living with MS. Comprehensive wellness plans need to start with education, support, and assisting the patient and their care partners in removing barriers to care. We regularly monitor the wellness data points and confirm our patients have a primary care physician. We review the lifestyle practices that are detrimental to short- and long-term brain health in the general population and likely in MS including excessive alcohol, nicotine in all forms, physical immobility, obesity, and social isolation.[112,113,128] We work with patients and their care partners to educate, find resources, and support them in achieving their wellness goals. We routinely clarify current patient wellness goals and use shared decision making and motivational interviewing to help them achieve those goals.

Nutritional planning is a common topic of concern among patients with MS. The optimal nutritional scheme for patients with MS remains elusive, but ongoing research in this arena is encouraging.[129] Nutrition-based interventions have been considered for decades as a part of MS management with variable success. Some research has supported the notion that healthier diets might decrease the risk of MS while more unhealthy diets may increase MS risk.[130,131] Randomized controlled trials comparing a modified anti-inflammatory diet to a standard Western diet showed significant positive changes in MS disease outcomes and immune markers with the anti-inflammatory diet.[132] Small studies of caloric restriction and intermittent fasting have been associated with positive alterations in immune balance, lipid markers, and emotional health.[133,134] Interestingly, limited studies showed a negative impact of bariatric surgery in patients with MS with increased disability progression, although relapse rates were stable, with nutritional levels being thought to contribute to these findings.[135] Proposals to combine the ketogenic diet, which has been successful in epilepsy, with the Mediterranean diet have been raised but not yet confirmed as helpful for long-term MS outcomes.[136] Multiple studies are ongoing to clarify the optimal nutritional plan needed for those living with MS.

Exercise and physical activity have widespread benefits in MS, including with respect to immune cellular balance, neurotrophic factors, brain structure and function, walking, cognitive performance, fatigue, depression, pain, and quality of life. Regardless, there is much to be learned to guide comprehensive lifestyle choices in those living with MS.[137] The level of exercise needed likely varies according to many factors. Education, employment, clinical course, cognitive ability, depression, anxiety, fatigue, disease duration, and disability status are all associated with the intensity and the quantity of movement in those living with MS.[138] Further, patients with MS move significantly less than those without MS.[139–141] Exercise may also benefit cognitive functioning, although some studies suggest the primary benefit is limited to processing speed.[142] Resistance training is likely an important component of the MS exercise regimen, having been shown to be beneficial not only for strength, but also functional capacity, balance, and fatigue.[143] Patients can receive guidance from primary care, their neurologic care team, physical therapy, and occupational therapy in establishing, maintaining, and adjusting the amount of movement in their well-being plans.

Sleep efficacy can influence general health and wellness of patients with MS as well as their MS symptoms. Fatigue is one of the most common symptoms in those living with MS and routine monitoring of wellness data points should include factors that impact sleep hygiene such as mood disorders, lifestyle behaviors, tobacco smoking, alcohol use, medications, nutrition, and exercise.[144,145] Loneliness and lack of social support can also impact mood disorder risk, sleep quality, and overall MS outcomes.[146] Patients' social networks should regularly be monitored and considered a modifiable factor that may need to be fortified with social workers and other means of connecting patients to their communities.

### *Vitamin D*

Vitamin D status appears to be important in patients with MS, but there remains uncertainty about its therapeutic role for the disease.[147] Lower vitamin D levels are a risk factor of MS and clinically isolated syndrome,[148] whereas higher levels have been correlated with a lower risk of relapse.[149] Vitamin D may also improve response to steroids during MS relapses.[150] MS care should include oral supplementation of vitamin

**Table 4**
**Multiple sclerosis wellness strategies**

| | Office Visit Screening Modalities | Monitor | Recommendations | Resources |
|---|---|---|---|---|
| Mental health well-being | PHQ-9<br>GAD<br>QOL | History<br>Examination<br>Screening tests<br>Medications<br>Consultants | Screen for mood disorder each visit and address findings<br>Consultation and medication as indicated<br>Address wellness goals and barriers | Psychology<br>Psychiatry<br>Behavioral medicine<br>Social work<br>Counselors<br>Patient advocacy groups<br>Medications<br>PCP |
| Comorbidity prevention | | Vitals<br>History<br>Examination<br>PCP<br>Nutrition<br>Sleep<br>Alcohol use<br>Tobacco use<br>Social connection<br>Medication use<br>Illicit drug use<br>Wellness goals<br>Wellness barriers | Primary care intervention<br>Education on brain reserve while living with MS<br>Address wellness goals and barriers | Patient advocacy groups |
| Vital signs | Vital signs | | Primary care intervention<br>Educate on brain reserve while living with MS<br>Address wellness goals and barriers | |

(*continued on next page*)

**Table 4**
***(continued)***

| | Office Visit Screening Modalities | Monitor | Recommendations | Resources |
|---|---|---|---|---|
| Comorbidity management | Medical history<br>Medication review<br>Lab review | Address comorbidities | Primary care intervention<br>Educate on brain reserve while living with MS<br>Address wellness goals and barriers<br>Specialist intervention as needed | PCP<br>Specialist |
| Social well-being | QOL<br>History<br>Examination<br>Care provider review | Social resource needs<br>History<br>Examination<br>Care providers | Intervene and connect patient and care providers to social resources | PCP<br>Psychologist<br>Social work<br>Counselors<br>Occupational therapist<br>Patient advocacy groups |
| Nutrition | Vitals<br>History<br>Examination | Weight management goals<br>Nutritional goals and needs<br>Barriers to healthy nutrition | Primary care intervention | Nutritionist<br>Speech pathology<br>Patient advocacy groups |
| Exercise | Movement/week<br>Stretching history<br>ADLs | Regular exercise<br>Review resources and barriers | Regular exercise as tolerated<br>Address resources and barriers | Rehabilitation<br>Physical therapist<br>Occupational therapist<br>Patient advocacy groups |
| Tobacco/smoking/vaping<br>Moderate alcohol use | History<br>Examination | Smoking<br>Vaping<br>Chew | Cessation of all tobacco<br>Avoid excessive alcohol use<br>Primary care intervention | Psychology<br>Social work<br>Primary care providers<br>Health coach<br>Tobacco cessation programs<br>Community programs |

| | | | | |
|---|---|---|---|---|
| Weight management | History<br>Weight<br>Height<br>BMI<br>Goals | Normal BMI | Support healthy weight management<br>Set wellness goals<br>Address resources and barriers | Psychology<br>Social work<br>Primary care providers<br>Endocrinology<br>Health coach |
| Vitamin D | Vitamin D3 dose | Annual vitamin D levels | Maintain normal vitamin D level | Address vitamin D levels and maintain in the normal range |
| Sleep efficacy | Sleep hygiene<br>Fatigue<br>Sleep disorders<br>QOL | Efficient sleep | Efficient sleep | PCP<br>Sleep medicine<br>PT<br>OT<br>Behavioral medicine |

*Abbreviations:* PHQ-9, Patient Health Questionnaire 9; GAD-7, Generalized Anxiety Disorder 7; QOL, quality of life; PCP, primary care provider; ADLs, activities of daily living; PT, physical therapy; OT, occupational therapy.

D3 to maintain a normal vitamin D level, typically greater than 30 and less than 80 ng/mL, and to institute an annual vitamin D blood test to be sure the patient's levels remain in the normal range. An average adult may require daily supplementation of 2000 international units of vitamin D3 to maintain normal levels.[10] However, prospective clinical trials investigating vitamin D as a treatment have not confirmed its benefits.[151]

### *Wellness Management Considerations*

A comprehensive wellness strategy is needed in MS to address the preventable and modifiable risks that will positively affect long-term outcomes (**Table 4**). Educating patients about the concept of brain reserve and the need for lifelong wellness practices at the time of diagnosis is a key starting point. Following this, continuous monitoring of wellness data points, reinforcement of current wellness priorities, and assistance in removing care barriers are needed to successfully promote long-term well-being. Preventive care in the absence of mood disorders and physical comorbidities is the preferred method of wellness. However, if comorbidities are present, aggressive management to lessen their long-term impact on brain health and overall level of functioning is essential. Comprehensive wellness strategies are an important tool in combating the neurodegenerative aspect of MS and to help optimize long-term functional outcomes in patients with MS.

## SUMMARY

Management of mental health, physical comorbidities, and wellness practices are all important aspects of MS care. Mental health disorders are common in MS and can influence the well-being and mortality rates of those living with MS. Mental health disorders need to be routinely screened for and addressed due to increased prevalence in the MS population. Physical comorbidities are frequent in patients with MS and can affect quality of life, well-being, and mortality rates. Assuring that mental and physical comorbidities are routinely screened for and addressed early and successfully is imperative to functional outcomes in MS. Wellness concepts should be introduced at the time of diagnosis and routinely reassessed through capture of wellness data points. Patient priorities should be clarified and supported with tools such as shared decision making and motivational interviewing used to educate, support, and counsel patients with MS. A comprehensive team-based approach to MS care has the opportunity to enhance and engage both those living with MS and their caregivers for optimal living.

## DISCLOSURE

D.S. Conway has received research support paid to his institution from Novartis Pharmaceuticals, Biogen, United States, Bristol Myers Squibbs, EMD Serono, United States, and Arena Pharmaceuticals. He has received consulting fees from Novartis, Bristol Myers Squibbs, and Horizon Therapeutics and speaking fees from Biogen. Amy Sullivan has received consulting fees from Novartis, Switzerland, Biogen, Genentech, United States, Bristol Myers Squibb and EMD Serono. Mary Rensel has received research funding (PPD, Novartis, Biogen, Genentech, Connor B Judge (CBJ) Foundation and National Multiple Sclerosis), patient education funds (Genzyme, CBJ Foundation) she also served on Data Safety Monitoring Committee (DSMC) for Biogen was a speaker or consultant for (Serono, Novartis, Genentech, Genzyme, United States, Horizon, TG Therapeutics, Improve Consulting, Bristol Myers Squibb (BMS and Cycle), Kijia and Multiple Sclerosis Association of America (MSAA) and is Founder of Brain Fresh LLC and Co-Founder of Brain Ops Group.

## CLINICS CARE POINTS

- Patients with MS are at high risk for mood disorders including depression, anxiety, and BPD. Stress is an important factor that may worsen MS symptoms and have an effect on the immune system. Powerful interventions exist, including CBT, and should be considered for patients with MS, particularly during stressful periods such as at the time of diagnosis.
- Comorbidities affect patients with MS in a number of ways, including more rapid disability accumulation with certain coexisting health conditions. Individuals with MS also experience some comorbidities at higher rates than the general population and DMT can increase the risk of some health conditions. Appropriate counseling and management is an essential part of MS care and is likely to require a multidisciplinary team that includes primary care and relevant specialists.
- Wellness is a multifaceted concept that is highly relevant to patients with MS. Addressing modifiable factors including tobacco cessation, maintaining a healthy diet, and exercise are likely to maximize wellness and also brain reserve, which may lead to improved outcomes in patients with MS. Engagement with patients and their families through techniques such as shared decision making is an important strategy to help promote wellness.
- DMT is an important aspect of MS care, but numerous other opportunities exist for improving quality of life in patients with MS. Addressing deleterious patient characteristics that are modifiable through treatment and lifestyle changes, especially when done in concert with DMT, are likely to lead to the best long-term outcomes for patients.

## REFERENCES


1. Olek MJ. Multiple Sclerosis. Ann Intern Med 2021;174(6):ITC81–96.
2. Higuera L, Carlin CS, Anderson S. Adherence to Disease-Modifying Therapies for Multiple Sclerosis. J Manag care Spec Pharm 2016;22(12):1394–401.
3. Fruewald S, Loeffler-Stastka H, Eher R, et al. Depression and quality of life in multiple sclerosis. Acta Neurol Scand 2001;104(5):257–61.
4. Wood B, Van Der Mei IAF, Ponsonby AL, et al. Prevalence and concurrence of anxiety, depression and fatigue over time in multiple sclerosis. Mult Scler 2013; 19(2):217–24.
5. Alschuler KN, Ehde DM, Jensen MP. Co-occurring depression and pain in multiple sclerosis. Phys Med Rehabil Clin N Am 2013;24(4):703–15.
6. Thormann A, Sorensen PS, Koch-Henriksen N, et al. Comorbidity in multiple sclerosis is associated with diagnostic delays and increased mortality. Neurology 2017;89(16):1668–75.
7. Dossi DE, Chaves H, Heck ES, et al. Effects of Systolic Blood Pressure on Brain Integrity in Multiple Sclerosis. Front Neurol 2018;9(JUN). https://doi.org/10.3389/FNEUR.2018.00487.
8. Schreiner TG, Genes TM. Obesity and Multiple Sclerosis-A Multifaceted Association. J Clin Med 2021;10(12). https://doi.org/10.3390/JCM10122689.
9. Weinstock-Guttman B, Zivadinov R, Mahfooz N, et al. Serum lipid profiles are associated with disability and MRI outcomes in multiple sclerosis. J Neuroinflammation 2011;8:127.
10. Moss BP, Rensel MR, Hersh CM. Wellness and the Role of Comorbidities in Multiple Sclerosis. Neurotherapeutics 2017;14(4):999–1017.
11. Motl RW, Sandroff BM, Kwakkel G, et al. Exercise in patients with multiple sclerosis. Pers View Lancet Neurol 2017;16:848–56. Available at: www.thelancet.com/neurology. Accessed December 29, 2022.

12. Di Cara M, Grezzo D, Palmeri R, et al. Psychological well-being in people with multiple sclerosis: a descriptive review of the effects obtained with mindfulness interventions. Neurol Sci 2022;43(1):211–7.
13. Stoiloudis P, Kesidou E, Bakirtzis C, et al. The Role of Diet and Interventions on Multiple Sclerosis: A Review. Nutrients 2022;14(6). https://doi.org/10.3390/NU14061150.
14. Yusuf FLA, Ng BC, Wijnands JMA, et al. A systematic review of morbidities suggestive of the multiple sclerosis prodrome. Expert Rev Neurother 2020;20(8):799–819.
15. Fischer A, Heesen C, Gold SM. Biological outcome measurements for behavioral interventions in multiple sclerosis. Ther Adv Neurol Disord 2011;4(4):217–29.
16. Marrie RA, Reingold S, Cohen J, et al. The incidence and prevalence of psychiatric disorders in multiple sclerosis: a systematic review. Mult Scler 2015;21(3):305–17.
17. Schiffer RB, Arnett P, Ben-Zacharia A, et al. The Goldman Consensus statement on depression in multiple sclerosis. Mult Scler 2005;11(3):328–37.
18. Taylor L, Wicks P, Leigh PN, et al. Prevalence of depression in amyotrophic lateral sclerosis and other motor disorders. Eur J Neurol 2010;17(8):1047–53.
19. Sadovnick AD, Eisen K, Ebers GC, et al. Cause of death in patients attending multiple sclerosis clinics. Neurology 1991;41(8):1193–6.
20. Pompili M, Forte A, Palermo M, et al. Suicide risk in multiple sclerosis: a systematic review of current literature. J Psychosom Res 2012;73(6):411–7.
21. Kellerman QD, Hartoonian N, Beier ML, et al. Risk Factors for Suicide in a National Sample of Veterans With Multiple Sclerosis. Arch Phys Med Rehabil 2020;101(7):1138–43.
22. Mikula P, Timkova V, Linkova M, et al. Fatigue and Suicidal Ideation in People With Multiple Sclerosis: The Role of Social Support. Front Psychol 2020;11.
23. Ploughman M, Downer MB, Pretty RW, et al. The impact of resilience on healthy aging with multiple sclerosis. Qual Life Res 2020;29(10):2769–79.
24. Zettl UK, Schreiber H, Bauer-Steinhusen U, et al. Baseline predictors of persistence to first disease-modifying treatment in multiple sclerosis. Acta Neurol Scand 2017;136(2):116–21.
25. Chrousos GP. Stress and disorders of the stress system. Nat Rev Endocrinol 2009;5(7):374–81.
26. Reynard AK, Sullivan AB, Rae-Grant A. A systematic review of stress-management interventions for multiple sclerosis patients. Int J MS Care 2014;16(3):140–4.
27. Artemiadis AK, Anagnostouli MC, Alexopoulos EC. Stress as a risk factor for multiple sclerosis onset or relapse: a systematic review. Neuroepidemiology 2011;36(2):109–20.
28. Bennett JL, Stüve O. Update on inflammation, neurodegeneration, and immunoregulation in multiple sclerosis: therapeutic implications. Clin Neuropharmacol 2009;32(3):121–32.
29. Flachenecker P, Reiners K, Krauser M, et al. Autonomic dysfunction in multiple sclerosis is related to disease activity and progression of disability. Mult Scler 2001;7(5):327–34.
30. Flachenecker P, Rufer A, Bihler I, et al. Fatigue in MS is related to sympathetic vasomotor dysfunction. Neurology 2003;61(6):851–3.
31. Gunal DI, Afsar N, Tanridag T, et al. Autonomic dysfunction in multiple sclerosis: correlation with disease-related parameters. Eur Neurol 2002;48(1):1–5.

32. Pittion-Vouyovitch S, Debouverie M, Guillemin F, et al. Fatigue in multiple sclerosis is related to disability, depression and quality of life. J Neurol Sci 2006;243(1–2):39–45.
33. Selye H. The general adaptation syndrome and the diseases of adaptation. J Clin Endocrinol Metab 1946;6:117–230.
34. Sapolsky RM, Romero LM, Munck AU. How do glucocorticoids influence stress responses? Integrating permissive, suppressive, stimulatory, and preparative actions. Endocr Rev 2000;21(1):55–89.
35. Selye H. The stresses of life. New York: Mc Graw Hill; 1956. p. 516.
36. Diamond BJ, Johnson SK, Kaufman M, et al. Relationships between information processing, depression, fatigue and cognition in multiple sclerosis. Arch Clin Neuropsychol 2008;23(2):189–99.
37. Dennison L, Moss-Morris R, Chalder T. A review of psychological correlates of adjustment in patients with multiple sclerosis. Clin Psychol Rev 2009;29(2):141–53.
38. Dennison L, Moss-Morris R. Cognitive-behavioral therapy: what benefits can it offer people with multiple sclerosis? Expert Rev Neurother 2010;10(9):1383–90.
39. Chwastiak L, Ehde DM, Gibbons LE, et al. Depressive symptoms and severity of illness in multiple sclerosis: epidemiologic study of a large community sample. Am J Psychiatr 2002;159(11):1862–8.
40. Greenberg B, Fan Y, Carriere L, et al. Depression and Age at First Neurology Appointment Associated with Receipt of Behavioral Medicine Services Within 1 Year in a Multiple Sclerosis Population. Int J MS Care 2017;19(4):199–207.
41. Mohr DC, Lovera J, Brown T, et al. A randomized trial of stress management for the prevention of new brain lesions in MS. Neurology 2012;79(5):412–9.
42. Van Kessel K, Moss-Morris R, Willoughby E, et al. A randomized controlled trial of cognitive behavior therapy for multiple sclerosis fatigue. Psychosom Med 2008;70(2):205–13.
43. Sung C, Chiu CY, Lee EJ, et al. Exercise, Diet, and Stress Management as Mediators Between Functional Disability and Health-Related Quality of Life in Multiple Sclerosis. Rehabil Counsel Bull 2013;56(2):85–95.
44. Minden SL, Feinstein A, Kalb RC, et al. Evidence-based guideline: assessment and management of psychiatric disorders in individuals with MS: report of the Guideline Development Subcommittee of the American Academy of Neurology. Neurology 2014;82(2):174–81.
45. Spitzer RL, Kroenke K, Williams JB. Validation and utility of a self-report version of PRIME-MD: the PHQ primary care study. Primary Care Evaluation of Mental Disorders. Patient Health Questionnaire. JAMA 1999;282(18):1737–44. Available at: http://www.ncbi.nlm.nih.gov/entrez/query.fcgi?cmd=Retrieve&db=PubMed&dopt=Citation&list_uids=10568646.
46. Terrill AL, Hartoonian N, Beier M, et al. The 7-item generalized anxiety disorder scale as a tool for measuring generalized anxiety in multiple sclerosis. Int J MS Care 2015;17(2):49–56.
47. Patrick S, Connick P. Psychometric properties of the PHQ-9 depression scale in people with multiple sclerosis: A systematic review. PLoS One 2019;14(2). https://doi.org/10.1371/JOURNAL.PONE.0197943.
48. Hughes AJ, Dunn KM, Chaffee T, et al. Diagnostic and Clinical Utility of the GAD-2 for Screening Anxiety Symptoms in Individuals With Multiple Sclerosis. Arch Phys Med Rehabil 2018;99(10):2045–9.
49. Mowry EM, Bermel RA, Williams JR, et al. Harnessing Real-World Data to Inform Decision-Making: Multiple Sclerosis Partners Advancing Technology and Health

Solutions (MS PATHS). Front Neurol 2020;11. https://doi.org/10.3389/FNEUR.2020.00632.
50. Raissi A, Bulloch AGM, Fiest KM, et al. Exploration of Undertreatment and Patterns of Treatment of Depression in Multiple Sclerosis. Int J MS Care 2015;17(6):292–300.
51. Nathoo N, Mackie A. Treating depression in multiple sclerosis with antidepressants: A brief review of clinical trials and exploration of clinical symptoms to guide treatment decisions. Mult Scler Relat Disord 2017;18:177–80.
52. Davidson JRT. Major depressive disorder treatment guidelines in America and Europe. J Clin Psychiatry 2010;71(Suppl E1).
53. Thomas PW, Thomas S, Hillier C, et al. Psychological interventions for multiple sclerosis. Cochrane Database Syst Rev 2006;2006(1). https://doi.org/10.1002/14651858.CD004431.PUB2.
54. Plow MA, Finlayson M, Rezac M. A scoping review of self-management interventions for adults with multiple sclerosis. Pharm Manag PM R 2011;3(3):251–62.
55. Kabat-Zinn J, Massion AO, Kristeller J, et al. Effectiveness of a meditation-based stress reduction program in the treatment of anxiety disorders. Am J Psychiatr 1992;149(7):936–43.
56. Feinstein A, Magalhaes S, Richard JF, et al. The link between multiple sclerosis and depression. Nat Rev Neurol 2014;10(9):507–17.
57. Marrie RA, Horwitz R, Cutter G, et al. Comorbidity delays diagnosis and increases disability at diagnosis in MS. Neurology 2009;72(2):117–24, 5f [doi].
58. Conway DS, Thompson NR, Cohen JA. Influence of hypertension, diabetes, hyperlipidemia, and obstructive lung disease on multiple sclerosis disease course. Mult Scler 2017;23(2):277–85.
59. Marrie RA, Elliott L, Marriott J, et al. Effect of comorbidity on mortality in multiple sclerosis. Neurology 2015;85(3):240–7.
60. Sierra C. Essential hypertension, cerebral white matter pathology and ischemic stroke. Curr Med Chem 2014;21(19):2156–64.
61. Moroni F, Ammirati E, Rocca MA, et al. Cardiovascular disease and brain health: Focus on white matter hyperintensities. IJC Hear Vasc 2018;19:63–9.
62. Marrie RA, Fisk J, Tremlett H, et al. Differing trends in the incidence of vascular comorbidity in MS and the general population. Neurol Clin Pract 2016;6(2):120–8.
63. Conrad N, Verbeke G, Molenberghs G, et al. Autoimmune diseases and cardiovascular risk: a population-based study on 19 autoimmune diseases and 12 cardiovascular diseases in 22 million individuals in the UK. Lancet (London, England) 2022;400(10354):733–43.
64. Marrie RA, Reider N, Cohen J, et al. A systematic review of the incidence and prevalence of cancer in multiple sclerosis. Mult Scler 2015;21(3):294–304.
65. Marrie RA, Rudick R, Horwitz R, et al. Vascular comorbidity is associated with more rapid disability progression in multiple sclerosis. Neurology 2010;74(13):1041–7 [doi].
66. Salter A, Kowalec K, Fitzgerald KC, et al. Comorbidity is associated with disease activity in MS: Findings from the CombiRx trial. Neurology 2020;95(5):E446–56.
67. Kowalec K, McKay KA, Patten SB, et al. Comorbidity increases the risk of relapse in multiple sclerosis: A prospective study. Neurology 2017;89(24):2455–61.
68. O'Gorman C, Bukhari W, Todd A, et al. Smoking increases the risk of multiple sclerosis in Queensland, Australia. J Clin Neurosci 2014;21(10):1730–3.

69. Asadollahi S, Fakhri M, Heidari K, et al. Cigarette smoking and associated risk of multiple sclerosis in the Iranian population. J Clin Neurosci 2013;20(12): 1747–50.
70. Degelman ML, Herman KM. Smoking and multiple sclerosis: A systematic review and meta-analysis using the Bradford Hill criteria for causation. Mult Scler Relat Disord 2017;17:207–16.
71. Nourbakhsh B, Mowry EM. Multiple Sclerosis Risk Factors and Pathogenesis. Continuum 2019;25(3):596–610.
72. Olsson T, Barcellos LF, Alfredsson L. Interactions between genetic, lifestyle and environmental risk factors for multiple sclerosis. Nat Rev Neurol 2017;13(1): 26–36.
73. Hersh CM, Harris H, Ayers M, et al. Effect of tobacco use on disease activity and DMT discontinuation in multiple sclerosis patients treated with dimethyl fumarate or fingolimod. Mult Scler J - Exp Transl Clin. 2020;6(4). 205521732095981.
74. Healy BC, Ali EN, Guttmann CRG, et al. Smoking and disease progression in multiple sclerosis. Arch Neurol 2009;66(7):858–64.
75. Roudbari SA, Ansar MM, Yousefzad A. Smoking as a risk factor for development of Secondary Progressive Multiple Sclerosis: A study in IRAN, Guilan. J Neurol Sci 2013;330(1–2):52–5.
76. Cohen JA, Tenenbaum N, Bhatt A, et al. Extended treatment with fingolimod for relapsing multiple sclerosis:the 14-year LONGTERMS study results. Ther Adv Neurol Disord 2019;12.
77. Teriflunomide (AUBAGIO. Multiple sclerosis: just a metabolite of leflunomide. Prescrire Int 2015;24(158):61–4. Available at: https://pubmed.ncbi.nlm.nih.gov/25897452/. Accessed May 11, 2023.
78. Shosha E, Casserly C, Tomkinson C, et al. Blood pressure changes during alemtuzumab infusion for multiple sclerosis patients. Eur J Neurol 2021;28(4): 1396–400.
79. Briggs FBS, Hill E, Abboud H. The prevalence of hypertension in multiple sclerosis based on 37 million electronic health records from the United States. Eur J Neurol 2021;28(2):558–66.
80. Briggs FBS, Krill D, Hill E, et al. Age of hypertension onset in multiple sclerosis patients. Mult Scler 2021;27(13):2108–11.
81. Marrie RA, Kosowan L, Singer A. Management of diabetes and hypertension in people with multiple sclerosis. Mult Scler Relat Disord 2020;40.
82. Conway DS, Briggs FB, Mowry EM, et al. Racial disparities in hypertension management among multiple sclerosis patients. Mult Scler Relat Disord 2022;64: 103972.
83. Robers M, Chan C, Vajdi B, et al. Hypertension and hypertension severity in Hispanics/LatinX with MS. Mult Scler J 2021;(12):1894–901.
84. Conway DS, Marck CH. Comorbidities require special attention in minorities with multiple sclerosis. Mult Scler 2021;27(12):1811–3.
85. Geraldes R, Esiri MM, Perera R, et al. Vascular disease and multiple sclerosis: a post-mortem study exploring their relationships. Brain 2020;143(10):2998–3012.
86. Melamed E, Lee MW. Multiple Sclerosis and Cancer: The Ying-Yang Effect of Disease Modifying Therapies. Front Immunol 2020;10. https://doi.org/10.3389/FIMMU.2019.02954.
87. Poirier AE, Ruan Y, Volesky KD, et al. The current and future burden of cancer attributable to modifiable risk factors in Canada: Summary of results. Prev Med 2019;122:140–7.

88. Salzer J, Hallmans G, Nyström M, et al. Smoking as a risk factor for multiple sclerosis. Mult Scler 2013;19(8):1022–7.
89. Munger KL, Chitnis T, Ascherio A. Body size and risk of MS in two cohorts of US women. Neurology 2009;73(19):1543–50.
90. Marrie RA, Maxwell C, Mahar A, et al. Cancer Incidence and Mortality Rates in Multiple Sclerosis: A Matched Cohort Study. Neurology 2021;96(4):e501–12.
91. Marrie RA, Cohen J, Stuve O, et al. A systematic review of the incidence and prevalence of comorbidity in multiple sclerosis: overview. Mult Scler 2015; 21(3):263–81.
92. Marrie RA, Maxwell C, Mahar A, et al. Breast Cancer Survival in Multiple Sclerosis: A Matched Cohort Study. Neurology 2021;97(1):e13–22.
93. Ge F, Huo Z, Li C, et al. Lung cancer risk in patients with multiple sclerosis: a Mendelian randomization analysis. Mult Scler Relat Disord 2021;51. https://doi.org/10.1016/J.MSARD.2021.102927.
94. Nørgaard M, Veres K, Didden EM, et al. Multiple sclerosis and cancer incidence: A Danish nationwide cohort study. Mult Scler Relat Disord 2019;28:81–5.
95. Giovannoni G, Comi G, Cook S, et al. A Placebo-Controlled Trial of Oral Cladribine for Relapsing Multiple Sclerosis. N Engl J Med 2010;362(5):416–26. Available at: http://www.ncbi.nlm.nih.gov/entrez/query.fcgi?cmd=Retrieve&db=PubMed&dopt=Citation&list_uids=20089960.
96. Giovannoni G, Soelberg Sorensen P, Cook S, et al. Safety and efficacy of cladribine tablets in patients with relapsing–remitting multiple sclerosis: Results from the randomized extension trial of the CLARITY study. Mult Scler J 2018;24(12): 1594–604.
97. Pakpoor J, Disanto G, Altmann DR, et al. No evidence for higher risk of cancer in patients with multiple sclerosis taking cladribine. Neurol Neuroimmunol neuroinflammation 2015;2(6). https://doi.org/10.1212/NXI.0000000000000158.
98. Hauser SL, Bar-Or A, Comi G, et al. Ocrelizumab versus Interferon Beta-1a in Relapsing Multiple Sclerosis. N Engl J Med 2017;376(3):221–34 [doi].
99. Montalban X, Hauser SL, Kappos L, et al. Ocrelizumab versus Placebo in Primary Progressive Multiple Sclerosis. N Engl J Med 2017;376(3):209–20 [doi].
100. Hauser SL, Kappos L, Montalban X, et al. Safety of Ocrelizumab in Patients With Relapsing and Primary Progressive Multiple Sclerosis. Neurology 2021;97(16): E1546–59.
101. Stamatellos VP, Rigas A, Stamoula E, et al. S1P receptor modulators in Multiple Sclerosis: Detecting a potential skin cancer safety signal. Mult Scler Relat Disord 2022;59.
102. Velter C, Thomas M, Cavalcanti A, et al. Melanoma during fingolimod treatment for multiple sclerosis. Eur J Cancer 2019;113:75–7.
103. Carbone ML, Lacal PM, Messinese S, et al. Multiple Sclerosis Treatment and Melanoma Development. Int J Mol Sci 2020;21(8). https://doi.org/10.3390/IJMS21082950.
104. Hill E, Abboud H, Briggs FBS. Prevalence of asthma in multiple sclerosis: A United States population-based study. Mult Scler Relat Disord 2019;28:69–74.
105. Sorensen A, Conway DS, Briggs FBS. Characterizing relapsing remitting multiple sclerosis patients burdened with hypertension, hyperlipidemia, and asthma. Mult Scler Relat Disord 2021;53:103040.
106. Wang L, Zhang J, Deng ZR, et al. The epidemiology of primary headaches in patients with multiple sclerosis. Brain Behav 2021;11(1). https://doi.org/10.1002/BRB3.1830.

107. Fragoso YD, Adoni T, Gomes S, et al. Persistent headache in patients with multiple sclerosis starting treatment with fingolimod. Headache 2015;55(4):578–9.
108. Mrabet S, Wafa M, Giovannoni G. Multiple sclerosis and migraine: Links, management and implications. Mult Scler Relat Disord 2022;68. https://doi.org/10.1016/J.MSARD.2022.104152.
109. Dobson R, Giovannoni G. Autoimmune disease in people with multiple sclerosis and their relatives: a systematic review and meta-analysis. J Neurol 2013; 260(5):1272–85.
110. Marrie RA, Horwitz R, Cutter G, et al. Comorbidity, socioeconomic status and multiple sclerosis. Mult Scler 2008;14(8):1091–8.
111. Lo LMP, Taylor BV, Winzenberg T, et al. Comorbidity patterns in people with multiple sclerosis: A latent class analysis of the Australian Multiple Sclerosis Longitudinal Study. Eur J Neurol 2021;28(7):2269–79.
112. Cecchini M, Sassi F, Lauer JA, et al. Tackling of unhealthy diets, physical inactivity, and obesity: health effects and cost-effectiveness. Lancet (London, England) 2010;376(9754):1775–84.
113. Livingston G, Huntley J, Sommerlad A, et al. Dementia prevention, intervention, and care: 2020 report of the Lancet Commission. Lancet (London, England) 2020;396(10248):413–46.
114. Pan Y, Li H, Wardlaw JM, et al. A new dawn of preventing dementia by preventing cerebrovascular diseases. BMJ 2020;371. https://doi.org/10.1136/BMJ.M3692.
115. Giovannoni G, Butzkueven H, Dhib-Jalbut S, et al. Brain health: time matters in multiple sclerosis. Mult Scler Relat Disord 2016;9(Suppl 1):S5–48 [doi].
116. Motl RW, Mowry EM, Ehde DM, et al. Wellness and multiple sclerosis: The National MS Society establishes a Wellness Research Working Group and research priorities. Mult Scler 2018;24(3):262–7.
117. Sumowski JF, Chiaravalloti N, DeLuca J. Cognitive reserve protects against cognitive dysfunction in multiple sclerosis. J Clin Exp Neuropsychol 2009; 31(8):913–26.
118. Christova P, Joseph J, Georgopoulos AP. Human Connectome Project: heritability of brain volumes in young healthy adults. Exp Brain Res 2021;239(4): 1273–86.
119. Sumowski JF, Rocca MA, Leavitt VM, et al. Brain reserve and cognitive reserve in multiple sclerosis: what you've got and how you use it. Neurology 2013; 80(24):2186–93.
120. Brandstadter R, Katz Sand I, Sumowski JF. Beyond rehabilitation: A prevention model of reserve and brain maintenance in multiple sclerosis. Mult Scler 2019; 25(10):1372–8.
121. Faraclas E, Merlo A, Lynn J, et al. Perceived facilitators, needs, and barriers to health related quality of life in people with multiple sclerosis: a qualitative investigation. J patient-reported outcomes 2022;6(1). https://doi.org/10.1186/S41687-022-00496-1.
122. Wang Y, Bos SD, Harbo HF, et al. Genetic overlap between multiple sclerosis and several cardiovascular disease risk factors. Mult Scler 2016;22(14): 1783–93.
123. Wens I, Dalgas U, Deckx N, et al. Does multiple sclerosis affect glucose tolerance? Mult Scler 2014;20(9):1273–6.
124. Keytsman C, Eijnde BO, Hansen D, et al. Elevated cardiovascular risk factors in multiple sclerosis. Mult Scler Relat Disord 2017;17:220–3.

125. Hardcastle S, Hagger MS. "You Can't Do It on Your Own": Experiences of a motivational interviewing intervention on physical activity and dietary behaviour. Psychol Sport Exerc 2011;12(3):314–23.
126. Dorstyn DS, Mathias JL, Bombardier CH, et al. Motivational interviewing to promote health outcomes and behaviour change in multiple sclerosis: a systematic review. Clin Rehabil 2020;34(3):299–309.
127. Ben-Zacharia A, Adamson M, Boyd A, et al. Impact of Shared Decision Making on Disease-Modifying Drug Adherence in Multiple Sclerosis. Int J MS Care 2018;20(6):287–97.
128. Barnes DE, Yaffe K. The projected effect of risk factor reduction on Alzheimer's disease prevalence. Lancet Neurol 2011;10(9):819–28.
129. Russell RD, Black LJ, Begley A. Nutrition Education Programs for Adults with Neurological Diseases Are Lacking: A Scoping Review. Nutrients 2022;14(8). https://doi.org/10.3390/NU14081577.
130. Keykhaei F, Norouzy S, Froughipour M, et al. Adherence to healthy dietary pattern is associated with lower risk of multiple sclerosis. J Cent Nerv Syst Dis 2022;14. https://doi.org/10.1177/11795735221092516. 117957352210925.
131. Hajianfar H, Mirmossayeb O, Mollaghasemi N, et al. Association between dietary inflammatory index and risk of demyelinating autoimmune diseases. Int J Vitam Nutr Res 2022. https://doi.org/10.1024/0300-9831/A000754.
132. Mousavi-Shirazi-Fard Z, Mazloom Z, Izadi S, et al. The effects of modified anti-inflammatory diet on fatigue, quality of life, and inflammatory biomarkers in relapsing-remitting multiple sclerosis patients: a randomized clinical trial. Int J Neurosci 2021;131(7):657–65.
133. Fitzgerald KC, Bhargava P, Smith MD, et al. Intermittent calorie restriction alters T cell subsets and metabolic markers in people with multiple sclerosis. EBioMedicine 2022;82. https://doi.org/10.1016/J.EBIOM.2022.104124.
134. Fitzgerald KC, Tyry T, Salter A, et al. Diet quality is associated with disability and symptom severity in multiple sclerosis. Neurology 2018;90(1):E1–11.
135. Anna Karin H, Erik S, Tim S, et al. The impact of bariatric surgery on disease activity and progression of multiple sclerosis: A nationwide matched cohort study. Mult Scler 2022;28(13):2099–105.
136. Di Majo D, Cacciabaudo F, Accardi G, et al. Ketogenic and Modified Mediterranean Diet as a Tool to Counteract Neuroinflammation in Multiple Sclerosis: Nutritional Suggestions. Nutrients 2022;14(12). https://doi.org/10.3390/NU14122384.
137. Motl RW, Fernhall B, McCully KK, et al. Lessons learned from clinical trials of exercise and physical activity in people with MS - guidance for improving the quality of future research. Mult Scler Relat Disord 2022;68. https://doi.org/10.1016/J.MSARD.2022.104088.
138. Motl RW, Sandroff BM. Benefits of Exercise Training in Multiple Sclerosis. Curr Neurol Neurosci Rep 2015;15(9):1–9.
139. Klaren RE, Motl RW, Dlugonski D, et al. Objectively quantified physical activity in persons with multiple sclerosis. Arch Phys Med Rehabil 2013;94(12):2342–8.
140. Huynh TLT, Silveira SL, Jeng B, et al. Association of disease outcomes with physical activity in multiple sclerosis: A cross-sectional study. Rehabil Psychol 2022;67(3):421–9.
141. Sullivan AB, Covington E, Scheman J. Immediate benefits of a brief 10-minute exercise protocol in a chronic pain population: a pilot study. Pain Med 2010;11(4):524–9.
142. Motl RW, Sandroff BM, Benedict RHB. Moderate-to-vigorous physical activity is associated with processing speed, but not learning and memory, in cognitively

impaired persons with multiple sclerosis. Mult Scler Relat Disord 2022;63. https://doi.org/10.1016/J.MSARD.2022.103833.
143. Andreu-Caravaca L, Ramos-Campo DJ, Chung LH, et al. Effects and optimal dosage of resistance training on strength, functional capacity, balance, general health perception, and fatigue in people with multiple sclerosis: a systematic review and meta-analysis. Disabil Rehabil 2022. https://doi.org/10.1080/09638288.2022.2069295.
144. Novak AM, Lev-Ari S. Resilience, Stress, Well-Being, and Sleep Quality in Multiple Sclerosis. J Clin Med 2023;12(2). https://doi.org/10.3390/JCM12020716.
145. Newland P, Lorenz RA, Smith JM, et al. The Relationship Among Multiple Sclerosis-Related Symptoms, Sleep Quality, and Sleep Hygiene Behaviors. J Neurosci Nurs 2019;51(1):37–42.
146. Reyes S, Suarez S, Allen-Philbey K, et al. The impact of social capital on patients with multiple sclerosis. Acta Neurol Scand 2020;142(1):58–65.
147. Miclea A, Bagnoud M, Chan A, et al. A Brief Review of the Effects of Vitamin D on Multiple Sclerosis. Front Immunol 2020;11. https://doi.org/10.3389/FIMMU.2020.00781.
148. Munger KL, Levin LI, Hollis BW, et al. Serum 25-hydroxyvitamin D levels and risk of multiple sclerosis. JAMA 2006;296(23):2832–8.
149. Simpson S, Taylor B, Blizzard L, et al. Higher 25-hydroxyvitamin D is associated with lower relapse risk in multiple sclerosis. Ann Neurol 2010;68(2):193–203.
150. Hoepner R, Bagnoud M, Pistor M, et al. Vitamin D increases glucocorticoid efficacy via inhibition of mTORC1 in experimental models of multiple sclerosis. Acta Neuropathol 2019;138(3):443–56.
151. Fatima M, Lamis A, Siddiqui SW, et al. Therapeutic Role of Vitamin D in Multiple Sclerosis: An Essentially Contested Concept. Cureus 2022;14(6). https://doi.org/10.7759/CUREUS.26186.

# Clinical and Treatment Considerations for the Pediatric and Aging Patients with Multiple Sclerosis

Areeba Siddiqui, MD[a,1], Jennifer H. Yang, MD[b,c,1], Le H. Hua, MD[a,*], Jennifer S. Graves, MD, PhD, MAS[b,c]

**KEYWORDS**

• Treatment • Management • Pediatric • Aging • Elderly • Progressive
• Multiple sclerosis

**KEY POINTS**

- Approximately 5% of patients with MS will have an initial onset before age 18 (pediatric-onset MS), while 2-12% will have onset after age 50 (late-onset MS).
- Sex hormone interactions with the immune system during times of puberty plays an important role in MS pathogenesis.
- While chronologic age is associated with clinical phenotypes of relapsing vs progressive MS, biological age measurements may be more useful in understanding non-relapse-related progression.
- The two age extremes (<18 and >50) offers unique insights into the complex interplay between neuroinflammation, senescence, environmental and epigenetic factors that influence risk of developing MS and disease course.

## INTRODUCTION

### *Epidemiology*

Most of the patients presenting with multiple sclerosis (MS) are in young or middle adulthood. However, approximately 5% have pediatric-onset MS (POMS), and with increasingly effective disease-modifying therapies (DMTs) and increasing age of the general population, the prevalence of MS has shifted to older ages. There is an estimated global prevalence of 2.8 million people living with MS, with an estimated

[a] Cleveland Clinic Lou Ruvo Center for Brain Health, 888 W. Bonneville Avenue, Las Vegas, NV 89106, USA; [b] Department of Neurosciences, University of California San Diego, 9500 Gilman Drive, Mail Code 0662, La Jolla, CA 92093, USA; [c] Division of Pediatric Neurology, Rady Children's Hospital, 3020 Children's Way MC 5009, San Diego, CA 92123, USA
[1] These authors share equal contributions.
* Corresponding author. Cleveland Clinic Lou Ruvo Center for Brain Health, 888 W Bonneville Avenue, Las Vegas, NV 89106
*E-mail address:* hual@ccf.org

Neurol Clin 42 (2024) 255–274
https://doi.org/10.1016/j.ncl.2023.07.003
neurologic.theclinics.com

913,925 persons affected in the United States. The peak prevalence is observed at ages 55 to 64 years in both females (656 per 100,000 individuals) and males (249.4 per 100,000 individuals).[1] The incidence of POMS is estimated to be 0.87 per 100,000 persons annually per data pooled from 18 studies globally.[2] At the end of the age spectrum, 2% to 12% of MS patients present with late-onset MS (LOMS; disease onset after 50 years of age).[3] The proportion of primary progressive MS cases in LOMS ranges from 50% to 80% based on multiple retrospective studies, and the sex ratio of women to men with LOMS is lower (1.4:1) than in patients with adult-onset MS (onset >18 years and ≤50 years; 2–3:1).[3–8]

The risk for developing MS is a complex interaction between genetic susceptibility and environmental influences. Based on monozygotic twin studies, the heritability of MS is approximately 25%.[9] Almost 50% of this heritability has now been explained by over 200 risk alleles for MS identified by genome-wide association studies, with *HLA-DRB1*15:01* being the strongest genetic risk factor. For both adults and children, carrying one copy of this risk allele confers threefold higher odds to have MS.[10] Although there is a high prevalence of MS in patients with northern European ancestries, MS impacts all populations around the world. The *HLA-DRB1*15:01* haplotype is the strongest risk allele in patients across different ancestries including African Americans, Hispanic, and Asian Americans.[11] Additional human leukocyte antigen (HLA) risk alleles have been identified for African Americans (HLA-DRB1*03:01, HLA-A*02:01, HLA-DRB1*14:01, HLA-B*38:01, HLA-DRB1*15:03). Lastly, a significant number of the less than 200 single-nucleotide polymorphisms associated with adult-onset MS have now been replicated in POMS,[10,12] lending further evidence to support the concept that POMS is the same disease as adult-onset MS.

The remainder of the risk for MS is related to environmental factors, gene environment interactions, and gene–gene interactions. Environmental factors for MS include infectious and noninfectious etiologies. Required but not sufficient to cause MS, Epstein–Barr virus (EBV) infection is a well-established risk factor for pediatric and adult MS.[12] A longitudinal cohort study of 10 million young adults enrolled in the US military before any diagnosis of neurologic disease followed their EBV infection status and MS diagnosis. The study found that EBV infection has a 32-fold increased risk for developing MS.[13] A case-control study in POMS found an increased risk for MS with EBV seropositivity with an odds ratio of 3.78 (95% CI 1.52–9.38).[14] Other environmental risk factors identified for MS include low vitamin D level, cigarette smoking and passive smoke exposure, obesity, gut microbiome, and perinatal factors.[12] High serum 25-hydroxy vitamin D levels in adolescence are associated with lower risk of MS later in life, though the studies did not account for ultraviolet radiation exposure.[15] To determine a more direct causal relationship, several Mendelian randomization studies demonstrated specific genetic variants affecting serum vitamin D levels that are associated with risk for MS, including genes that encode the vitamin D receptor.[16] Cigarette smoking and passive smoke exposure are associated with an increased risk of MS. Parental smoking is associated with POMS in a dose–responsive manner based on a population case-control study.[17] Obesity in childhood and adolescence is associated with MS risk in both children and adults with an increased risk observed in female patients.[18] The association between obesity and onset of MS is complicated by its interaction with other environmental and genetic factors. The risk for developing POMS has also been implicated with exposure to ozone pollution,[19] household chemicals,[20] and pesticides.[21] Conversely, there is a 60% lower odds of developing MS with maternal C-section suggesting that perinatal exposures, potentially its interactions with the gut microbiome, may play a role in MS susceptibility.[21]

Genetic and environmental and lifestyle factors may also influence MS disease course. Genetic ancestry may impact disease outcomes, but these associations are complex as health outcomes may be influenced by racism and social determinants of health.[22] In a study of pediatric MS, genetic ancestry was not associated with relapse rate in children.[23] Self-identified African American race has been associated with more severe MS progression, but these results require further inquiry into effects related to ancestry versus systemic issues in health care systems with regard to race.[22] Genetic polymorphism at the MS susceptibility loci for the gene *AHI1* was associated with relapse rate in children and adults[24] and in a genome wide search, polymorphism within *LRP2* gene was also associated with risk to relapse in children and adults.[25] Very recently, the first gene associated with disability progression was reported.[26] For environmental factors, low 25-hydroxyvitamin D levels are associated with higher rates of relapse and disability progression.[27] Higher vitamin D levels have been associated with decreased relapse risk in POMS patients who carry a risk allele for *HLA-DRB1*15:01 or 15:03*.[23] In a multicenter cohort study of pediatric patients, a 10% higher dietary fat intake increased the hazard for relapse by 56% and an additional cup of vegetables per day decreased relapse risk by 50%.[28] In a longitudinal study of patients with MS and clinically isolated syndrome, each 1 g/m$^2$ higher body mass index was associated with reduced normalized gray matter volume on MRI even after adjusting for vitamin D level, age, sex, ethnicity, smoking status, and DMT exposure.[29] A cross-sectional study demonstrated that higher physical activity in pediatric MS patients is associated with lower T2 lesion burden and relapse rates, though many factors play a role in this association.[30]

### *Influence of Sex Hormones on Disease Course*

Sex hormones also play an important role in MS pathogenesis. The overall sex ratio is 2 to 3:1 female to male in pediatric patients, although this ratio is closer to 1:1 in the prepubertal age group.[31] Only about 15% to 20% of pediatric MS patients have onset in prepuberty. Sex differences are more apparent after age 12 years, around the onset of menarche.[31] There is also an increased relapse rate during the peri-menarche period (within 1 year of menarche) compared with the post-menarche period.[32] Even among boys with MS, those who present during peri-puberty had over twofold increased relapse risk compared with those who presented postpuberty,[33] suggesting that sex hormone interactions with the immune system during times of developmental maturity drive disease processes in both sexes. Sexual dimorphism is well-recognized in adult-onset MS as well. Although the overall female-to-male ratio is closer to 3:1, in LOMS (>50 years) the incidence sex ratio is closer to 1:1.[34] Men may exhibit a progressive clinical picture earlier and more frequently than women.[35] In male patients, there is increased disability accumulation with less time to progression,[36] whereas female patients may experience a more inflammatory disease course with up to 20% more relapses than men.[37] However, postmenopausal women may be at higher risk of developing progressive disease, with a decline in circulating levels of estrogen.[38,39] In addition, testosterone has been shown to exert anti-inflammatory effects, with low levels of testosterone being associated with risk to have MS and possibly with worse disability.[40,41]

## CLINICAL DIAGNOSIS AND DISEASE PHENOTYPES ACROSS THE LIFESPAN

Chronologic age is one of the foremost determinants of clinical phenotype in MS.[39] Although onset of MS is primarily in young adulthood with a large majority manifesting an initial inflammatory relapsing-remitting course, an eventual predominance of

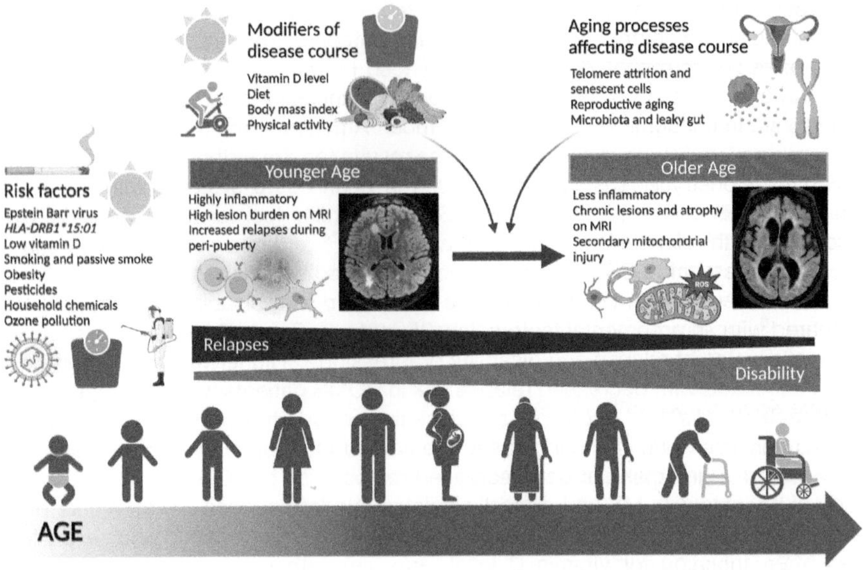


**Fig. 1.** MS phenotype and disease course across the lifespan. (*Adapted from* BioRender.com.)

progressive disability is observed with advancing age. Although neurodegenerative processes start at disease onset, disability progression may not be clinically apparent until decades later. Age may influence not only different proportions of types of MS-related central nervous system (CNS) injury but also resilience to this injury and capacity for repair and remyelination.[42]

## *Pediatric Multiple Sclerosis*

POMS has a predominant inflammatory phenotype with more than three times higher relapse rates compared with patients with adult-onset MS (**Fig. 1**).[43] Acute clinical presentations include optic neuritis, myelitis, cerebral, cerebellar, and brainstem syndromes. Children can present with a monofocal or polyfocal acquired demyelinating syndrome at disease onset and sometimes with high lesion burden on imaging that may be confused for acute disseminated encephalomyelitis-like syndromes.[44] It is important to distinguish clinical features that make MS more likely than other types of demyelinating disorders such as myelin oligodendrocyte glycoprotein-associated disease and neuromyelitis optica spectrum disorders.[45,46] Genetic white matter disorders such as leukodystrophy or mitochondrial disease should be considered in cases with an indolent clinical course rather than relapsing-remitting, atypical MRI features for MS (confluent, symmetric T2 changes, or bilateral basal ganglia involvement), and atypical systemic involvement (failure to thrive, cardiomyopathy, diabetes). A prospective cohort study evaluating initial cerebrospinal fluid (CSF) studies and MRI scans and applying the 2010 and 2017 McDonald criteria demonstrated 70% sensitivity and 95% specificity for the 2017 McDonald criteria in the pediatric population, suggesting that the existing international criteria for diagnosis of MS perform well when applied to pediatric cases.[47]

Despite higher relapse rates, children recover well from relapses compared with adult patients with MS, even in cases where patients present with high lesion burden and severe ambulatory deficits after the initial attack. The mechanisms attributed to this observation include greater neurologic reserve and resilience of younger patients to withstand inflammatory damage. Regardless of clinical relapse recovery, there is evidence of loss of attainment of expected brain growth[48] and/or progressive volume loss on MRI characterized by lower than expected brain volume for age and early gray matter atrophy.[49] Although pediatric-onset cases have overall slower disability accumulation compared with adult-onset MS, sustained higher Expanded Disability Status Scale (EDSS) milestones may be reached at younger ages with longer overall lifespan lived with ambulatory disability. Pathology accumulated in childhood may be unmasked clinically in adulthood as neural compensatory mechanisms abate with age. A large European database of patients less than 16 years of age at onset of disease demonstrated delayed time (up to 10 years of disease duration) to reach EDSS 4.0 compared with an adult MS cohort, whereas the median age at which POMS patients reached EDSS 4.0 was 46.9 years compared with 60.8 years among the adult cohort.[50]

### *Multiple Sclerosis in the Aging Population*

With increasing chronologic age, relapse rates decrease while disability accumulation may accelerate. Independently, disease duration also contributes to disability accumulation, particularly ambulatory disability (see **Fig. 1**). Approximately 10% of all adult-onset MS will present with a progressive course, generally in the fifth decade of life.[51] For those over 50 years at onset, the frequency of progressive-onset disease is approximately 42%.[34] Secondary progressive disease features in those with relapsing onset often seem in the fifth decade as well, correlating with a decline in white matter integrity.[51] Age is also associated with incomplete recovery following relapses, furthering disability accumulation in older age groups.[52] This risk of incomplete recovery emphasizes the importance of preventing relapses even if they are less frequent in older patients with MS.[52] There has been no distinction in genetic susceptibility factors for relapsing versus progressive MS and much of the clinical, imaging, and pathologic features are similar to those who present with an initial clinical relapsing course. Pathologically, underlying disease mechanisms in phenotypically relapsing or progressive MS likely exist on a spectrum, ranging from actively inflamed white matter lesions to smoldering chronic lesions and gray matter atrophy, featuring infiltrative CD8+ T cells and B cells and pathologic resident CNS cells, dependent on chronologic age and duration of disease.[39]

### *Distinguishing Biological from Chronologic Age and Relevance to Disease Course*

Measuring biological age may be more precise in understanding the influence of age on pathophysiology and clinical disease expression in MS. Studying biological aging pathways may help elucidate the mechanisms of non-relapse-related progression. Several biological age markers have been evaluated in people with MS. A case-control study of DNA methylation from blood, a marker of epigenetic clock, demonstrated that age acceleration was higher in participants with MS.[53] Disability accumulation and brain atrophy have been associated with telomere attrition.[54] Telomere attrition activates downstream DNA damage responses and can drive aging-related changes in cells, including senescence. One study found that shorter leukocyte telomere lengths in participants with relapsing MS had a higher risk of converting to secondary progressive phenotypes in 10 years.[55] Greater telomere attrition was also found in bone marrow mesenchymal stem cells of MS participants compared with control participants, suggesting premature aging processes in MS.[56] Downstream of telomere attrition are senescence-associated secretory phenotypes[57] which have been implicated in other aging-related disorders, as the chronic low-grade inflammation caused from the senescent cells contributes to "inflammaging"

**Box 1**
**Summary of treatment approach in pediatric patients with multiple sclerosis**

Disease-Modifying Therapy (DMT)
- Initiate DMT early on favoring high efficacy therapies
- Update childhood vaccines before the initiation of immunosuppressive medication (at least 6 weeks before DMT for live vaccines and 2 weeks for inactive/mRNA vaccines)
- Consider factors contributing to medication adherence
- Follow weight-based dosing for younger children

Multidisciplinary Management
- Mental health screening and referral to therapist or psychiatrist if needed
- Address symptoms of fatigue, sleep, bowel/bladder dysfunction
- Diet: vegetable forward, low-saturated fat
- Physical activity: moderate to vigorous exercise
- School evaluation: individualized education plan or 504 plan
- Formal neuropsychological testing

processes.[58] With senescence, changes in immunomodulation may affect multiple aspects of disease, including MS phenotypic variability, subclinical disease activity, and pathophysiological processes.[59]

## TREATMENT AND MANAGEMENT CONSIDERATIONS

### *Treatment Strategies for Pediatric Multiple Sclerosis*

The approach to treatment of POMS in general aligns with approaches to treatment in adult-onset MS, which combines DMTs and symptomatic management (**Box 1**). In terms of DMT choice, unique considerations for pediatric patients include addressing higher relapse rates with patients starting with high lesion burden, timing of DMTs with childhood vaccines, and factors surrounding medication adherence. Historically, there are very few DMTs that have been evaluated in a randomized control trial for pediatric MS (**Table 1**). The first Food and Drug Administration (FDA)-approved DMT for pediatric MS was fingolimod in 2017 (PARADIGMS) for the use in patients ages 10 to 17 years.[60] In the trial, there was an annualized relapse rate (ARR) of 0.12 in patients treated with fingolimod compared with an ARR of 0.67 in patients in the interferon beta-1a (IFN beta-1a) arm.[60] The results from TERIKIDS, a phase 3 randomized controlled trial comparing teriflunomide to placebo did not show a difference in time to first relapse.[61] However, this may have resulted from earlier and more frequent switches from double-blind to open-label in the placebo group due to higher MRI activity that affected the power of the censored survival analysis.[61] Additional clinical trials are underway to investigate the efficacy of DMTs approved for use in adult patients (clinical trials.gov NCT04926818, NCT05123703). Despite limited clinical trial data in pediatric MS, observational data support the use of most available DMTs in children with increasing evidence that early treatment with high-efficacy DMTs may be better at lowering relapse rates and MRI changes.[62] Lastly, the effects of chronic immunosuppression on a developing immune system should be considered, particularly in younger children. Younger children have more frequent vaccinations and boosters, and this should be considered in treatment selection and treatment timing. On the other hand, neurodegeneration in MS is evident in the pediatric years, and although children have resilience and plasticity to compensate, this resilience may change with older age. Therefore, controlling the neuroinflammatory process early in the disease course may protect the developing brain against the neurodegenerative sequelae of MS.

**Table 1**
**Pivotal clinical trials and studies**

| Study or Trial | Study Type | Age Inclusion Criteria | Treatment Comparisons | Primary Outcomes | Notable findings |
|---|---|---|---|---|---|
| Pediatric MS Trials | | | | | |
| PARADIGMS[60] | RCT | 10–17 y | Fingolimod vs interferon beta-1a | 82% reduction in ARR in fingolimod group | Reduced brain volume loss in fingolimod group |
| TERIKIDS[61] | RCT | 10–17 y | Teriflunomide vs placebo | No significant difference in time to first relapse | Decreased T1 enhancing and T2 lesions in teriflunomide group |
| OPERETTA 1 and 2 | RCT | 10–17 y | Ocrelizumab vs fingolimod | Ongoing | – |
| NEOS | RCT | 10 to <18 y | Siponimod and ofatumumab vs fingolimod | Ongoing | – |
| Progressive MS Trials | | | | | |
| ORATORIO[69] | RCT | 18–55 y | Efficacy and safety of ocrelizumab vs placebo in adults with PPMS | 24-wk CDP; EDSS for ocrelizumab vs placebo; 51·7% vs 64·8% [95% CI 4·9–21·3] | Percent change from baseline in timed 25-foot walk (T25-FW), total volume of T2 brain lesions at week 120 |
| EXPAND[70] | RCT | 18–60 y | Siponimod vs placebo in SPMS | Time to 3-mo CDP: (26%) in siponimod group vs 32%in placebo had 3-mo CDP (hazard ratio 0·79, 95% CI 0·65–0·95; relative risk reduction 21%; $P = 0{\cdot}013$) | Adverse events occurred in 89%of siponimod group vs 82% receiving placebo |
| FenTREPID | RCT | 18–65 y | Fenebrutinib vs ocrelizumab PPMS | Time to onset of composite 12-wk confirmed disability progression | Awaiting completion |
| HERCULES | RCT | 18–65 y | Tolebrutinib vs placebo for SPMS | 6-mo confirmed disability progression | Awaiting completion |
| PERSEUS | RCT | 18–55 y | Tolebrutinib vs placebo for PPMS | 6-mo confirmed disability progression | Awaiting completion |

(*continued on next page*)

**Table 1**
***(continued)***

| Study or Trial | Study Type | Age Inclusion Criteria | Treatment Comparisons | Primary Outcomes | Notable findings |
|---|---|---|---|---|---|
| SPRINT-MS[90] | RCT | 21–65 y | Oral ibudilast (≤100 mg daily) or placebo in PPMS or SPMS | Rate of brain atrophy; −0.0010 per year with ibudilast and −0.0019 per year with placebo (difference, 0.0009; 95% CI 0.00004–0.0017; *P* = .04) | – |
| MS-STAT | RCT | 18–65 y | High-dose simvastatin vs placebo in SPMS | Mean annualized brain atrophy rate; lower in patients in the simvastatin group (0·288% per year [SD 0·521]) than in those in the placebo group (0·584% per year [0·498]). Adjusted difference in atrophy rate: −0·254% per year (95% CI −0·422 to −0·087; *P* = 0·003); 43% reduction in annualized rate | |

*Abbreviations:* RCT, randomized control trial; ARR, annualized relapse rate; CDP, confirmed disability progression; SD, standard deviation; PPMS, primary progressive multiple sclerosis; SPMS, secondary progressive multiple sclerosis.

Beyond DMTs, the treatment of POMS involves a multidisciplinary approach that addresses symptom management, lifestyle modifications, mental health, and scholastic achievement as well as promoting independence and resilience. Symptomatic management may include treatment for fatigue, neuropathic pain, spasticity, bladder/bowel symptoms, and visual support. Forming partnerships with other subspecialties such as primary care, urology, ophthalmology, and physiatry are encouraged. Addressing diet in a healthy way and promoting physical activity and wellness are integral parts of anticipatory guidance of POMS patients. There is no single diet preferred for MS, a vegetable forward diet may be protective against relapses, and a higher intake of saturated fats may increase the hazard to relapse.[28] In addition, diet quality (eg, more fruits and vegetables, healthy fats, and whole grains) is associated with lower disability and comorbid symptoms such as fatigue and cognitive impairment.[63] Patients with moderate to vigorous physical activity are found to have less fatigue and depression.[64] In a longitudinal study, an additional 15 to 30 minutes of moderate to vigorous physical activity per week was found to have a clinical difference in mood and fatigue.[64] Therefore, enlisting the help of pediatric dieticians and physical and occupational therapists, if available, can be greatly beneficial for the patient.

In terms of cognition, the three areas previously found to be affected in POMS include executive function, complex attention, and visuospatial reasoning and sequencing.[65] Language function and intelligence were thought to be affected because the disease presents at a time of critical brain development and these deficits become more apparent with increasing academic burden.[65] However, a more recent study evaluating neurocognitive function in pediatric MS patients compared with age-matched healthy controls does not suggest a significant difference in their performance in various cognitive domains.[66] This suggests that the observed cognitive deficits in pediatric MS may be influenced by factors other than the effect of the disease itself such as psychiatric comorbidities.

At least 30% of POMS patients report depression or anxiety.[65] Treatment approaches include engaging in counseling or psychotherapy, encouraging regular physical activity, connecting with local or national patient support groups, and pharmacologic treatment if needed. Although neurocognitive and psychiatric symptoms are also common in adult patients, it is important to recognize these features in the clinical evaluation of pediatric patients. Although poor quality sleep and concomitant fatigue can often confound or accentuate cognitive difficulties, a highly inflammatory pathophysiology characterized by lesion accumulation in an otherwise actively growing brain undergoing myelination and maturation, can further compound these issues. This may be extrapolated by neuropsychological studies among pediatric populations demonstrating a protective effect of well-controlled disease on cognition,[67] although larger studies are needed to definitively establish this causal relationship. As with adult MS patients, in the pediatric population, formal neuropsychological testing is recommended if access to a trained pediatric clinical neuropsychologist is available. Neuropsychological evaluation can be especially helpful in cases when cognitive symptoms may be influenced by concurrent psychiatric symptoms and in cases where there is a progressive decline in school performance. Formal neurocognitive treatment in POMS is still an area in need of more rigorous research and implementation especially in resource poor areas. Patients should be encouraged to work with school counselors and adopt a formal individualized education plan to optimize their academic support. Treating comorbid psychiatric, fatigue, and sleep issues may also help cognitive symptoms.

Another aspect unique to the care of pediatric patients is factoring in family dynamics and the mental health of caregivers. Children living with MS may face additional challenges in social relationships, particularly within academic domains. Studies focusing on health-related quality of life (HRQoL) in MS patients found that the HRQoL in POMS patients correlated with HRQoL scores in their family.[68] Thus, a multidisciplinary model addressing mental health and neuropsychological and academic aspects of the disease are the key in the comprehensive care of POMS.

### *Treatment Strategies for the Aging Population*

Immunosenescence with advancing age may be associated with poor response to DMTs and a higher risk of adverse events. There is an overall decline in overt inflammatory disease activity (indicated by reduced clinical relapses and gadolinium enhancing lesions), paralleling a decreased efficiency in inherent immune responses. Current DMTs primarily target active inflammatory disease activity and unfortunately have little proven efficacy in halting non-relapse-related progression (see **Table 1**).[52] For instance, although efficacy for progressive disease has been reported in some trials for ocrelizumab and siponimod (ORATORIO[69] and EXPAND,[70] respectively), treatment benefits were primarily observed in those with active disease (eg, enhancing lesions on MRI or clinical relapses). Traditionally, relapsing MS trials have harbored a lack of representation of older patients in clinical trials, hindering practical evaluation of efficacy and adverse events from DMTs in older MS patients as the upper age limit for most study populations is 55 to 60 years.[71] Furthermore, subgroup efficacy analyses of the phase 3 ORATORIO study demonstrated decreased efficacy of ocrelizumab in older patients (age >45 years) compared with the younger cohort less than 45 years of age, as evidenced by a decrease in rate of reduction of disability accumulation.[72] Although age limits may be set due to concerns with advancing age, including treatment-associated infection risks, lymphopenia, and compounded risk from preexisting comorbidities, these limits substantially diminish our ability to apply these medications to the most prevalent age group with MS.[73,74]

Periodic reevaluation of the risk–benefit ratio of DMTs in aging patients is an imperative aspect of MS management (**Box 2**). Consideration must be given to an increased risk of infections, needle fatigue, and financial feasibility of continuing DMTs, weighed against true benefit in the absence of active disease. In patients greater than 60 years of age without evidence of active disease in the 2 years prior, DMT discontinuation may be safely undertaken in a large majority.[75] The DISCO-MS study ("discontinuing"

**Box 2**
**Summary of treatment approach in aging patients with multiple sclerosis**

Disease-Modifying Therapy (DMT)
- Consider risk versus benefit of continuing DMT and potential adverse effects
- De-escalation or DMT discontinuation may be considered in patients with stable disease greater than 60 years of age
- Consider enrollment in clinical trials with immunomodulatory or neuroprotective therapies

Multidisciplinary Management
- Address vascular risk factors, sleep disturbances, bowel/bladder dysfunction, and psychiatric comorbidities
- Formal neuropsychological testing if concerns for cognitive impairment
- Mobility: physical therapy, assistive devices, home safety evaluation
- Diet: vegetable forward, low-saturated fat
- Physical activity: aerobic exercise
- Consider impacts of reproductive aging and menopause

DMT clinicaltrials.gov, NCT03073603) evaluated a cohort of MS patients age greater than 55 years without evidence of clinically or radiographically active disease for the prior 5 and 3 years, respectively, for non-inferiority of DMT discontinuation versus DMT continuation. However, these results were largely inconclusive; whereas clinical relapses were uncommon in the discontinuation group, the risk of minimally increased radiographic activity was about 7% higher in the discontinuation group, though the clinical significance of this point estimate was unclear.[76] A recent retrospective study explored effects of DMT de-escalation from high-/moderate-efficacy to low-efficacy therapies on ARRs, disability outcomes, and radiographic measures with a mean study population age of 57 years. The results suggest that de-escalation may be non-inferior; however, the outcomes of ARR and disability were not significant, whereas change in burden of T2 lesions met the prespecified non-inferiority threshold for significance.[77]

Cognitive impairment is well-recognized in the aging MS population, affecting up to 70% of adult MS patients based on population studies impacting various domains.[78] Specifically, patients may present with dysfunction in frontal and subcortical domains, ranging from deficits in processing speed, attention and concentration, and executive function.[78] Underlying inflammatory processes in MS can accentuate deterioration in higher executive function and working memory associated with advancing age.[79] Calabrese and colleagues provided a potential pathologic biomarker for the impact of aging on cognition by demonstrating augmented brain atrophy in affected cohorts compared with control groups.[79] Tremblay and colleagues conducted extensive neuropsychological evaluations in a small subset of elderly patients with MS, with decline in domains of information processing speed more than that expected for normal aging, suggesting accrual of myelin damage may indeed impair performance in tasks dependent on efficient synaptic transmission.[78] A small-scale study evaluating the effect of adaptive training on neuropsychological testing and fMRI activation patterns demonstrated that goal-directed cognitive training can positively impact cognitive recovery.[80] The idea is that through improving motor functioning and working memory, wellness strategies can further complement ongoing therapeutic efforts to minimize functional decline related to aging.

It is important to address healthy lifestyle habits, optimization of vascular risk factors, smoking cessation, and detailed assessment for depression as part of the clinic visit. The increased density of cerebral small vessel disease has been observed in postmortem analyses of patients with MS.[39] Vascular comorbidities, and obesity, are associated with greater disability accrual.[81] This becomes an important consideration when deciding on a treatment course and expectations. Ease of access to treatment for older adults should be elucidated by identifying and addressing barriers to care; including but not limited to obtaining prescriptions, arranging transportation for follow-up appointments, and ability to use available modalities of communication with their physician; a multidisciplinary approach with early involvement of a licensed social worker may be warranted. Assistive devices for safe mobilization can allow for greater independence and self-confidence in managing activities of daily living; indeed, progressive disability can worsen depression in this population. Exercise, particularly maintained cardiorespiratory fitness, may have a role in countering this aging associated white matter degeneration and stimulation of growth factors such as brain-derived neurotrophic factor.[82,83] Neurorehabilitation with the goal to improve physical endurance and reduce risk of falls can help improve quality of life for aging patients with MS. In addition, individuals with MS are at higher risk of developing vascular comorbidities—with observations of increased prevalence of cerebrovascular and cardiovascular disease in these cohorts compared with the general population.[39] Exercise training has been shown to be a highly effective non-pharmacologic tool for managing both physical and cognitive symptoms in MS.[84] Strategies, such as exercise training, physical therapy, and gait training, have demonstrated variable benefit on mobility disability in particular.[85] Recommendations by the Consortium of Multiple Sclerosis Centers include endorsing at least 150 minutes per week of exercise and/or $\ngeq$150 minutes per week of lifestyle physical activity, with a graduated progress toward these targets based on individual tolerance.[86,87]

### *Remyelination Strategies and Future Therapeutics*

Enhancing endogenous remyelination may prove to be an effective therapeutic strategy to theoretically allow for halting disease progression. Native remyelinating mechanisms are dependent on age (greatest potential <55 years) and disease duration (<10 years), and multiple challenges exist when practically attempting to demonstrate remyelination in living individuals, precluding development of a wholly successful remyelination agent.[88]

Remyelination strategies are currently under study; however, diminished responsiveness of adult oligodendrocyte progenitor cells (OPCs) with age poses a challenge to the efficacy of remyelination-enhancing agents.[88] Extrapolating from this phenomenon, it would be highly informative to observe the effects of these strategies at either end of the age spectrum, lending further to our understanding of the biological mechanisms underlying successful remyelination. In particular, these strategies will need to prove myelinating potential, not only in progressive disease, but particularly may need to do so in animal models of aging as well. Interestingly, Franklin and colleagues demonstrated that fasting or treatment of aged rodent OPCs with metformin may restore regenerative capacity by allowing pro-differentiation signals to improve remyelination capacity of OPCs.[89] Therefore, although recovery and repair strategies are most effective early on, aging particularly necessitates success of the same—whereas some strategies show promise, no definite clinically proven benefit is apparent at this time.

Prior therapies targeting neuroprotection and immunomodulation did not demonstrate clear efficacy in reducing brain volume loss or promoting remyelination. Investigational agents included ibudilast (phase II SPRINT-MS),[90] simvastatin (MS-STAT),[91] high-dose biotin,[92] and amiloride, fluoxetine, and riluzole (MS SMART).[93] Although simvastatin and ibulidast demonstrated some reduction in brain atrophy rates compared with placebo, the rest did not meet this primary endpoint. Of note, however, these studies were not conducted in pediatric and aging MS cohorts and remain an unmet need.

Bruton tyrosine kinase (BTK) inhibition and T-cell-based therapy targeting EBV have emerged as novel therapeutic strategies targeting multiple immunomodulatory mechanisms that affect CNS-driven neurodegeneration and progression in MS. BTK inhibitors (BTKis) modulate B-cell activation, along with myeloid (macrophages and microglia) cell activity.[94] Microglia, in particular, have demonstrated a central role in driving progression in chronic active lesions,[95] represented radiographically as paramagnetic rim lesions and slowly expanding lesions (SELs): an important imaging outcome measure in multiple BTKi trials in MS.[96] A phase II trial demonstrated efficacy of evobrutinib (clinicaltrials.gov, NCT02975349) in reducing SEL volume in a dose-dependent fashion, over 48 weeks.[97] Of note, older patients were included in this study, with upper age limit of 65 years. Further trials in process with similar older study populations include FENtrepid (efficacy of fenebrutinib vs ocrelizumab in primary progressive MS, clinicaltrials.gov, NCT04544449) and HERCULES and PERSEUS (tolebrutinib in nonrelapsing secondary progressive MS and primary progressive MS, clinicaltrials.gov, NCT04411641, NCT04458051). The ongoing EMBOLD phase 1/2 trial is evaluating safety and efficacy of a T-cell therapy targeting EBV (clinicaltrials.

gov, NCT03283826). Prior studies demonstrated that poor T-cell responses to EBV infections result in an accumulation of B cells that contribute to progressive MS phenotypes.[98] An early open-label phase 1 study with six progressive MS patients who received T-cell targeting EBV antigens showed improvement in neurologic function and quality of life.[98]

### *Role of Hormonal Therapy*

As discussed earlier, reproductive aging and menopause can contribute to multiple immunologic and neurologic processes that ultimately impact MS disease course.[39,99] Fluctuating levels of sex steroid hormones may influence the risk of adopting an increasingly progressive phenotype and disability accumulation. Estrogen levels have shown to impact neuroprotective processes relating to oligodendrocytes and neurons.[39] Higher estriol levels in particular may be associated with diminished cortical gray matter atrophy.[100] Multiple studies assessing the impact of menopause on disability progression have shown a statistically significant mean increase in the EDSS from before to after menopause—ranging from an increase of 0.08 points over 10 years to a 0.4-point increase up to 3.5 years after menopause.[101,102] However, these results are limited by the use of self-reported menopause, which may not necessarily coincide with innate biological fluctuations in sex hormones, marking earlier onset of ovarian functional decline.

Anti-Mullerian hormone levels showed a strong correlation with disability level in the cross-sectional and longitudinal analyses of over 400 women with MS, implicating ovarian aging and perimenopause as possible contributors to progressive disease.[99] In addition to potential pathologic effects on MS, perimenopause creates symptoms that mimic MS symptoms and can complicate management. These include body temperature dysregulation, cognition, sleep, and genitourinary functions. Extra attention should be paid to improve quality of life.

Few studies have explored the impact of estrogen or combined estrogen-progesterone treatment—hormonal therapy (HT) —on the MS disease course with mixed results. In a study of 164 women (18–50 years) with relapsing MS who received combination glatiramer acetate and the pregnancy estrogen (estriol) treatment, a reduced ARR was demonstrated. There were 0.25 relapses per year (95% CI 0.17–0.37) in the treatment group compared with 0.37 relapses per year (95% CI 0.25–0.53) in the placebo group with an adjusted rate ratio of 0.63 (95% CI 0.37–1·05, $P = 0{\cdot}077$).[103] However, the study did not meet its primary endpoint of ARR reduction over 24 months.[103] In another trial of 150 women ages 18 to 45 years with relapsing MS comparing IFN beta-1a and oral contraceptives (ethinylestradiol 40 μg/desogestrel 125 μg) in combination to IFN beta-1a alone, there was up to a 26% reduction in the number of active lesions on brain MRI as well as a lower probability of developing gadolinium enhancing lesions ($P = .03$).[104] However, in another prospective cohort study of 495 women with MS and clinically isolated syndrome, exposure to oral contraceptives was not associated with risk of a second attack (hazard ratio [HR] 0.73, 95% CI 0.33–1.61) or disability accumulation (HR 0.81, 95% CI 0.17–3.76), although this was a cross-sectional survey-based study.[105]

Unfortunately, the use of HT, in particular combination progesterone and estrogen, does portend risks including venous thromboembolism and breast cancer. A randomized controlled trial through the Women's Health Initiative Memory Study reported an increased risk of stroke and dementia with the administration of HT to women beyond menopause.[106] Symptomatic treatment for menopausal symptoms can be undertaken when HT is contraindicated; for instance, selective serotonin reuptake inhibitors and norepinephrine reuptake inhibitors can be used to manage vasomotor symptoms,[107] and urinary dysfunction may be treated with intra-detrusor botulinum toxin injection and pelvic floor exercises.[108] In a pilot randomized placebo-controlled study using bazedoxifene + conjugated estrogen evaluating effects of HT on hot flashes in menopause, recruitment was protracted due to safety concerns with continued HT use; the Hot Flash Related Daily Interference scale performed at 2 months was lower in the HT treatment group.[109]

## SUMMARY

The clinical features of the two extreme age populations—pediatric and aging—in MS offer unique insights into the complex interplay between neuroinflammatory mechanisms and the effects of chronologic and biological aging as well as their interactions with environmental and epigenetic factors that influence risk for disease and disease course. An additional important aspect of biological age is reproductive age and its effects on the immune system from the pro-inflammatory phenotype during periods of sexual maturity to disability accumulation during times of ovarian aging. A proactive, comprehensive approach to address age-specific considerations with DMT and symptomatic management is critical for holistic care. Additional age extreme management considerations include recognizing the cognitive impacts and social relationships with caregivers on the well-being of children and older adults living with MS.

## CLINIC CARE POINTS

- Pediatric-onset multiple sclerosis (MS) presents with highly inflammatory disease with higher rates of relapses compared with adult-onset MS.
- The treatment for pediatric-onset MS includes early initiation of high-efficacy disease-modifying therapy to reduce accumulation of CNS injury from recurring relapses as well as a multidisciplinary approach to address mental health, neuropsychological, and cognitive aspects of the disease.
- Chronologic age and immunosenescence are associated with decreased disease-modifying therapy efficacy and increased adverse events including infections.
- Although treatments targeting aging-related pathologic changes are not available, these are a potential future area of MS therapeutics. For now, a holistic approach targeting lifestyle habits and comorbidities should be undertaken when managing MS in the aging patient population.
- Reproductive milestones should be considered in MS management including potential increase in relapse activity around puberty and increased disability accumulation in perimenopause. In addition, perimenopause symptoms may overlap with features of a progressive MS course; a thorough clinical evaluation can help direct symptomatic therapy and help improve quality of life for this patient population.

## DISCLOSURE

A. Siddiqui and J.H. Yang do not have any disclosures to report. L.H. Hua has received personal fees for speaking, consulting, and advisory board activities from Alexion, Bristol Myers Squibb, EMD Serono, Genentech, Genzyme, Greenwich Biosciences, Horizon, and Novartis and has received research support paid to her institution from Biogen. J.S. Graves has received grant or clinical trial funding from the NMSS, UCSD, United States, Octave, Biogen, United States, EMD Serono, United States and ABM. She serves on a steering committee for a clinical trial with Novartis and served on advisory boards for TG therapeutics, Genentech, and Bayer unrelated to the current work.

## REFERENCES


1. Wallin MT, Culpepper WJ, Campbell JD, et al. The prevalence of MS in the United States: A population-based estimate using health claims data. Neurology 2019;92(10):e1029–40.
2. Yan K, Balijepalli C, Desai K, et al. Epidemiology of pediatric multiple sclerosis: A systematic literature review and meta-analysis. Mult Scler Relat Disord 2020; 44:102260.
3. Polliack ML, Barak Y, Achiron A. Late-onset multiple sclerosis. J Am Geriatr Soc 2001;49(2):168–71.
4. Awad A, Stüve O. Multiple Sclerosis in the Elderly Patient. Drugs Aging 2010; 27(4):283–94.
5. Tremlett H, Devonshire V. Is late-onset multiple sclerosis associated with a worse outcome? Neurology 2006;67(6):954–9.
6. Kis B, Rumberg B, Berlit P. Clinical characteristics of patients with late-onset multiple sclerosis. J Neurol 2008;255(5):697–702.
7. Thompson AJ, Polman CH, Miller DH, et al. Primary progressive multiple sclerosis. Brain 1997;120(Pt 6):1085–96.
8. Mirmosayyeb O, Brand S, Barzegar M, et al. Clinical Characteristics and Disability Progression of Early- and Late-Onset Multiple Sclerosis Compared to Adult-Onset Multiple Sclerosis. J Clin Med 2020;9(5):1326.
9. Esposito F, Guaschino C, Sorosina M, et al. Impact of MS genetic loci on familial aggregation, clinical phenotype, and disease prediction. Neurol Neuroimmunol Neuroinflamm 2015;2(4):e129.
10. Gianfrancesco MA, Stridh P, Shao X, et al. Genetic risk factors for pediatric–onset multiple sclerosis. Mult Scler 2018;24(14):1825–34.
11. Chi C, Shao X, Rhead B, et al. Admixture mapping reveals evidence of differential multiple sclerosis risk by genetic ancestry. PLoS Genet 2019;15(1): e1007808.
12. Waubant E, Ponsonby AL, Pugliatti M, et al. Environmental and genetic factors in pediatric inflammatory demyelinating diseases. Neurology 2016;87(9 Suppl 2): S20–7.
13. Bjornevik K, Cortese M, Healy BC, et al. Longitudinal analysis reveals high prevalence of Epstein-Barr virus associated with multiple sclerosis. Science 2022; 375(6578):296–301.
14. Waubant E, Mowry EM, Krupp L, et al. Common viruses associated with lower pediatric multiple sclerosis risk. Neurology 2011;76(23):1989–95.
15. Munger KL, Levin LI, Hollis BW, et al. Serum 25-hydroxyvitamin D levels and risk of multiple sclerosis. JAMA 2006;296(23):2832–8.
16. Rhead B, Bäärnhielm M, Gianfrancesco M, et al. Mendelian randomization shows a causal effect of low vitamin D on multiple sclerosis risk. Neurol Genet 2016;2(5):e97.
17. Lavery AM, Collins BN, Waldman AT, et al. The contribution of secondhand tobacco smoke exposure to pediatric multiple sclerosis risk. Mult Scler 2019; 25(4):515–22.
18. Jacobs BM, Noyce AJ, Bestwick J, et al. Gene-Environment Interactions in Multiple Sclerosis: A UK Biobank Study. Neurol Neuroimmunol Neuroinflamm 2021; 8(4):e1007.

19. Ziaei A, Lavery AM, Shao XM, et al. Gene-environment interactions increase the risk of pediatric-onset multiple sclerosis associated with ozone pollution. Mult Scler 2022;28(9):1330–9.
20. Nasr Z, Schoeps VA, Ziaei A, et al. Gene-environment interactions increase the risk of paediatric-onset multiple sclerosis associated with household chemical exposures. J Neurol Neurosurg Psychiatry 2023. https://doi.org/10.1136/jnnp-2022-330713. jnnp-2022-330713.
21. Graves JS, Chitnis T, Weinstock-Guttman B, et al. Maternal and Perinatal Exposures Are Associated With Risk for Pediatric-Onset Multiple Sclerosis. Pediatrics 2017;139(4):e20162838.
22. Amezcua L, Rivera VM, Vazquez TC, et al. Health Disparities, Inequities, and Social Determinants of Health in Multiple Sclerosis and Related Disorders in the US: A Review. JAMA Neurol 2021;78(12):1515–24.
23. Graves JS, Barcellos LF, Shao X, et al. Genetic predictors of relapse rate in pediatric MS. Mult Scler 2016;22(12):1528.
24. Graves JS, Barcellos LF, Simpson S, et al. The multiple sclerosis risk allele within the AHI1 gene is associated with relapses in children and adults. Mult Scler Relat Disord 2018;19:161–5.
25. Zhou Y, Graves JS, Simpson S, et al. Genetic variation in the gene LRP2 increases relapse risk in multiple sclerosis. J Neurol Neurosurg Psychiatry 2017;88(10):864–8.
26. International Multiple Sclerosis Genetics Consortium. MultipleMS Consortium. Locus for severity implicates CNS resilience in progression of multiple sclerosis. Nature 2023. https://doi.org/10.1038/s41586-023-06250-x.
27. Mowry EM, Krupp LB, Milazzo M, et al. Vitamin D status is associated with relapse rate in pediatric-onset multiple sclerosis. Ann Neurol 2010;67(5):618–24.
28. Azary S, Schreiner T, Graves J, et al. Contribution of dietary intake to relapse rate in early paediatric multiple sclerosis. J Neurol Neurosurg Psychiatry 2018;89(1):28–33.
29. Mowry EM, Azevedo CJ, McCulloch CE, et al. Body mass index, but not vitamin D status, is associated with brain volume change in MS. Neurology 2018;91(24):e2256–64.
30. Grover SA, Aubert-Broche B, Fetco D, et al. Lower physical activity is associated with higher disease burden in pediatric multiple sclerosis. Neurology 2015;85(19):1663–9.
31. Belman AL, Krupp LB, Olsen CS, et al. Characteristics of Children and Adolescents With Multiple Sclerosis. Pediatrics 2016;138(1):e20160120.
32. Lulu S, Graves J, Waubant E. Menarche increases relapse risk in pediatric multiple sclerosis. Mult Scler 2016;22(2):193–200.
33. Young B, Waubant E, Lulu S, et al. Puberty onset and pediatric multiple sclerosis activity in boys. Mult Scler Relat Disord 2019;27:184–7.
34. Naseri A, Nasiri E, Sahraian MA, et al. Clinical Features of Late-Onset Multiple Sclerosis: a Systematic Review and Meta-analysis. Mult Scler Relat Disord 2021;50:102816.
35. Miclea A, Salmen A, Zoehner G, et al. Age-dependent variation of female preponderance across different phenotypes of multiple sclerosis: A retrospective cross-sectional study. CNS Neurosci Ther 2018;25(4):527–31.
36. Confavreux C, Vukusic S, Moreau T, et al. Relapses and progression of disability in multiple sclerosis. N Engl J Med 2000;343(20):1430–8.

37. Ribbons KA, McElduff P, Boz C, et al. Male Sex Is Independently Associated with Faster Disability Accumulation in Relapse-Onset MS but Not in Primary Progressive MS. PLoS One 2015;10(6):e0122686.
38. Bove R, Healy BC, Musallam A, et al. Exploration of changes in disability after menopause in a longitudinal multiple sclerosis cohort. Mult Scler 2016;22(7): 935–43.
39. Graves JS, Krysko KM, Hua LH, et al. Ageing and multiple sclerosis. Lancet Neurol 2023;22(1):66–77.
40. Bove R, Musallam A, Healy BC, et al. Low testosterone is associated with disability in men with multiple sclerosis. Mult Scler 2014;20(12):1584–92.
41. Gilli F, DiSano KD, Pachner AR. SeXX Matters in Multiple Sclerosis. Front Neurol 2020;11:616.
42. Kuhlmann T, Moccia M, Coetzee T, et al. Multiple sclerosis progression: time for a new mechanism-driven framework. Lancet Neurol 2023;22(1):78–88.
43. Gorman MP, Healy BC, Polgar-Turcsanyi M, et al. Increased relapse rate in pediatric-onset compared with adult-onset multiple sclerosis. Arch Neurol 2009;66(1):54–9.
44. Chitnis T. Pediatric Central Nervous System Demyelinating Diseases. Continuum 2019;25(3):793–814.
45. Fadda G, Armangue T, Hacohen Y, et al. Paediatric multiple sclerosis and antibody-associated demyelination: clinical, imaging, and biological considerations for diagnosis and care. Lancet Neurol 2021;20(2):136–49.
46. Banwell B, Bennett JL, Marignier R, et al. Diagnosis of myelin oligodendrocyte glycoprotein antibody-associated disease: International MOGAD Panel proposed criteria. Lancet Neurol 2023. https://doi.org/10.1016/S1474-4422(22)00431-8.
47. Fadda G, Brown RA, Longoni G, et al. MRI and laboratory features and the performance of international criteria in the diagnosis of multiple sclerosis in children and adolescents: a prospective cohort study. Lancet Child Adolesc Health 2018;2(3):191–204.
48. Fadda G, Cardenas de la Parra A, O'Mahony J, et al. Deviation From Normative Whole Brain and Deep Gray Matter Growth in Children With MOGAD, MS, and Monophasic Seronegative Demyelination. Neurology 2023. https://doi.org/10.1212/WNL.0000000000207429.
49. De Meo E, Portaccio E, Giorgio A, et al. Identifying the Distinct Cognitive Phenotypes in Multiple Sclerosis. JAMA Neurol 2021;78(4):414–25.
50. Renoux C, Vukusic S, Mikaeloff Y, et al. Natural history of multiple sclerosis with childhood onset. N Engl J Med 2007;356(25):2603–13.
51. Conway BL, Zeydan B, Uygunoğlu U, et al. Age is a critical determinant in recovery from multiple sclerosis relapses. Mult Scler 2019;25(13):1754–63.
52. Zeydan B, Kantarci OH. Impact of Age on Multiple Sclerosis Disease Activity and Progression. Curr Neurol Neurosci Rep 2020;20(7):24.
53. Theodoropoulou E, Alfredsson L, Piehl F, et al. Different epigenetic clocks reflect distinct pathophysiological features of multiple sclerosis. Epigenomics 2019; 11(12):1429–39.
54. Habib R, Ocklenburg S, Hoffjan S, et al. Association between shorter leukocyte telomeres and multiple sclerosis. J Neuroimmunol 2020;341:577187.
55. Hecker M, Fitzner B, Jäger K, et al. Leukocyte Telomere Length in Patients with Multiple Sclerosis and Its Association with Clinical Phenotypes. Mol Neurobiol 2021;58(6):2886–96.

56. Redondo J, Sarkar P, Kemp K, et al. Reduced cellularity of bone marrow in multiple sclerosis with decreased MSC expansion potential and premature ageing in vitro. Mult Scler 2018;24(7):919–31.
57. Tchkonia T, Zhu Y, van Deursen J, et al. Cellular senescence and the senescent secretory phenotype: therapeutic opportunities. J Clin Invest 2013;123(3): 966–72.
58. Giardini MA, Segatto M, da Silva MS, et al. Telomere and telomerase biology. Prog Mol Biol Transl Sci 2014;125:1–40.
59. Krysko KM, Henry RG, Cree BAC, et al. Telomere Length Is Associated with Disability Progression in Multiple Sclerosis. Ann Neurol 2019;86(5):671–82.
60. Chitnis T, Arnold DL, Banwell B, et al. Trial of Fingolimod versus Interferon Beta-1a in Pediatric Multiple Sclerosis. N Engl J Med 2018;379(11):1017–27.
61. Chitnis T, Banwell B, Kappos L, et al. Safety and efficacy of teriflunomide in paediatric multiple sclerosis (TERIKIDS): a multicentre, double-blind, phase 3, randomised, placebo-controlled trial. Lancet Neurol 2021;20(12):1001–11.
62. Krysko KM, Graves JS, Rensel M, et al. Real-World Effectiveness of Initial Disease-Modifying Therapies in Pediatric Multiple Sclerosis. Ann Neurol 2020; 88(1):42–55.
63. Fitzgerald KC, Tyry T, Salter A, et al. Diet quality is associated with disability and symptom severity in multiple sclerosis. Neurology 2018;90(1):e1–11.
64. Stephens S, Shams S, Lee J, et al. Benefits of Physical Activity for Depression and Fatigue in Multiple Sclerosis: A Longitudinal Analysis. J Pediatr 2019;209: 226–32.e2.
65. Amato MP, Krupp LB, Charvet LE, et al. Pediatric multiple sclerosis: Cognition and mood. Neurology 2016;87(9 Supplement 2):S82–7.
66. Krupp LB, Waubant E, Waltz M, et al. A new look at cognitive functioning in pediatric MS. Mult Scler 2023;29(1):140–9.
67. Johnen A, Elpers C, Riepl E, et al. Early effective treatment may protect from cognitive decline in paediatric multiple sclerosis. Eur J Paediatr Neurol 2019; 23(6):783–91.
68. O'Mahony J, Salter A, Ciftci B, et al. Physical and Mental Health-Related Quality of Life Trajectories Among People With Multiple Sclerosis. Neurology 2022; 99(14):e1538–48.
69. Fox EJ, Markowitz C, Applebee A, et al. Ocrelizumab reduces progression of upper extremity impairment in patients with primary progressive multiple sclerosis: Findings from the phase III randomized ORATORIO trial. Mult Scler 2018;24(14):1862–70.
70. Kappos L, Bar-Or A, Cree BAC, et al. Siponimod versus placebo in secondary progressive multiple sclerosis (EXPAND): a double-blind, randomised, phase 3 study. Lancet 2018;391(10127):1263–73.
71. Schweitzer F, Laurent S, Fink GR, et al. Age and the risks of high-efficacy disease modifying drugs in multiple sclerosis. Curr Opin Neurol 2019;32(3): 305–12.
72. Hauser SL, Bar-Or A, Weber MS, et al. Association of Higher Ocrelizumab Exposure With Reduced Disability Progression in Multiple Sclerosis. Neurology - Neuroimmunology Neuroinflammation 2023;10(2).
73. Grebenciucova E, Berger JR. Immunosenescence: the Role of Aging in the Predisposition to Neuro-Infectious Complications Arising from the Treatment of Multiple Sclerosis. Curr Neurol Neurosci Rep 2017;17(8):61.
74. Vaughn CB, Jakimovski D, Kavak KS, et al. Epidemiology and treatment of multiple sclerosis in elderly populations. Nat Rev Neurol 2019;15(6):329–42.

75. Hua LH, Fan TH, Conway D, et al. Discontinuation of disease-modifying therapy in patients with multiple sclerosis over age 60. Mult Scler 2019;25(5):699–708.
76. Hartung HP, Meuth SG, Miller DM, et al. Stopping disease-modifying therapy in relapsing and progressive multiple sclerosis. Curr Opin Neurol 2021;34(4): 598–603.
77. Goldschmidt CH, Glassman J, Ly B, et al. A Retrospective Study on the Effects of De-Escalation of Disease Modifying Therapy in Patients with Multiple Sclerosis. *Platform Presentation.* Consortium of Multiple Sclerosis Centers 2023 Annual Meeting, Denver, CO. International Journal of MS Care 2023;25(s1):6.
78. Tremblay A, Charest K, Brando E, et al. The effects of aging and disease duration on cognition in multiple sclerosis. Brain Cognit 2020;146:105650.
79. Calabrese M, Filippi M, Gallo P. Cortical lesions in multiple sclerosis. Nat Rev Neurol 2010;6(8):438–44.
80. Bonzano L, Pedullà L, Pardini M, et al. Brain activity pattern changes after adaptive working memory training in multiple sclerosis. Brain Imaging Behav 2020; 14(1):142–54.
81. Geraldes R, Esiri MM, Perera R, et al. Vascular disease and multiple sclerosis: a post-mortem study exploring their relationships. Brain 2020;143(10):2998–3012.
82. Hayes SM, Salat DH, Forman DE, et al. Cardiorespiratory fitness is associated with white matter integrity in aging. Ann Clin Transl Neurol 2015;2(6):688–98.
83. Shobeiri P, Karimi A, Momtazmanesh S, et al. Exercise-induced increase in blood-based brain-derived neurotrophic factor (BDNF) in people with multiple sclerosis: A systematic review and meta-analysis of exercise intervention trials. PLoS One 2022;17(3):e0264557.
84. Dalgas U, Stenager E. Exercise and disease progression in multiple sclerosis: can exercise slow down the progression of multiple sclerosis? Ther Adv Neurol Disord 2012;5(2):81–95.
85. Benito-León J, Morales JM, Rivera-Navarro J, et al. A review about the impact of multiple sclerosis on health-related quality of life. Disabil Rehabil 2003;25(23): 1291–303.
86. Baird JF, Sandroff BM, Motl RW. Therapies for mobility disability in persons with multiple sclerosis. Expert Rev Neurother 2018;18(6):493–502.
87. Kalb R, Brown TR, Coote S, et al. Exercise and lifestyle physical activity recommendations for people with multiple sclerosis throughout the disease course. Mult Scler 2020;26(12):1459–69.
88. Chari DM. Remyelination In Multiple Sclerosis. Int Rev Neurobiol 2007;79: 589–620.
89. Neumann B, Baror R, Zhao C, et al. Metformin Restores CNS Remyelination Capacity by Rejuvenating Aged Stem Cells. Cell Stem Cell 2019;25(4):473–85.e8.
90. Fox RJ, Coffey CS, Conwit R, et al. Phase 2 Trial of Ibudilast in Progressive Multiple Sclerosis. N Engl J Med 2018;379(9):846–55.
91. Chataway J, Schuerer N, Alsanousi A, et al. Effect of high-dose simvastatin on brain atrophy and disability in secondary progressive multiple sclerosis (MS-STAT): a randomised, placebo-controlled, phase 2 trial. Lancet 2014; 383(9936):2213–21.
92. Cree BAC, Cutter G, Wolinsky JS, et al. Safety and efficacy of MD1003 (high-dose biotin) in patients with progressive multiple sclerosis (SPI2): a randomised, double-blind, placebo-controlled, phase 3 trial. Lancet Neurol 2020;19(12): 988–97.
93. Chataway J, De Angelis F, Connick P, et al. Efficacy of three neuroprotective drugs in secondary progressive multiple sclerosis (MS-SMART): a phase 2b,

multiarm, double-blind, randomised placebo-controlled trial. Lancet Neurol 2020;19(3):214–25.
94. Geladaris A, Torke S, Weber MS. Bruton's Tyrosine Kinase Inhibitors in Multiple Sclerosis: Pioneering the Path Towards Treatment of Progression? CNS Drugs 2022;36(10):1019–30.
95. Schneider R, Oh J. Bruton's Tyrosine Kinase Inhibition in Multiple Sclerosis. Curr Neurol Neurosci Rep 2022;22(11):721–34.
96. Marcille M, Hurtado Rúa S, Tyshkov C, et al. Disease correlates of rim lesions on quantitative susceptibility mapping in multiple sclerosis. Sci Rep 2022;12(1): 4411.
97. Arnold D, Elliott C, Montalban X, et al. Effects of Evobrutinib, a Bruton's Tyrosine Kinase Inhibitor, on Slowly Expanding Lesions: An Emerging Imaging Marker of Chronic Tissue Loss in Multiple Sclerosis (S14.009). Neurology 2022;98(18 Supplement). Available at: https://n.neurology.org/content/98/18_Supplement/2674. Accessed June 22, 2023.
98. Pender MP, Csurhes PA, Smith C, et al. Epstein-Barr virus-specific adoptive immunotherapy for progressive multiple sclerosis. Mult Scler 2014;20(11): 1541–4.
99. Graves JS, Henry RG, Cree BAC, et al. Ovarian aging is associated with gray matter volume and disability in women with MS. Neurology 2018;90(3):e254–60.
100. MacKenzie-Graham A, Brook J, Kurth F, et al. Estriol-mediated neuroprotection in multiple sclerosis localized by voxel-based morphometry. Brain Behav 2018; 8(9):e01086.
101. Baroncini D, Annovazzi PO, De Rossi N, et al. Impact of natural menopause on multiple sclerosis: a multicentre study. J Neurol Neurosurg Psychiatry 2019; 90(11):1201–6.
102. Bove R, Okai A, Houtchens M, et al. Effects of Menopause in Women With Multiple Sclerosis: An Evidence-Based Review. Front Neurol 2021;12:554375.
103. Voskuhl RR, Wang H, Wu TCJ, et al. Estriol combined with glatiramer acetate for women with relapsing-remitting multiple sclerosis: a randomised, placebo-controlled, phase 2 trial. Lancet Neurol 2016;15(1):35–46.
104. Pozzilli C, De Giglio L, Barletta VT, et al. Oral contraceptives combined with interferon β in multiple sclerosis. Neurol Neuroimmunol Neuroinflamm 2015; 2(4):e120.
105. Otero-Romero S, Carbonell-Mirabent P, Midaglia L, et al. Oral contraceptives do not modify the risk of a second attack and disability accrual in a prospective cohort of women with a clinically isolated syndrome and early multiple sclerosis. Mult Scler 2022;28(6):950–7.
106. Shumaker SA, Legault C, Rapp SR, et al. Estrogen plus progestin and the incidence of dementia and mild cognitive impairment in postmenopausal women: the Women's Health Initiative Memory Study: a randomized controlled trial. JAMA 2003;289(20):2651–62.
107. Hall E, Frey BN, Soares CN. Non-hormonal treatment strategies for vasomotor symptoms: a critical review. Drugs 2011;71(3):287–304.
108. Çetinel B, Tarcan T, Demirkesen O, et al. Management of lower urinary tract dysfunction in multiple sclerosis: a systematic review and Turkish consensus report. Neurourol Urodyn 2013;32(8):1047–57.
109. Bove R, Anderson A, Rowles W, et al. A hormonal therapy for menopausal women with MS: A phase Ib/IIa randomized controlled trial. Mult Scler Relat Disord 2022;61:103747.

# Women's Health and Pregnancy in Multiple Sclerosis

Riley Bove, MD, MSc[a], Paige Sutton, MD[b,*],
Jacqueline Nicholas, MD, MPH[b]

**KEYWORDS**

- Multiple sclerosis • Pregnancy • Disease-modifying therapies • Neuroimmunology
- Women's health

**KEY POINTS**

- Multiple sclerosis (MS) is influenced by hormonal changes throughout women's lives. Puberty is a risk factor for developing MS, relapses tend to decrease during pregnancy, and transition to secondary progressive MS seems to coincide with menopause.
- MS most commonly presents in young adult women, and it is therefore vital to consider family planning and other issues surrounding women's health.
- Certain disease-modifying therapies (DMTs) may impact the health of the fetus and there has been a recent expansion of knowledge surrounding DMT use in family planning.
- Postpartum care of women with MS should be comprehensive and include a focus on the health of the patient and newborn to optimize psychosocial functioning and to prevent new MS disease activity.

## INTRODUCTION

Multiple sclerosis (MS) is an autoimmune, inflammatory, demyelinating, neurodegenerative disease of the central nervous system with numerous treatment options dependent on disease phenotype. MS has a 3:1 female-to-male predominance[1] in the approximately 95% cases with onset after puberty,[2,3] implicating a role of gonadal hormones, such as estrogen and progesterone, on this elevated risk in females.

Because MS predominantly arises in females between the ages of 20 to 45, health care professionals must be equipped to guide women on appropriate treatment options to optimize maternal health throughout the reproductive years and minimize

[a] UCSF Weill Institute for Neurosciences, 1651 Fourth Street, San Francisco, CA 94158, USA;
[b] OhioHealth Multiple Sclerosis Center, 3535 Olentangy River Road, Columbus, OH 43214, USA
* Corresponding author.
*E-mail address:* Paige.Sutton@ohiohealth.com

Neurol Clin 42 (2024) 275–293
https://doi.org/10.1016/j.ncl.2023.07.004
neurologic.theclinics.com

any risk to a potential fetus. Asking patients if they plan to become pregnant in the next 1 to 2 years at each visit can aid in proactive planning. MS does not affect fertility or pregnancy itself. Patients and neurologists alike are concerned about fetal exposure to MS disease-modifying therapies (DMTs), and conflicting reports in labeling of MS DMTs can make appropriate recommendations challenging. As a result, many women discontinue MS DMTs before attempts at conception or are not offered counseling on effective MS DMT options surrounding pregnancy and the postpartum period. This can result in women being unprotected from MS disease activity during attempts at conception or being offered less effective MS DMT options due to perceived greater safety. This may lead to an increased risk of relapse and worse outcomes for both mother and baby.

Prior studies demonstrated that the risk of MS relapse decreases during pregnancy and is less with each successive trimester; however, this reduction in risk is insufficient to rely on in all women with MS.[4] The discontinuation of certain DMTs such as fingolimod and natalizumab (NTZ) can increase risk of relapse from disease rebound.[5,6] In the postpartum period, however, the risk of MS relapse increases. The greatest predictors for relapse risk postpartum are prepregnancy inflammatory activity (annualized relapse rate (ARR) or active MRI),[4,7] as well as discontinuation of highly active DMTs. As a result, many MS specialists recommend stabilizing disease activity before attempts at conception when possible as well as mitigating strategies if discontinuing DMTs with rebound effects.

## WOMEN'S HEALTH

### *Puberty*

Puberty in females is a risk factor for the development of MS. Interestingly, an earlier age of onset of menarche seems to be associated with an increased risk of MS and also an earlier onset of MS symptoms.[8,9] Earlier age at puberty is associated with childhood adiposity; Mendelian randomization studies have shown that genes regulating both childhood obesity and pubertal age independently confer MS susceptibility.[10]

The course of MS is heterogeneous; however, female sex is considered a favorable prognostic factor in MS until the age of menopause.[11] Reproductive hormones have heterogeneous effects on MS risk and course. For example, estrogens seem to have a biphasic dose effect: immunostimulatory effects at low levels consistent with menstrual cycling, but at high levels of pregnancy seem to reduce immune activation.[12]

### *Contraception Considerations*

The use of contraception in women has not been shown to increase the risk of MS.[13,14] The importance of contraception should be regularly discussed with patients to prevent unplanned pregnancies while on DMTs that potentially carry fetal risks. Should pregnancies not be planned in the immediate future, the use of highly effective, long-acting and reversible options for contraception, such as intrauterine devices or implants, is ideal. Closer to a planned pregnancy, hormonal contraceptives can be discontinued to allow ovulatory cycles to resume, with the use of mechanical/barrier methods until planned conception. Special consideration to contraception selection should be made in women with decreased mobility, as combined hormonal contraceptives may increase the risk of thromboembolism. A common medication used off label for MS-related fatigue, modafinil, may decrease the effectiveness of hormonal contraceptives.[15]

### *Pregnancy in Multiple Sclerosis*

Women with MS are increasingly choosing to become pregnant after MS diagnosis and are increasingly receiving guidance from their neurologists in this choice. Although specific details are discussed below, an overview of the MS course during pregnancy is helpful in framing the following sections. During the immunotolerant state of pregnancy, most women with MS experience a lowered risk of relapses, followed by a risk of relapses postpartum (*vide infra*). For this reason, in many cases on the balance, it is preferable to discontinue DMTs when planning conception with specific guidance varying by DMT class and to resume high-efficacy DMTs with short therapeutic lag early postpartum (*vide infra*). MS symptoms also anecdotally are improved during pregnancy. MS is not in itself a high-risk condition during pregnancy, and therefore obstetrical considerations guide most management including comorbidities and delivery plan, but maternofetal medicine experts may be consulted for specific concerns or in the case of unintended exposure to DMTs (*vide infra*). Pregnancy loss—whether from spontaneous abortion, elective termination, miscarriage, or stillbirth—also seems to be associated with elevated risk of relapses.

Having MS overall does not seem to influence women's ability to become pregnant or their pregnancy outcomes. Obstetrical anesthesia is not considered a risk factor for MS relapses. There may be some slightly increased risk of having smaller babies and of elective cesarean or assisted deliveries, but no specific guidance is warranted. Specific care should be taken when advising women who are minoritized (due to race, ethnicity, or other sociocultural factors) or who have moderate to severe disability, as they may experience disparities in MS-related and pregnancy-related care. For these patients, collaborative care models—whereby neurologists actively collaborate with patients and their other clinicians to provide comprehensive care may be beneficial.

Before a planned conception, women with MS should be counseled about general health behaviors, such as smoking cessation, physical activity, and prenatal vitamins. Achieving normal vitamin D levels could be associated with the reduced risk of MS in their offspring.[16] A prepregnancy MRI could serve as a "baseline." In the event of new neurologic symptoms during pregnancy, when gadolinium use is not advised, a new non-contrast MRI could be compared against this baseline.

### *Fertility Treatment*

Women with MS may use various fertility treatments to support their fertility goals. These treatments include in vitro fertilization (IVF), that is, controlled ovarian stimulation (COS), egg retrieval and embryo transfer, COS and egg retrieval for fertility preservation, embryo transfer from frozen or donated eggs, and intrauterine insemination (IUI). Earlier, small studies reported increased relapse risk after fertility treatment; recent larger studies indicate that most women with MS do not experience this elevated risk, possibly as a result of more of them being treated with DMTs until embryo transfer.[17–19] If a woman with MS is undergoing IVF or IUI, DMT should be continued or discontinued similar to spontaneous pregnancies.[20] For men with MS providing sperm, DMT should be discontinued if it is known to be transferred in sperm (teriflunomide). Women with MS also seem to have similar chances of a live birth with assistive reproductive technologies compared with women without MS.[21] A multidisciplinary approach with inclusion of an MS specialist and a reproductive endocrinology obstetrician is best to ensure safety in these cases.

***General Principles for Disease-Modifying Therapy Management in Family Planning***

To avoid any presence of DMT in a patient's blood at the time of conception, the general principle of waiting five maximal half-lives should be followed. However, the decision of how to approach DMT continuation or cessation in preparation for conception should be guided by physiological principles, evolving evidence of risk in animal or human studies, evolving regulatory guidance, and patients' clinical profiles and preferences. Although specific decision-making should be individualized according to updated evidence, at present the currently available DMTs can be categorized as follows with respect to pregnancy planning (summarized in **Table 1**). In the postpartum period, the risk of relapses could be mitigated by resuming effective treatments with minimal therapeutic lag either within the first days postpartum, or in the

**Table 1**
**Overview of guidance on disease-modifying therapy cessation relative to conception**

| Agent | General Guidance on Product Discontinuation |
|---|---|
| First-line self-injectables | |
| Interferons | Short half-life, extensive data with no evidence of fetotoxicity, could continue until positive pregnancy test, through first trimester or even pregnancy |
| Glatiramer | Short half-life, extensive data with no evidence of fetotoxicity, could continue until positive pregnancy test or through pregnancy |
| IgG monoclonal antibodies | Minimal placental transfer until second trimester (week 20); for products with t1/2 between 12 and 24 d, based on the principle of 5 half-lives, a mAb administered near time of conception would be eliminated by the time product might cross the placenta |
| Anti-B-cell therapy | Persistent B-cell depletion at least 6 mo after treatment provides optimized pharmacokinetic/pharmacodynamic parameters if conception occurs 1–3 mo after treatment. Ofatumumab has slightly shorter half-life and could be "timed to menses," ie, injected monthly after confirmation of menses in nonpregnant state and discontinued at the time of pregnancy and missed period. |
| Natalizumab | Risk of rebound; consider either bridge to anti-CD20 before conception, or continue at extended interval dosing (every 6 weeks) until week 34 and check newborn cord blood/serum for complete blood count |
| Alemtuzumab | Conception 4 mo after second annual treatment; monitor monthly for thyroid abnormalities during pregnancy |
| Oral agents | |
| Fumarates | Discontinue at the time of positive pregnancy test |
| S1P receptor modulators | Risk of rebound; consider anti-CD20 "bridge" to reduce the risk of rebound; discontinue before conception depending on specific product half-life: ozanimod 3 mo, fingolimod 2 mo, ponesimod and siponimod: 2 wk |
| Teriflunomide | Discontinue 2 y before conception or undergo accelerated protocol to ensure maternal serum concentration of <0.02 mcg/mL |
| Cladribine | Conception 6 mo after second annual treatment |

Based on Bove and Houtchens, *Neurology Continuum* 2022 and Krysko, Dobson et al, *Lancet Neurology* 2023.

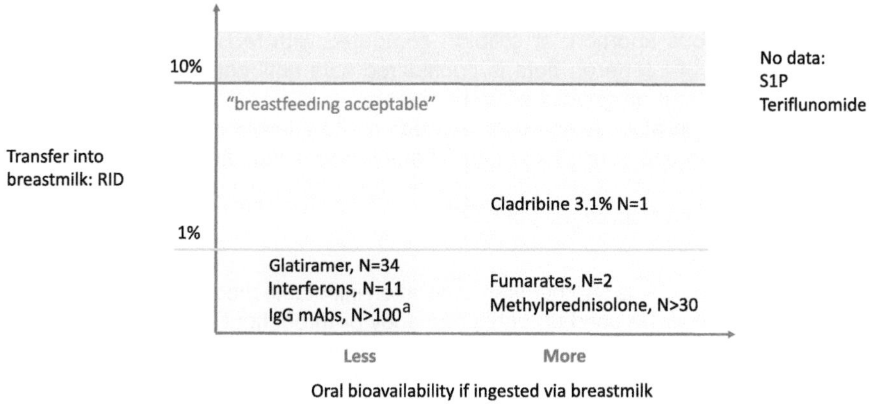


**Fig. 1.** Summary of data available on breast milk transfer of MS disease-modifying therapies. The currently available evidence, as summarized on LactMed.gov on 6/5/2023, is presented. For each product category, the relative infant disease (RID) is presented as well as the number of individual patients contributing to this observation. Typically, an RID < 10% is considered compatible with breastfeeding. Products are further categorized into lower and greater likelihood of oral bioavailability should these be ingested via breast milk. Several IgG monoclonal antibodies have been evaluated including those used for MS (ocrelizumab, rituximab, natalizumab) as well as for other conditions,[83] and levels are consistently <1%. [a]There is minimal transfer of maternal endogenous IgG into breast milk; transfer of IgG monoclonal antibodiess has been evaluated for several products, all demonstrating RID <1% (LaHue et al, N2 2022). Caution with alemtuzumab given risk of thyroid dysfunction.

case of breastfeeding, once the mature milk is established (2 weeks postpartum). The current evidence basis for transfer of products is summarized in **Fig. 1**.

- *First-line DMTs (interferons, glatiramers) and fumarates*: continue until conception attempts or missed period
- *Teriflunomide:* accelerated washout protocol or wait 2 years before conception for women
- *Medications with rebound risk (S1Ps, NTZ):* bridge to anti-CD20 therapy or, for NTZ, continue at extended interval dosing (6 weeks) until gestational age 34 weeks
- *"Induction" therapies (alemtuzumab and cladribine):* complete full course, then wait 6 months
- *Anti-B-cell monoclonals (ofatumumab, ocrelizumab, rituximab, ublituximab):* wait 1 to 3 months after last treatment and continue conception attempts while B cells remain undetectable

In the case of unplanned conception while on a DMT, a maternofetal medicine expert can be consulted.

## SPECIFIC DISEASE-MODIFYING THERAPIES

### *First-Line Disease-Modifying Therapies*

#### *Interferon beta*

Interferon beta 1a and 1b injections are polypeptides with large molecular weights that do not cross the placenta.[22] In a large cohort study, treatment of MS patients with interferon beta resulted in no increase of major congenital anomalies, ectopic pregnancy, spontaneous abortion, or stillbirth compared with MS patients off of treatment.[23] The use of interferon beta is considered safe until conception and can be continued throughout pregnancy when necessary.

Interferon beta is also detected at exceedingly low levels in breast milk and is considered safe to use during lactation.[24] Safety of breastfeeding on interferon beta has been shown in infants at 1 year who did not have increased risk of hospitalization, antibiotic use, or developmental delays.[25]

#### Glatiramer acetate

Glatiramer acetate (GA) is another first-generation injectable medication. Different formulations of GA may be used up until pregnancy or throughout pregnancy. In fact, it was the most used DMT during pregnancy in women with MS in the United States from 2016 to 2021.[26] Studies have shown that GA use during pregnancy does not result in any increased rate of spontaneous abortion, premature births, low birth weight, or congenital abnormalities.[27,28]

Because GA is a large molecule, it is unlikely to be excreted in breast milk.[24] Labels for generic GA 20 mg and 40 mg support the use of this medication during breastfeeding. At 18 months of age, infants exposed to GA through breast milk had no increase in hospitalizations, antibiotic use, or incidence of developmental delay or abnormal growth parameters.[29]

#### Fumarates

The fumarates include dimethyl fumarate, diroximel fumarate, and monomethyl fumarate. Because of their short half-life and lack of rebound disease activity, fumarates can be discontinued for family planning or potentially at the time of a positive pregnancy test. No washout period is required. An international registry recently reported on cases of exposure to dimethyl fumarate during the first trimester and found an expected proportion of spontaneous abortions (10.9%) compared with the general MS population and no congenital anomalies or malformations.[30] No published data are available on monomethyl fumarate or diroximel fumarate in pregnancy.

In lactating women taking dimethyl fumarate, the relative infant doses of the metabolite monomethyl fumarate were significantly lower than the theoretical threshold of concern in two measured cases.[31] Larger studies are needed to confirm these findings, and current recommendations are to avoid use during lactation.

### Therapies with Specific Discontinuation Parameters

#### Teriflunomide

Because of animal studies showing teratogenicity and embryotoxicity, teriflunomide is contraindicated for use during pregnancy or in women of childbearing potential not on effective contraception. In cases of unplanned pregnancy on teriflunomide, the medication should immediately be stopped, and rapid elimination protocol should be initiated with activated charcoal or cholestyramine.

Because it is contraindicated during pregnancy, limited data are available about outcomes of infants exposed to teriflunomide in utero. There have not been clear reports of increased spontaneous abortion, preterm delivery, or congenital malformations when compared with the general population.[32,33] However, more data are needed and those with unplanned pregnancies on teriflunomide should undergo accelerated elimination of the drug. A unique characteristic to consider with teriflunomide is the transmission of drug via semen with potential for fetal toxicity.[34] Therefore, the use of barrier contraception for men on this treatment is recommended. Men and women considering pregnancy should be treated with an alternate DMT.

Teriflunomide is a small molecule that is likely to be excreted in breast milk and is therefore also contraindicated in breastfeeding women.[35]

### *Therapies with Discontinuation Rebound Risk*

#### *Natalizumab*

Because of its pharmacokinetics, NTZs effects begin to reverse at 8 weeks post-infusion[36] and there is risk of rebound disease activity with discontinuation. This presents unique challenges, as the use of NTZ before conception predicted increased relapse rate during pregnancy.[37]

An Italian cohort of pregnant women with relapsing remitting multiple sclerosis (RRMS) treated with NTZ found that those with long exposure during pregnancy had significantly lower ARRs compared with those with short (30–90 days after LMP) or no exposure.[38] No differences were found in infant gestational age and size in those exposed to NTZ in utero versus other groups or in congenital anomalies compared with the general population.[38] However, a German registry found that NTZ exposure during the third trimester increased risk of anemia in newborns.[39] It may be best to hold NTZ after 30 to 34 weeks gestation and reinitiate after delivery. Multiple studies have shown that early resumption postpartum results in reduced relapse risk.[38,39]

Early resumption for women planning to breastfeed is recommended as well. Transfer in breast milk is below the threshold for concern, and there are no known adverse effects on infants.[40]

#### *Sphingosine 1-phosphate receptor modulators*

The sphingosine 1-phosphate (S1P) receptor modulators are oral pills that include fingolimod, siponimod, ponesimod, and ozanimod. A somewhat unique characteristic of the S1P receptor modulators is the risk of rebound MS disease activity with abrupt discontinuation. Women who stopped fingolimod for family planning purposes experienced rebound disease activity at a level higher than pretreatment.[41] When stopping fingolimod before conception or within the first trimester, there was increased disease activity during pregnancy despite pregnancy's protective effects on MS relapse.[37,42]

Because these medications are contraindicated during pregnancy, there are limited data on outcomes of fetuses exposed to S1P receptor modulators. Preclinical animal data in rats and rabbits suggested teratogenicity of fingolimod, and one study in humans also showed a higher rate of abnormal fetal development than would be expected.[43] A later study of women who stopped fingolimod during the first trimester found no increase in spontaneous abortions or congenital malformations, though the medication was discontinued at a median of 6 weeks gestation.[44] Data are not available on the safety of newer S1P modulators (siponimod, ozanimod, ponesimod) during pregnancy but would be expected to have similar risks.

Owing to the potential teratogenic risks and risks of rebound with cessation, an alternate class of DMT should be considered in women of reproductive potential and especially in those planning for future pregnancy.

Based on elimination times, ozanimod should be discontinued at least 3 months before pregnancy and fingolimod should be discontinued at least 2 months before pregnancy. Siponimod and ponesimod have shorter half-lives and waiting at least 10 days to conceive should allow reasonable clearance before conceiving. To prevent rebound disease activity with discontinuation, a "bridge" can be considered with anti-CD20 infusion at the time of S1P receptor modulator discontinuation.[45]

It is unknown if the S1P receptor modulators are excreted in human breast milk, though fingolimod is excreted in rat milk.[46] These medications should be avoided during breastfeeding due to the potential cardiovascular toxic effects for the infant.

### *Therapies with Optimized Pharmacokinetic and Pharmacodynamic Parameters: "Induction Therapies" and Anti-B-Cell Monoclonals*

#### *Cladribine*

Cladribine is dosed in two treatment courses over 2 years with sustained results in many patients for years 3 and 4 without further courses.[47] Because of its short treatment course, cladribine may be initiated in those who desire future, but not current, pregnancy. Owing to cladribine's ability to damage genetic information in cells, current recommendations are to avoid pregnancy for 6 months after a male or female patient is treated with cladribine.

Analysis of unplanned pregnancies within 6 months of administration of cladribine resulted in comparable birth weight, gestational age,[48] and no increase in spontaneous abortion rates.[49] No cases of major congenital anomalies or stillbirths have been reported in a worldwide surveillance program.[50] There was also no increased risk of adverse fetal outcomes in fathers treated with cladribine during this at-risk window.[50] Although these results are generally positive, continued counseling about the importance of contraception for 6 months following treatment is necessary.

Current prescribing recommendations are to wait 10 days to resume breastfeeding after cladribine in the United States. A case report supported the safety of this washout period by demonstrating rapid decline in cladribine levels 12 to 24 hours after drug administration and undetectable levels by 48 hours.[51] Further data on breast milk transfer and infant outcomes are needed.

#### *B-cell depletion*

Ocrelizumab, rituximab, ofatumumab, and ublituximab are anti-CD20 monoclonal immunoglobulin 1 (IgG1) antibodies. Transplacental transfer of IgG1 from mother to fetus is negligible in the first trimester and higher in the second and third. Based on half-lives of each of these medications, it is expected that most anti-CD20 monoclonal antibodies, if administered around the time of conception, would be cleared from the patient's body by the time they could begin to be transferred across the placenta at 17 to 20 weeks gestation. Because of the long-lasting effects of these medications and ability to dose up until conception, the use of B-cell depletion therapy for family planning is rapidly increasing. As of March 2022, there were over 2000 pregnancies in women treated with ocrelizumab,[52] and it was the second most used DMT in women planning for pregnancy, during pregnancy and in the postpartum period from 2017 to 2021.[26] Women who used ocrelizumab during pregnancy had expected rates of preterm deliveries, ectopic pregnancy, spontaneous abortions, and fetuses with major congenital anomalies compared with unexposed women.[52] A washout period of approximately 2 months for ocrelizumab and rituximab before attempting to conceive can optimize both disease stability (through persistent B-cell depletion) and fetal safety (by ensuring minimal concentration in maternal serum by the second trimester). Similarly, there were no increased rates of spontaneous abortions or congenital anomalies reported in pregnancies after maternal ofatumumab treatment and no increase in serious infections in infants during the first year of life.[53] Given the slightly shorter half-life of ofatumumab, with an approximate 12-week clearance, it may be reasonable to continue ofatumumab in patients attempting to conceive with a pregnancy test before each dose, with treatment discontinuation when pregnancy is confirmed. Ublituximab has not been studied during pregnancy at this point, and the label recommends a negative pregnancy test before each infusion.

Monoclonal antibodies have high molecular weights and therefore have minimal transfer to breast milk. The relative infant doses of ocrelizumab and rituximab in mature breast milk are on average less than 1% which is far below the theoretically acceptable level of 10% or less.[54] There were also normal rates of infections and normal CD19 levels in those infants.[54] Maximum concentrations occurred 1 to 7 days after infusion. There are no published studies on the use of ofatumumab or ublituximab in breastfeeding to date. Because more antibodies may be transferred in colostrum, it may be reasonable to wait until mature milk is established (1–2 weeks postpartum) before restarting B-cell depleting treatments in breastfeeding mothers.

#### *Alemtuzumab*

Alemtuzumab is an infusion treatment given over two courses with re-dosing as needed. In some cases, efficacy for relapse prevention and preventing disability can be maintained for up to 12 years.[55] Levels of alemtuzumab are low or undetectable within 30 days of administration,[56] but to avoid fetal exposure, the drug label recommends avoiding pregnancy for 4 months after infusion. Rates of spontaneous abortions, congenital anomalies, and birth defects were not increased in infants of women treated with alemtuzumab before or during pregnancy.[57] ARRs of pregnant women treated with alemtuzumab were also low during pregnancy, increased slightly after delivery and were similar in those treated with one versus two courses.[57] However, most patients undergoing treatment with alemtuzumab are considered highly active, and two courses are recommended followed by a 4-month washout period for optimal disease control before trying to conceive.

Ideally, patients would have completed both annual courses with alemtuzumab before a pregnancy. Alemtuzumab is expected to be minimally excreted in breast milk, but given possible transfer also of thyroid antibodies, it is not recommended for lactating women.[35]

## RELAPSES DURING PREGNANCY

Should a woman experience new neurologic symptoms during pregnancy to distinguish an MS relapse from other causes of neurologic symptoms (eg, entrapment neuropathy such as carpal tunnel syndrome or meralgia paresthetica), an MRI without gadolinium can be used to assess for new lesions relative to the preconception baseline MRI. For relapses resulting in functional impairments, the steroids methylprednisolone or prednisone can be used after the first trimester, and often in the first trimester, if in consensus with the patient's obstetrician.[58] Plasmapheresis has been used for severe relapses, as well.

### *Postpartum Multiple Sclerosis Management*

The postpartum period represents a time of high risk for women with MS in several ways; they experience many care gaps, especially in countries such as the United States with low support for parental leave. This risk includes an elevated risk of hospital readmission for severe maternal conditions,[59] elevated risk of relapses and new inflammatory activity on MRI,[60] and elevated risk of depression.[61] Postpartum care planning should begin well before delivery to aid in the best outcomes and involve the mother, family, and when necessary other health care professionals. If possible, insurance authorizations and referral scheduling should occur before the patient delivers and is occupied with the newborn.

One critical decision in the postpartum period is discussion around breastfeeding and timing of DMT resumption. This individualized shared decision between the neurologist and the patient can engage, as warranted: a patient's partner, obstetrical clinician, and pediatrician. Commonly, patients with MS receive mixed messages from their various clinicians who may not be up to date on latest management guidelines, and this can affect their birth experience and mood. Breastfeeding has numerous benefits for the dyad (eg, bonding), the newborn (nutrition, decreased infection, decreased long-term risk of autoimmune, and cardiometabolic conditions), the mother (cancer and cardiometabolic condition prevention), and in the case of mothers with MS, exclusive breastfeeding in the first 6 months also reduces risk of relapses.[62–64] If patients wish to breastfeed and are able to, then early referral to a lactation consultant can help support them and optimize ability.

There is emerging evidence that early resumption of highly effective therapies with minimal therapeutic lag (ie, onset of efficacy) can also help to reduce postpartum relapse risk. Rather than counsel patients to choose between breastfeeding and resuming DMTs, there is evidence of minimal transfer of some DMTs into breast milk, which could support decisions to both breastfeed and resume DMT if clinically indicated.

In the event of a postpartum relapses, steroids have minimal transfer into breast milk.[65] An MRI to monitor disease activity may be helpful to guide timing of DMT reinitiation in women who have delayed DMT reinitiation for breastfeeding. Gadolinium is considered compatible with lactation and holding breastfeeds following administration is not recommended.[66]

Beyond DMT reinitiation, comprehensive care involves assessment for rehabilitation-amenable symptoms including focal weakness, balance difficulties, and bladder dysfunction. It also involves screening and monitoring for postpartum depression which occurs in about one in five women with MS postpartum[67] and screening for thyroid or other metabolic conditions. Empirically, sleep disruption is a major factor affecting postpartum wellness in MS and guidance that patients achieve at least 4 to 5 hours of uninterrupted sleep could be beneficial. Social workers may be beneficial in supporting patients with social support needs and logistical concerns including time off work, medical resources, and resources for childcare. The overarching goals of postpartum care are to provide comprehensive care to support the health of the patient with MS and the newborn to prevent new disease activity and to optimize psychosocial functioning.

### *Lesbian, gay, bisexual, transgender, queer/questioning, intersex, asexual, plus (LBTQIA+)*

Neurologists overall require more training in caring for sexual and gender minorities,[68] who face a number of unmet clinical and social needs (**Fig. 2**). A North American Research Committe on Multiple Sclerosis (NARCOMS) study of over 5000 individuals with MS found that 0.45% of participants identified as transgender (TGD) and 4.6% as nonheterosexual. As compared with cisgender heterosexual individuals with MS, those who identified as TGD or nonheterosexual reported less comfort in discussing sexual health with their doctor,[69] pointing to an unmet need for awareness and discussion of their unique needs, gender-inclusive language, and comprehensive assessment of physical and mental health. TGD individuals may use exogenous hormones as part of gender-affirming care, including testosterone for trans men and estrogens, progestins, and/or antiandrogens for trans women. These hormones could influence the risk of autoimmunity, mental health, and laboratory values, and their possible impact on MS risk or course is not well understood.[70] For example, a single study demonstrated an

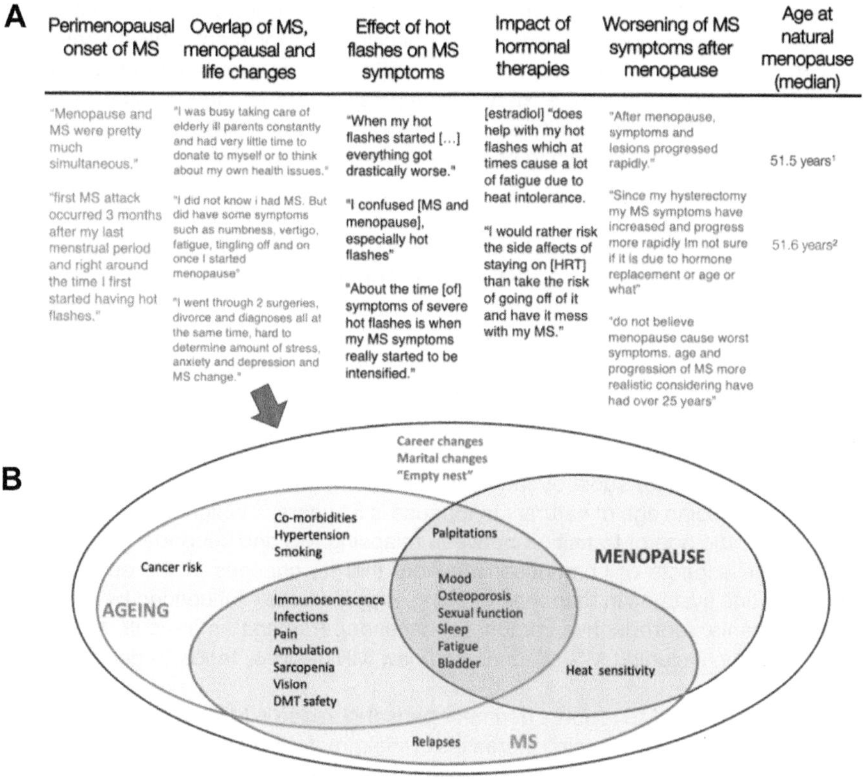


**Fig. 2.** Overview of commonly reported experiences of women with MS during the menopausal transition.

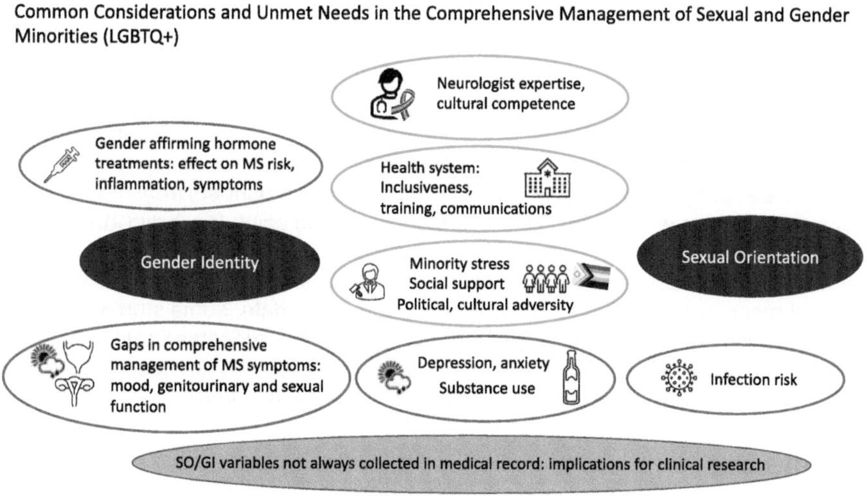


**Fig. 3.** Common considerations and unmet needs in the comprehensive management of sexual and gender minorities (LGBTQIA+) individuals.

increased risk of MS in trans women relative to cis men, possibly related to a shift in estrogen:androgen ratios.[71] There is also specific need for mental health screening and care, because persons with MS have a 50% lifetime prevalence of depression and in TGD persons, rates of anxiety and depression are as high as 39%.[70] Finally, care should be taken to identify sources of social support for individuals who are both minoritized and experiencing neurologic symptoms and impairments.[72]

### *Menopause*

The menopausal transition is a normal physiological transition with several implications for women with MS (**Fig. 3**). In the general population, the final menstrual period, which by definition characterizes the age of menopause, usually occurs in the sixth decade. Before this final menstrual period, progesterone levels begin to decrease during the 30s, and estrogen levels peak in the late 40s before their perimenopausal decline.[73] Ovarian aging is reflected by levels of anti-Müllerian hormone, which peaks around age 25 years and is undetectable by menopause.[74] The perimenopausal period refers to the few years before and immediately after the final menstrual period, after which women are subsequently considered postmenopausal.

In MS, the median age of natural menopause is 51 years,[75] which coincides with the mean diagnostic age of transition between relapsing MS and secondary progressive MS.[11] Some aspects of immunosenescence, that is, changes in the adaptive and innate immune systems in response to aging, may be further influenced by reproductive changes (ie, reproductive immunosenescence). Perhaps as a result, MS inflammatory activity, including MS relapses and new MRI lesions, tends to decrease after menopause.[76]

Many women with MS report a perimenopausal increase in MS-related symptoms,[77] even if they are not experiencing increases in inflammatory activity. Some of this worsening can be attributed to vasomotor symptoms (hot flashes). Some symptomatic worsening can also be related to worsening in "overlap symptoms" (sleep, fatigue, mood, pain, and bladder function), facets of both MS and menopause, and which can synergistically worsen function. Historically, overinterpretation of risk from data in older women treated with HRT in the Women's Health Initiative led to a dramatic reduction in HRT use and as a consequence, vasomotor symptoms are undertreated in the modern era. More recently, the benefits and risks of HRT use in women during their menopausal transition have been reevaluated, and in women with MS, treating these vasomotor symptoms could alleviate symptomatic fluctuations and worsening. When hormones are contraindicated, vasomotor symptoms can also be treated with selective norepinephrine reuptake inhibitors and neurokinin 3 receptor antagonists.

Beyond these symptomatic changes, it can be diagnostically challenging to differentiate between progression from MS, normal aging, and confounders from other comorbidities associated with aging. Biomarkers of neurologic aging (eg, brain atrophy) are known to associate with both biomarkers of general aging (eg, telomere length) and biomarkers of ovarian aging in both the general population and in MS.[78] With respect to an effect of menopause itself on the MS disease course, to date, some studies have reported an acceleration in worsening of the Expanded Disability Status Scale,[79] whereas others have not.[76] More studies using more sensitive outcomes are needed to further determine whether menopause might influence MS disease course.

## HEALTHY AGING

Although half of all individuals living with MS are in their sixth decade or beyond,[80] most DMT RCTs exclude participants older than 55 years, substantially limiting the availability of trial data—and understanding of the treatment effects or side effects—in postmenopausal females.[81] Optimizing overall health by early detection and management of comorbidities is important for brain health. Comorbidities associated with aging are important to screen following menopause. These include, but are not limited to, blood pressure, thyroid disease, bone density, and substance use such as alcohol and tobacco use.[82] Given immunosenescence patterns, vaccines should also be updated including pneumonia, shingles, and respiratory syncytial virus (RSV)—the latest Centers for Disease Control and Prevention (CDC) guidelines should be followed. Further, it is important to overcome diagnostic neglect and ensure that postmenopausal females receive age-appropriate cancer screening including gynecological and breast cancers and dermatological and gastrointestinal cancers. These screenings can be done in coordination with primary care and ob-gyn specialists. More research is needed on patient experiences with cancer as well as MS outcomes after cancer treatment in women with MS. To ensure healthy aging and well-being, patients should be screened for affective disorders, rehabilitation needs, home safety needs, and social support. It has been shown that social support is integral to health in aging women.

## SUMMARY

The care of women with MS is complex and should be carried out under the guidance of a neurologist with expertise in MS disease and symptom management in this population during the reproductive years and beyond. Fortunately, in the past 50 years, research has helped to inform an improved approach to the care of females with MS. Women with MS can now feel comfortable that pregnancy does not impact the MS disease course negatively and that disease modification can be optimized to protect women from ongoing neurologic injury during their reproductive years.

It is vital to consider reproductive safety when starting any DMTs in women of childbearing potential—and long before conception. Some MS therapies can be continued until conception (fumarates) or even into/throughout pregnancy (interferons, GA). Certain DMTs such as S1P receptor modulators, teriflunomide, cladribine, and alemtuzumab should not be used in women who may become pregnant in the near future. Cladribine and alemtuzumab may be used as induction therapies in those on effective birth control who are planning a future pregnancy. Timing of discontinuation or completion of treatment courses before conception is vital and details about washout periods are recommended in this review. B-cell depletion infusion therapies have become a common therapy used in women who are planning to conceive due to optimized pharmacokinetic and pharmacodynamic properties—that is, conception attempts just a few months after infusion. NTZ should be either transitioned to B-cell depleting therapies before conception attempts or continued until 30 to 34 weeks in cases of high MS disease activity. Timing of restarting DMTs is also important due to the increased risk of relapses following delivery. In general, to protect against postpartum relapses, high-efficacy DMTs with short therapeutic lag should be started early after delivery, and ideally, DMTs compatible with lactation if patients plan to breastfeed. This should be planned while the patient is still in the early stages of pregnancy, and timing will depend on the patient's plans to breastfeed.

The goal of MS care is to enable women with MS to adequately control their MS disease activity and manage symptoms while feeling empowered to make their own personal choices regarding reproductive decisions. Furthermore, future research is needed to better understand the impact of menopause on women with MS and to improve quality of life throughout the lifespan.

## CLINICS CARE POINTS

- Although the risk of MS relapse is lower during pregnancy, this is not sufficient protection for many women with MS.
- Some MS therapies should be discontinued before attempts to conceive (S1P receptor modulators, teriflunomide); some can be continued until conception (fumarates) or even into/throughout pregnancy (interferons, GA). Cladribine and alemtuzumab may be used as induction therapies in those on effective birth control planning a future pregnancy. NTZ should be transitioned to a B-cell depleting therapy before conception or continued until 30 to 34 weeks gestation. A B-cell depleting therapy can be used during family planning by using timed windows for conception after infusions.
- There is also an increased risk of relapse following delivery, and high-efficacy therapy should be resumed as soon as possible with consideration of transfer in milk for breastfeeding mothers.
- Breastfeeding has many benefits for mother and newborn and can help reduce postpartum relapse risk. Consider a DMT with data regarding safe use and minimal transfer during breastfeeding (interferon beta, GA, fumarates, NTZ, B-cell depleting therapy).

## DISCLOSURES

R. Bove is funded by the NIH, DOD, and the National Multiple Sclerosis Society Harry Weaver Award, as well as by Biogen, Novartis, and Roche-Genentech. She has received consulting/advisory board fees from Alexion, EMD Serono, Horizon, Janssen and TG Therapeutics. P. Sutton has received honoraria for consulting from: Genentech, Horizon Therapeutics and Octave Bioscience. J. Nicholas has received research grants from: Biogen, Novartis, PCORI, Genentech, University of Buffalo; honoraria for consulting from: EMD Serono, Genentech, Greenwich Biosciences, Novartis, TG Therapeutics, Sanofi, Octave Bioscience; and speaking honoraria from BMS, EMD Serono, Horizon and TG Therapeutics.

## REFERENCES

1. Koch-Henricksen N, Magyari M. Apparent changes in the epidemiology and severity of multiple sclerosis. Nat Rev Neurol 2021;17:676–88.
2. Banwell BL. Multiple sclerosis in children. Handb Clin Neurol 2014;122. 427-241.
3. Chitnis T. Paediatric MS is the same disease as adult MS. Mult Scler 2013;19(10): 1255–6. https://doi.org/10.1177/1352458513488842.
4. Confavreux C, Hutchinson M, Hours MM, et al. Rate of pregnancy –related relapse in multiple sclerosis. Pregnancy in multiple sclerosis group. N Engl J Med 1998;339:285–91.
5. Alroughani R, Alowayesh MS, Ahmed SF, et al. Relapse occurrence in women with multiple sclerosis during pregnancy in the new treatment era. Neurology 2018;90:e840–6.
6. Hellwig K, Tokic M, Thiel S, et al. Multiple sclerosis disease activity and disability following discontinuation of natalizumab for pregnancy. JAMA Netw Open 2022; 5:e2144750.
7. Hughes SE, Spelman T, Gray OM, et al. Predictors and dynamics of post-partum relapses in women with multiple sclerosis. Mult Scler 2014;20:739–46.
8. Ramagopalan SV, Valdar W, Criscuoli M, et al. Age of puberty and the risk of multiple sclerosis: a population based study. Eur J Neurol 2009;16:342–7.

9. Sloka JS, Pryse-Phillips WEM, Stefanelli M. The relation between menarche and the age of first symptoms in a multiple sclerosis cohort. Mult Scler 2006;12:333–9.
10. Harroud A, Mitchell RE, Richardson TG, et al. Childhood obesity and multiple sclerosis: A Mendelian randomization study. Mult Scler 2021;27(14):2150–8.
11. Krysko KM, Graves JS, Dobson R, et al. Sex effects across the lifespan in women with multiple sclerosis. Ther Adv Neurol Disord 2020;13. 1756286420936166.
12. Soldan SS, Alvarez Retuerto AI, Sicotte NL, et al. Immune modulation in multiple sclerosis patients treated with the pregnancy hormone estriol. J Immunol 2003; 171:6267–74.
13. Ghajarzadeh M, Mohammadi A, Shahraki Z, et al. Pregnancy history, oral contraceptive pills consumption (OCPs), and risk of multiple sclerosis: a systematic review and meta-analysis. Int J Prev Med 2022;13:89.
14. Otero-Romero S, Carbonell-Mirabent P, Midaglia L, et al. Oral contraceptives do not modify the risk of a second attack and disability accrual in a prospective cohort of women with a clinically isolated syndrome and early multiple sclerosis. Mult Scler 2022;28(6):950–7.
15. Houtchens MK, Zapata LB, Curtis KM, et al. Contraception for women with multiple sclerosis: guidance for healthcare providers. Mult Scler 2017;23:757–64.
16. Mansur JL, Oliveri B, Giacoia E, et al. Vitamin D: Before, during and after pregnancy: effect on neonates and children. Nutrients 2022;14(9):1900.
17. Dobson R, Bove R. In vitro fertilization and multiple sclerosis: evolving treatments and reducing relapse risk. Neurology 2022;99(17):737–8.
18. Mainguy M, Tillaut H, Degremont A, et al. Assessing the risk of relapse requiring corticosteroids after in vitro fertilization in women with multiple sclerosis. Neurology 2022;11. https://doi.org/10.1212/WNL.0000000000201027.
19. Graham EL, Bakkensen JB, Anderson A, et al. Inflammatory activity after diverse fertility treatments: a multicenter analysis in the modern multiple sclerosis treatment era. Neurology(R) neuroimmunology & neuroinflammation 2023;10:1–13.
20. Oreja-Guevara C, Rabanal A, Rodríguez CH, et al. Assisted reproductive techniques in multiple sclerosis: recommendations from an expert panel. Neurol Ther 2023;12(2):427–39.
21. Riis Jølving L, Due Larsen M, Fedder J, et al. Live birth in women with multiple sclerosis receiving assisted reproduction. Reprod Biomed Online 2020;40(5): 711–8.
22. Cree BA. Update on reproductive safety of current and emerging disease-modifying therapies for multiple sclerosis. Mult Scler 2013;19(7):835–43.
23. Hakkarainen KM, Juuti R, Burkill S, et al. Pregnancy outcomes after exposure to interferon beta: a register-based cohort study among women with MS in Finland and Sweden. Ther Adv Neurol Disord 2020;13. 1756286420951072.
24. Bove RM, Houtchens MK. Pregnancy management in multiple sclerosis and other demyelinating diseases. Continuum 2022;28(1):12–33.
25. Ciplea AI, Langer-Gould A, Stahl A, et al. Safety of potential breast milk exposure to IFN-β or glatiramer acetate: one-year infant outcomes. Neurol Neuroimmunol Neuroinflamm 2020;7(4):e757.
26. Graham E, Chaudhary N, Sun D, Liu C, Pasquarelli N. Trends in the Use of Disease-Modifying Therapies in Pre-Pregnant, Pregnant and Postpartum Women With Multiple Sclerosis in the United States: 2016–2021. Poster presented at: 38th Congress of the European Committee for Treatment and Research in Multiple Sclerosis (ECTRIMS); 2022 October 26-28; Amsterdam, the Netherlands.

27. Sandberg-Wollheim M, Neudorfer O, Grinspan A, et al. Pregnancy outcomes from the branded glatiramer acetate pregnancy database. Int J MS Care 2018; 20(1):9–14.
28. Kaplan S, Zeygarnik M, Stern T. Pregnancy, fetal, and infant outcomes following maternal exposure to glatiramer acetate during pregnancy and breastfeeding. Drug Saf 2022;45(4):345–57.
29. Ciplea AI, Kurzeja A, Thiel S, et al. Eighteen-month safety analysis of offspring breastfed by mothers receiving glatiramer acetate therapy for relapsing multiple sclerosis - COBRA study. Mult Scler 2022;28(10):1641–50.
30. Hellwig K, Rog D, McGuigan C, et al. Interim analysis of pregnancy outcomes after exposure to dimethyl fumarate in a prospective international registry. Neurol Neuroimmunol Neuroinflamm 2021;9(1):e1114.
31. Ciplea AI, Datta P, Rewers-Felkins K, et al. Dimethyl fumarate transfer into human milk. Ther Adv Neurol Disord 2020;13. 1756286420968414.
32. Andersen JB, Moberg JY, Spelman T, et al. Pregnancy outcomes in men and women treated with teriflunomide. A population-based nationwide danish register study. Front Immunol 2018;9:2706.
33. Vukusic S, Coyle PK, Jurgensen S, et al. Pregnancy outcomes in patients with multiple sclerosis treated with teriflunomide: Clinical study data and 5 years of post-marketing experience. Mult Scler 2020;26(7):829–36.
34. Guarnaccia JB, Cabot A, Garten LL, et al. Teriflunomide levels in women whose male sexual partner is on teriflunomide for relapsing multiple sclerosis. Mult Scler Relat Disord 2022;57:103347.
35. Varytė G, Arlauskienė A, Ramašauskaitė D. Pregnancy and multiple sclerosis: an update. Curr Opin Obstet Gynecol 2021;33(5):378–83.
36. Plavina T, Muralidharan KK, Kuesters G, et al. Reversibility of the effects of natalizumab on peripheral immune cell dynamics in MS patients. Neurology 2017; 89(15):1584–93 [Epub 2017 Sep 15. Erratum in: Neurology. 2020 Oct 6;95(14): 661. PMID: 28916537; PMCID: PMC5634662].
37. Yeh WZ, Widyastuti PA, Van der Walt A, et al, MSBase Study Group. Natalizumab, fingolimod and dimethyl fumarate use and pregnancy-related relapse and disability in women with multiple sclerosis. Neurology 2021;96(24):e2989–3002.
38. Landi D, Bovis F, Grimaldi A, et al. Exposure to natalizumab throughout pregnancy: effectiveness and safety in an Italian cohort of women with multiple sclerosis. J Neurol Neurosurg Psychiatr 2022. https://doi.org/10.1136/jnnp-2022-329657. jnnp-2022-329657.
39. Thiel S, Litvin N, Haben S, Ciplea A, Gold R, Hellwig K. 2022. Disease activity and Pregnancy outcomes after long-term Exposure to Natlizumab during Pregnancy. [Poster]. 38th Congress of the European Committee for Treatment and Research in Multiple Sclerosis (ECTRIMS), 26-28 October, Amsterdam.
40. Proschmann U, Haase R, Inojosa H, et al. Drug and neurofilament levels in serum and breastmilk of women with multiple sclerosis exposed to natalizumab during pregnancy and lactation. Front Immunol 2021;12:715195.
41. Callens A, Leblanc S, Le Page E, et al. Disease reactivation after fingolimod cessation in Multiple Sclerosis patients with pregnancy desire: a retrospective study. Mult Scler Relat Disord 2022;66:104066.
42. Bianco A, Lucchini M, Totaro R, et al. Disease reactivation after fingolimod discontinuation in pregnant multiple sclerosis patients. Neurotherapeutics 2021; 18:2598–607.

43. Karlsson G, Francis G, Koren G, et al. Pregnancy outcomes in the clinical development program of fingolimod in multiple sclerosis. Neurology 2014;82(8): 674–80.
44. Pauliat E, Onken M, Weber-Schoendorfer C, et al. Pregnancy outcome following first-trimester exposure to fingolimod: a collaborative ENTIS study. Mult Scler 2021;27(3):475–8.
45. Rowles WM, Hsu WY, McPolin K, et al. Transitioning from S1P receptor modulators to B cell-depleting therapies in multiple sclerosis: clinical, radiographic, and laboratory data. Neurol Neuroimmunol Neuroinflamm 2022;9(4):e1183.
46. Almas S, Vance J, Baker T, et al. Management of multiple sclerosis in the breastfeeding mother. Mult Scler Int 2016;2016:6527458.
47. Giovannoni G, Soelberg Sorensen P, Cook S, et al. Safety and efficacy of cladribine tablets in patients with relapsing–remitting multiple sclerosis: Results from the randomized extension trial of the CLARITY study. Multiple Sclerosis Journal 2018;24(12):1594–604.
48. Dost-Kovalsky K, Thiel S, Ciplea AI, et al. Cladribine and pregnancy in women with multiple sclerosis: the first cohort study. Mult Scler 2023;29(3):461–5.
49. Giovannoni G, Galazka A, Schick R, et al. Pregnancy outcomes during the clinical development program of cladribine in multiple sclerosis: an integrated analysis of safety. Drug Saf 2020;43(7):635–43.
50. Hellwig K, Tilson H H, Seebeck J, Aydemir A, Sabido M. Pregnancy and Infant Outcomes From an Ongoing Worldwide Surveillance Program of Cladribine Tablets: 5-year Pharmacovigilance Results from MAPLE-MS. [Poster]. 9th Annual Americas Committee for Treatment and Research in Multiple Sclerosis (ACTRIMS) Forum 2023, 23-25 February, San Diego, California.
51. Datta P, Ciplea AI, Rewers-Felkins K, et al. Cladribine transfer into human milk: a case report. Mult Scler 2021;27(5):799–801.
52. Oreja-Guevara C, Vukusic S, Bove B, Dobson R, McElrath T, Pietrasanta C, Lin CJ, Ferreira G, Craveiro L, Zecevic D, Pasquarelli N, Hellwig K. Pregnancy and Infant Outcomes in Women Receiving Ocrelizumab for the Treatment of Multiple Sclerosis. Poster session presented at: 38th Congress of the European Committee for Treatment and Research in Multiple Sclerosis (ECTRIMS); 2022 October 26-28; Amsterdam, the Netherlands.
53. Hellwig K, Yamout B, Bove R, Gummuluri KS, Schulze-Topphoff U, Fantaccini S, Zielman R, Sullivan R, Amato MP, Dobson R, Houtchens MK. Pregnancy Outcomes in Ofatumumab-treated Patients with Multiple Sclerosis. [Poster]. Consortium of Multiple Sclerosis Centers, 2022, 1-4 June, National Harbor, Maryland.
54. Anderson A, Poole S, Rowles W, Balan A, Jacobs D, Ciplea A, Brandstater R, Fabian M, Kakara M, Krysko KM, Rutatangwa A, Marcus J, Bevan C, Longbrake E, Repovic P, Romeo A, West T, Cooper J, Riley C, Hale TW, Hellwig K, Lahue SC, Bove R. Anti-CD20 monoclonal antibody therapy after 59 pregnancies in women with neurological conditions: Low breastmilk transfer and normal infant development in a multicenter cohort. Poster presented at: 38th Congress of the European Committee for Treatment and Research in Multiple Sclerosis (ECTRIMS); 2022 October 26-28; Amsterdam, the Netherlands.
55. Steingo B, Al Malik Y, Bass AD, et al, CAMMS223, CAMMS03409, and TOPAZ Investigators. Long-term efficacy and safety of alemtuzumab in patients with RRMS: 12-year follow-up of CAMMS223. J Neurol 2020;267(11):3343–53.
56. Li Z, Richards S, Surks HK, et al. Clinical pharmacology of alemtuzumab, an anti-CD52 immunomodulator, in multiple sclerosis. Clin Exp Immunol 2018;194(3): 295–314.

57. Oh J, Achiron A, Celius EG, et al. CAMMS223, CARE-MS I, CARE-MS II, CAMMS03409, and TOPAZ Investigators. Pregnancy outcomes and postpartum relapse rates in women with RRMS treated with alemtuzumab in the phase 2 and 3 clinical development program over 16 years. Mult Scler Relat Disord 2020;43: 102146.
58. Canibaño B, Deleu D, Mesraoua B, et al. Pregnancy-related issues in women with multiple sclerosis: an evidence-based review with practical recommendations. J Drug Assess 2020;9(1):20–36.
59. Decker BM, Thibault D, Davis KA, et al. Population-based study of nonelective postpartum readmissions in women with stroke, migraine, multiple sclerosis, and myasthenia gravis. Neurology 2022;98:e1545–54.
60. Anderson A, Krysko KM, Rutatangwa A, et al. Clinical and Radiologic Disease Activity in Pregnancy and Postpartum in MS. Neurol Neuroimmunol Neuroinflamm 2021;8(2):e959.
61. Krysko KM, Anderson A, Singh J, et al. Risk factors for peripartum depression in women with multiple sclerosis. Mult Scler 2022;28(6):970–9. https://doi.org/10.1177/13524585211041108.
62. Krol KM, Grossmann T. Psychological effects of breastfeeding on children and mothers. Bundesgesundheitsblatt - Gesundheitsforsch - Gesundheitsschutz 2018;61(8):977–85.
63. Vieira Borba V, Sharif K, Shoenfeld Y. Breastfeeding and autoimmunity: programing health from the beginning. Am J Reprod Immunol 2018;79(1). https://doi.org/10.1111/aji.12778.
64. Dobson R, Mowry EM. Breastfeeding may reduce postpartum relapse in some women with multiple sclerosis. Neurology 2020;94(18):769–70.
65. Drugs and lactation database (LactMed®). Bethesda (MD): National Institute of Child Health and Human Development; 2006. Methylprednisolone. 2021 May 17. PMID: 30000087.
66. Webb JA, Thomsen HS, Morcos SK, Members of Contrast Media Safety Committee of European Society of Urogenital Radiology (ESUR). The use of iodinated and gadolinium contrast media during pregnancy and lactation. Eur Radiol 2005;15(6):1234–40.
67. Eid K, Torkildsen ØF, Aarseth J, et al. Perinatal depression and anxiety in women with multiple sclerosis: a population-based cohort study. Neurology 2021;96: e2789–800.
68. Rosendale N, Ostendorf T, Evans DA, et al. American Academy of Neurology members' preparedness to treat sexual and gender minorities. Neurology 2019;93:159–66.
69. Khayambashi S, Salter A, Tyry T, et al. Gender identity and sexual orientation affect health care satisfaction, but not utilization, in persons with Multiple Sclerosis. Mult Scler Relat Disord 2020;37:101440.
70. Sullivan A, Kane A, Valentic G, et al. Recommendations to Address the Unique Clinical and Psychological Needs of Transgender Persons Living With Multiple Sclerosis. Int J MS Care 2022;24(1):35–40.
71. Pakpoor J, Wotton CJ, Schmierer K, et al. Gender identity disorders and multiple sclerosis risk: a national record-linkage study. Mult Scler 2016;22(13):1759–62.
72. Anderson A, Dierkhising J, Rush G, et al. Experiences of sexual and gender minority people living with multiple sclerosis in Northern California: An exploratory study. Multiple sclerosis and related disorders 2021;55:103214.

73. Ferrell RJ, O'connor KA, Rodríguez G, et al. Monitoring reproductive aging in a 5-year prospective study: aggregate and individual changes in steroid hormones and menstrual cycle lengths with age. Menopause 2005;12:567–77.
74. Kelsey TW, Wright P, Nelson SM, et al. A validated model of serum anti-Müllerian hormone from conception to menopause. PLoS One 2011;6:e22024.
75. Bove R, Chitnis T, Houtchens M. Menopause in multiple sclerosis: therapeutic considerations. J Neurol 2014;261(7):1257–68.
76. Ladeira F, Salavisa M, Caetano A, et al. The influence of menopause in multiple sclerosis course: a longitudinal cohort study. Eur Neurol 2018;80:223–7.
77. Bove R, Healy BC, Secor E, et al. Patients report worse MS symptoms after menopause: findings from an online cohort. Mult Scler Relat Disord 2015;4:18–24.
78. Graves JS, Henry RG, Cree BAC, et al. Ovarian aging is associated with gray matter volume and disability in women with MS. Neurology 2018;90:e254–60.
79. Bove R, Healy BC, Musallam A, et al. Exploration of changes in disability after menopause in a longitudinal multiple sclerosis cohort. Mult Scler 2016;22:935–43.
80. Wallin MT, Culpepper WJ, Campbell JD, et al, US Multiple Sclerosis Prevalence Workgroup. The prevalence of MS in the United States: a population-based estimate using health claims data. Neurology 2019;92(10):e1029–40 [Epub 2019 Feb 15. Erratum in: Neurology. 2019 Oct 8;93(15):688. PMID: 30770430; PMCID: PMC6442006].
81. Houtchens M, Bove R. A case for gender-based approach to multiple sclerosis therapeutics. Front Neuroendocrinol 2018;50:123–34.
82. Bove R, Okai A, Houtchens M, et al. Effects of menopause in women with multiple sclerosis: an evidence-based review. Front Neurol 2021;12:554375.
83. LaHue SC, Anderson A, Krysko KM, et al. Transfer of monoclonal antibodies into breastmilk in neurologic and non-neurologic diseases. Neurol Neuroimmunol Neuroinflamm 2020;7(4):e769.

# Multiple Sclerosis in Black and Hispanic Populations

## Serving the Underserved

Mitzi J. Williams, MD[a,*], Christopher Orlando, MD, MPH[b], Jemima Akisanya, DO, MD[c,1], Lilyana Amezcua, MD, MS[b]

**KEYWORDS**

- Multiple sclerosis • Underserved • Race • Ethnicity • Black • Hispanic
- Health disparities • Health equity

**KEY POINTS**

- The incidence and prevalence of multiple sclerosis in minoritized populations is much higher than previously thought.
- The mechanisms by which socioeconomic status and other social determinants of health influence disparate risk and disability accumulation among Black, Hispanic, and White persons with multiple sclerosis are likely complex, and at present they are incompletely understood.
- Continued efforts addressing the barriers to participation in clinical research are needed to best address low enrollment that could represent a bioethical concern in the care and treatment of multiple sclerosis.

## INTRODUCTION

Multiple sclerosis (MS) has historically been described as most prevalent in people who live farther away from the equator, namely those of White European ancestry. Recently MS in individuals of Black, Hispanic, Native American, and Asian background is better understood. Recent incidence reports suggest not only an increasing rate of MS among Black people compared with White people but also potentially higher risk among Black women.[1,2] MS-specific mortality trends demonstrate distinctive disparities by race, ethnicity, and age, suggesting that there is an unequal burden of disease.

[a] Joi Life Wellness Multiple Sclerosis Center, 767 Concord Road, SE, Smyrna, GA 30082, USA; [b] Department of Neurology, University of Southern California, Keck School of Medicine, 1520 San Pablo Street, Suite 3000, Los Angeles, CA, USA; [c] Georgetown Department of Neurology, 10401 Hospital Drive, Suite 102, Clinton, MD 20735, USA

[1] Present address: 10401 Hospital Drive, Suite 102, Clinton, MD 20735.

* Corresponding author. 1400 Veterans Memorial Highway Southeast, Suite 134-341, Mableton, GA 30126.

*E-mail address:* drmitzi@joilifewellness.com

Twitter: @NerdyNeuroMD (M.J.W.); @OrlandoMDMPH (C.O.); @MimasMyelin (J.A.)

Neurol Clin 42 (2024) 295–317
https://doi.org/10.1016/j.ncl.2023.06.005
neurologic.theclinics.com

Although there are many recognized social determinants affecting inequalities in health, we review clinical characteristics, genetic predispositions, and health disparities related to ethnicity in Black and Hispanic people that may be contributing to disease variability in these fast-growing populations in the United States.

## PREVALENCE, INCIDENCE, AND MORTALITY

The Multiple Sclerosis International Federation and the World Health Organization estimate the global median prevalence of MS to be 35.9 cases per 100,000 population and the incidence to be 2.1 cases per 100,000 person-years, reflecting a total of approximately 2.8 million persons living with MS (PwMS) throughout the world.[3] The 2010 prevalence of MS among persons living in the United States, including those of all racial and ethnic groups, has recently been estimated using a nationally representative collection of private, military, and public administrative health claim datasets to be 309.2 per 100,000, representing 727,344 total cases.[4] There are differences reported among West, Midwest, South, and Northeast regions, as well as racial and ethnic groups, challenging the idea that MS is primarily a disease of White people.

**Table 1** summarizes evidence that the incidence of MS is highest among Black persons followed by White persons, Hispanic persons, and Asian or American Indian and Alaska Native persons.[2,5] Notably, the reported incidence and prevalence of MS among Hispanic persons living in the United States is lower than those reported in Latin American countries[6]; this may reflect differences in social determinants of health (ie, access to a specialist), environmental and epigenetic factors such as the influence of latitude, or a combination of such, although methodological differences are also possible. A retrospective study of a multiethnic cohort of patients enrolled in the Kaiser Permanente Southern California (KPSC) plan reported an incidence of 2.9 per 100,000 person-years in Hispanic persons versus 6.9 in White persons, whereas the incidence for Black persons was 10.2, almost twice that of White persons (see **Table 1**).[2] Furthermore, the incidence of clinically isolated syndrome (CIS) is also lower among Hispanic persons when compared with White persons.[7] A similar incidence in CIS was found between Black persons and White persons, although Black persons had a higher incidence of MS. It is unclear whether this could be attributed to more rapid disease progression, delays in health care access, or other factors. Among veterans who served in the US military from 1990 to 2007 a significantly lower incidence of MS was again observed among Hispanic persons.[1] The estimated annual age-specific incidence rate for Hispanic persons was reported at 8.2%, significantly lower than White persons (9.3) and Black persons (12.1) (see **Table 1**).

Interestingly, the increased incidence among Black persons in the KPSC cohort was only observed among women.[2] Black women displayed a markedly higher incidence compared with White women (risk ratio [RR] 1.59, 95% confidence interval [CI] 1.27–1.99; $P = .0005$), whereas the incidence was similar among Black and White men (RR 1.04, 95% CI 0.67–1.5, $P = .87$). These researchers also separately demonstrated a greater female predominance in incidence of CIS among Black and Hispanic persons compared with White and Asian/Pacific Islander persons.[7]

The largest studies to date of differences in the prevalence of MS between racial and ethnic groups are retrospective reviews of electronic health record data from Sutter Health in Northern California and KPSC (**Table 2**).[8,9] Prevalence of MS among Black persons was markedly higher than that among White persons in the Sutter Health cohort, but similar in the KPSC cohort, except for those aged 18 to 24 years among whom the incidence was higher among Black persons. It is unclear whether this represents differences in sampling bias or whether environmental exposure,

**Table 1**
**Incidence of multiple sclerosis in diverse minority populations (cases per 100,000 person-years)**

| Study Group | Cohort | Period | White | Black[a] | Hispanic | Asian/Pacific Islander | American Indian/ Alaska Native |
|---|---|---|---|---|---|---|---|
| Langer-Gould,[2] 2013 | Kaiser Permanente Southern California | 2008–2010 | 6.9 | 10.2 | 2.9 | 1.4 | n/a |
| Wallin et al,[1] 2012 | US military-Veteran population | 1990–2007, 200–2007 for Hispanic persons | 9.3 | 12.1 | 8.2 | 3.3 | 3.1 |

[a] Black or African American.

**Table 2**
**Prevalence of multiple sclerosis in diverse minority populations (cases per 100,000 persons)**

| Prevalence of MS | Cohort | Period | White | Black[a] | Hispanic | Asian/Pacific Islander |
|---|---|---|---|---|---|---|
| Romanelli,[8] 2020 | Sutter Health | 2010–2016 | 384.6 | 521.3 | 183.7 | 63.9 |
| Langer-Gould,[2] 2013 | Kaiser Permanente Southern California | 2009–2010 | 234.8 | 233.2 | 66.2 | 23.5 |

[a] Black or African American.

differing socioeconomic inequity, or other factors give rise to true regional variation in prevalence. In parallel to the incidence data summarized earlier, the prevalence of MS in Hispanic persons is lower than that in White persons in both cohorts, and Asian/Pacific Islander persons are affected least frequently of all. A nearly 4-fold greater prevalence of MS among Hispanic women compared with men in the Northern California cohort was identified, a larger difference than among White, Black, or Asian/Pacific Islander groups.[4] The female:male ratio was highest at the ages of 35 to 64 years among White and Black persons but peaked at a younger age (25–34 years) among Hispanic and Asian/Pacific Islander individuals within the KPSC cohort.[9]

US population–based mortality studies in MS by race and ethnicity are limited. An analysis of deaths due to MS by race/ethnicity from 1990 to 2001 using national multiple cause of death data found that the overall age-adjusted mortality was 1.44/100,000 population, with mortalities highest among White persons followed by Black, Hispanic, American Indian/Alaska Native, and Asian/Pacific Islander individuals.[10] The increased MS mortality was uniform in both sexes, although higher in women than in men. Age-adjusted mortality per 100,000 population was 1.58 in White persons, 0.39 (95% CI 0.23–0.26) in Hispanic persons, and 1.28 (95% CI 0.78–0.83) in Black persons. Mortalities increase with age for all groups and decrease for individuals older than 85 years.[10] A study using the Compressed Mortality data file for 1999 to 2015 in the WONDER (Wide-ranging online Data for Epidemiologic Research) system developed by the Centers for Disease Control and Prevention reported that age-specific MS mortality patterns were highest among Black persons younger than 55 years, whereas White persons had the highest rate after age 55 years.[11] For both groups, MS mortality increased with age in both sexes and peaked at ages 55 to 64 years for Black persons and 65 to 74 years for non-Hispanic White persons before declining substantially, whereas for Hispanic White and Asian/Pacific Islander persons, the risk plateaued after age 55 years. It is unclear to what extent these differences may be related to a more severe disease course observed among Black and Hispanic persons, differences in incidence among groups, and/or disparate patterns of comorbid diseases. These questions warrant further investigation.

## COMORBIDITIES WITH MULTIPLE SCLEROSIS

There are multiple studies describing differences in disease course and health outcomes in Black and Hispanic people with MS. Social determinants of health (SDOH) and potential genetic underpinnings likely play a role in these differences. It is also well recognized that there is a higher incidence of comorbid conditions in individuals with MS, including depression, anxiety, and hypertension.[12] A 3-year longitudinal study examined the effects of several comorbidities and found that hypertension, diabetes, and obstructive lung disease adversely affected walking speed, self-reported disability, and depression.[13] Another study found that there is a higher incidence of uncontrolled hypertension in Black individuals with MS but also higher exposure to antihypertensive therapy than White individuals.[14] Comorbidities in Hispanic PwMS are also reported to be common. Studies range from 30% to 42% to have a comorbid condition.[15,16] Immigrants to the United States with MS reported more vascular risk factors, with hypercholesterolemia being the most common reported comorbid medical problem affecting them compared with US-born individuals ($P$ = .002).[15] Vascular comorbidities have been reported as high as 24.2% in Hispanic PwMS, with hypertension (7.3%) being the most common, particularly older than 40 years (12.6%). A cross-sectional assessment of headache as a comorbidity in individuals affected by MS found that chronic migraine was significantly more common among Hispanics (82%) than Whites (18%; $P$ = .012) and was noted to have significant impact on their daily life activities.[17]

## *Clinical Presentation*

### *Black and African Americans with multiple sclerosis*

Data concerning age of onset have been conflicting with studies reporting Black people develop MS at both an earlier [18,19] and at a later age[20] compared with White people. Although the discrepancies in age of onset have not been rectified, interestingly the studies seem to differ by region of ascertainment (East vs West of the US), which could suggest genetic and environmental differences within Black cohorts. Nevertheless, the observation that age of onset differs by geography could also be ascribed to differences in methodology and source population.[18,19]

Clinically, Black people are reported to suffer from more disabling symptoms, poorer recovery, shorter time to a second MS attack, and increased disease burden on MRI.[20–24] Relapse characteristics more common in Black people include cerebellar dysfunction, cognitive dysfunction, and opticospinal manifestations such as transverse myelitis.[21,22,25] A cross-sectional study using data from 7 US sites found greater disease burden with cognitive processing, walking, and manual dexterity when compared with White PwMS.[26,27] African ancestry has also been associated with higher risk of COVID-19 infection in PwMS.[28] Black people also have increased occurrence of multifocal signs and symptoms, which could indicate a poor prognosis from the start of disease. Although the cause of this variability from Whites is unknown, genetic, environmental, and disparities in care could be acting as risk factors.

MS is also characterized by intrathecal humoral inflammation, which has been shown to be greater in Black than in White PwMS,[29] although this was shown to not be a predictor of early disease progression. Elevated cerebrospinal fluid (CSF) immunoglobulin G (IgG) index was found to negatively correlate with brain gray matter volume in Black PwMS but not in White PwMS. The possibility of a more pronounced CSF humoral response in African Americans with MS warrants further investigation.

A consistent pattern of greater disability has been observed in Black compared with White PwMS.[18,19] The greater level of disability seen is in part explained by the higher degree of MRI involvement and clinical presentation.[30] MRI results indicate that Black PwMS have higher T2- and T1-weighted lesion volumes, lower N-acetylaspartate values, and lower brain magnetization transfer ratios (MTR). Fisniku and colleagues estimated the rate of T2 lesion volume growth per year is faster in secondary progressive MS than in relapsing-remitting MS (2.89 $cm^3$ compared with 0.80 $cm^3$ respectively).[31] Black PwMS with higher disability have greater T2 and T1 lesion volumes when compared with White PwMS ($P$ < .001–0.006).[24,30] The proportion of contrast-enhancing lesions has been shown to be similar in both Black and White PwMS.[30]

In regard to brain atrophy parameters, Black PwMS seem to suffer more severe diffuse tissue damage as measured by MTR.[30] One study found that when compared with non-Hispanic White American PwMS, Black PwMS had more rapid neurodegeneration with faster gray matter, white matter, nuclear thalamic, and retinal nerve fiber layer atrophy rates.[32] A cohort study of 209 MS patients found Black PwMS had lower pontine volumes and a greater rate of pontine volume change when compared with White PwMS; however, White PwMS demonstrated greater rates of medulla volume decrease than Black PwMS.[33] In a single-center prospective cohort study, Black PwMS were found to have more rapid rates of generalized atrophy of the medulla and upper cervical spinal cord when compared with White patients.[34] Greater lesion volume and atrophy may explain the rapid clinical progression in Black patients, but this has not been confirmed.

Black PwMS with acute optic neuritis have been reported to have more visual loss and poorer recovery and can often involve both optic nerves.[20,35] Studies using optical coherence tomography found that Black PwMS seem to have faster retinal nerve fiber loss (RNFL) and ganglion cell/inner plexiform layer (GCIP) thinning compared with White PwMS.[35] Kimbrough and colleagues, in addition, found that Black PwMS trended toward a greater loss of RNFL per year of disease duration ($P$ = .056) and had a significantly greater loss of GCIP per year of disease duration compared with otherwise similar White patients ($P$ = .015). In a similar study, Seraji-Bozorgzad and colleagues also show that the RNFL was significantly thinner in Black compared with White patients (87.2 μm vs 90.0 μm, $P$ = .004).[36] These findings, similar to MRI data and clinical disease course, support more aggressive disease progression in the Black population.

Reasons for these disparities in clinical outcomes seen in Black PwMS still prove to be evasive. Black patients with newly diagnosed MS/CIS have been found to have lower Symbol Digit Modalities Test (SDMT) scores when compared with White patients; however, Black controls also had lower SDMT scores when compared with White controls. This finding suggests that cognitive impairment seen in Black PwMS is possibly due to baseline population differences, namely racial and ethnic disparities due to systemic racism.[37] Another study evaluating disability outcomes compared self-identified Black and White PwMS with healthy controls. This study showed that Black PwMS had worse performances in manual dexterity and cognition after accounting for total income, education, body mass index, and comorbidities. They found that Black race and MS independently contributed to this finding.[38] Again, this study suggests that unmeasured social factors at the population level, such as systemic racism, influence the observed disparities seen in Black PwMS. The effects of systemic racism require an exponential increase in investigation to evaluate its impact on the clinical outcomes of patients.

***Hispanic Americans with multiple sclerosis***

Hispanic persons comprise one of the largest minority ethnic groups in the United States. By 2060, the number of Hispanic persons in the United States is projected to exceed 100,000,000, accounting for more than a quarter of the total population.[39] Mexican Americans make up the largest subgroup followed by Puerto Ricans and Cubans. An understanding of MS disease as experienced by Hispanic PwMS is crucial if clinicians are to provide optimal care to this growing population. The research summarized here must be interpreted with the understanding that there is tremendous heterogeneity in ancestry, culture, and lived experience among Hispanic persons in the United States, and the patterns of such may vary considerably among regions of the country.

Available research indicates that Hispanic PwMS, similar to Black PwMS, develop symptoms of and are diagnosed with MS at a younger age compared with White

PwMS[18,40–42]; this has been observed in study populations in multiple regions of the United States, and reported mean ages at symptom onset and diagnosis are summarized in **Table 3**. An early cross-sectional study compared 125 Hispanic PwMS with 100 non-Hispanic White PwMS in the Southern California region and reported a younger mean age at first symptom in the Hispanic group (28.4 ± 0.97 years) than in the White group (32.5 ± 1.37 years).[12] Hispanic PwMS were also diagnosed with MS at a younger age (29.7 ± 0.98 years) compared with White PwMS (32.9 ± 1.48 years), although after a longer period of time since symptom onset (1.2 ± 0.26 years among Hispanic PwMS compared with 0.3 ± 0.12 years among White PwMS). Interestingly, among the Hispanic PwMS, those who were born in the United States or migrated before the age of 15 years had a younger age at symptom onset (25.5 ± 1.42 years) and diagnosis (24.1 ± 1.47 years) compared with those who migrated after age 15 years (first symptom 35.7 ± 2.16 years, diagnosis 34.0 ± 2.31 years). A cross-sectional study from the Southeastern United States including Hispanic PwMS of primarily Caribbean ancestry noted a younger age at diagnosis, although not at symptom onset.[41] This study observed differences by place of birth complementary to the findings in the aforementioned study in Southern California, specifically a younger age at both symptom onset and diagnosis for Hispanic PwMS born in the United States compared with those born elsewhere. The association of younger onset with earlier arrival in the United States may be consistent with the well-described North-South gradient of MS risk, but the totality of the observed differences between White and Hispanic PwMS suggests that other factors such as genetic predisposition and social determinants may also be relevant.

Symptom profiles and the presence of syndromes referrable to demyelination in a specific anatomic region seem to differ between Hispanic PwMS and other groups. Reported comparisons are summarized in **Table 3**. In a more recent study, Hispanic and Black PwMS had higher scores (indicative of greater symptom severity) in all symptomatic domains measured, and Hispanic PwMS had even higher pain, cognition, depression, and anxiety scores compared with Black PwMS.[43] Interestingly, these differences may vary by region of the United States. Several reports from Western regions of the United States suggest that Hispanic PwMS experience optic neuritis as the initial manifestation of the disease more frequently than White and other groups of patients.[7,42,44] A comparison of White and Hispanic PwMS in the Southeastern United States, however, showed no difference in the frequency of optic neuritis or other syndromes.[41] It can be hypothesized that genetic risk differs between the 2 groups. Hispanic persons living in the Western United States are predominantly of Mexican ancestry and have been reported to have a greater proportion of non-European ancestry compared with other groups, and an association between Native American ancestry and optic neuritis has been reported.[45] Further research is required to elucidate the relative contributions of genetic risk, environmental exposures, social determinants, and other factors to patterns of MS clinical manifestations among Hispanic PwMS and other groups.

A previous report noted that opticospinal MS (OSMS) was present in 11% of the Hispanic PwMS examined, which is markedly higher than the published estimates of 1% to 3% among White PwMS who were available at the time of the study.[46] Of those with OSMS, about 20% were found to have spinal cord MRI features consistent with longitudinally extensive spinal cord lesions. Patients with longitudinally extensive lesions were 7 times more likely to have ambulatory disability than those without spinal cord lesions. OSMS was initially characterized as a separate entity from neuromyelitis optica, and the absence of antibody against aquaporin-4 was a defining characteristic. With updated diagnostic criteria, a syndrome of recurrent optic neuritis and

**Table 3**
**Age of multiple sclerosis symptom onset and diagnosis in minority populations**

| | | Mean Age at Symptom Onset (Years) | | | | Mean Age at Diagnosis (Years) | | | |
|---|---|---|---|---|---|---|---|---|---|
| **Study Group** | **Cohort or Geographic Region** | **White** | **Hispanic** | **Black[a]** | **Asian/Pacific Islander** | **White** | **Hispanic** | **Black[a]** | **Asian/Pacific Islander** |
| Buchanan et al,[40] 2010 | NARCOMS registry | 30.1 | 28.6 | 29.8 | NR | 37.4 | 34.5 | 35.8 | NR |
| Amezcua,[42] 2011 | Los Angeles County | 32.6 | 28.5 | NR | NR | 32.9 | 29.7 | NR | NR |
| Langer-Gould,[2] 2013 | Southern California (Kaiser Permanente) | 40.7 | 33.2 | 38.3 | 39.4 | 44.5 | 35.1 | 41.7 | 40.3 |
| Hadjixenofontos et al,[41] 2015 | South Florida | 35.21 | 33.62 | NR | NR | 40.87 | 38.09 | NR | NR |

Ventura et al.[18] also reported that Hispanic PwMS in their cohort from New York and New Jersey displayed a younger age at symptom onset compared with White PwMS and similar age at onset to African American PwMS, but mean ages were not specified.

[a] Black or African American.

myelitis attacks with minimal brain involvement in a patient negative for aquaporin-4 antibody now falls within the category of neuromyelitis optica spectrum disorders (NMOSD).[47] It is also unclear how many of these patients might have had myelin oligodendrocyte glycoprotein (MOG) antibody-associated disease, given that widespread antibody testing for MOG-IgG has only recently become available.[48] Given the risk of ambulatory disability with the extensive spinal cord involvement often seen in NMOSD, the previous finding that such may be more common in Hispanic patients should direct clinicians to consider these disorders in the differential of MS.

Hispanic PwMS may experience more severe disease and become more disabled compared with White PwMS. Two studies in populations from the Northeastern United States reported indicators of greater MS disease severity[18] and associated disability[43] among Hispanic and Black groups compared with White counterparts. Another study in the Southeastern United States noted that Hispanic PwMS displayed greater ambulatory disability than White PwMS, especially those with relapsing disease.[41] An aforementioned study in Southern California did not demonstrate a difference between Hispanic and White patients in terms of disability but again demonstrated a difference between groups of Hispanic PwMS as defined by age at migration, namely that migration at age greater than 15 years was associated with greater risk of disability.[42] Again, it remains unclear to what extent these differences between racial and ethnic groups and between regions are attributable to genetic, environmental, social, and other factors.

### *Genetic Underpinnings in Black and Hispanic Persons with Multiple Sclerosis*

Black people are an ethnic group of Americans with ancestral roots to the original peoples of Africa in combination with European genetic admixture as a result of the transatlantic slave trade.[49] Hispanic people are also a complex ethnic group where both genetic and cultural admixture derives mostly from the original indigenous inhabitants of America, its European settlers, and to some degree Africans.[50] Variation in MS disease presentation (clinical or MRI), severity, and course could be influenced by environmental, social, and genetic factors. Although there is considerable genetic heterogeneity within Black[51] and Hispanic people, it is the European genetic ancestry that is thought to contribute to the risk of MS in this population. [52–55] Genome-wide association studies done in Black individuals have shown that known MS genetic risk variants in White people partially overlaps with that of Black individuals.[55] However, it is important to note that an admixture study by Beecham and colleagues found less replication of European MS risk alleles among their sample of Black PwMS than expected based on power analysis, highlighting the genetic heterogeneity in the Black population, and possibly indicating that not all of these risk alleles are relevant.[56] Similar observations were seen in the replication capacity for Hispanic PwMS.

An admixture study found that in 899 Black MS cases and 1155 Black controls, those who inherited segments of European ancestry at a chromosome 1 locus (a signal associated with the CD58 and FCRL3 genes) were at a 1.44 times increased risk of MS.[57] The HLA region is the most important MS susceptibility locus genome wide, with a primary signal arising from DRB1*15 alleles.[53,58] In a study performed by Johnson and colleagues they analyzed 1574 Black individuals, including 918 MS cases and 656 unrelated control individuals.[59] Seven single-nucleotide polymorphisms (SNPs) in 5 genes of interest (CD6, CLEC16a, EV15, GPC5, TYK2) were found to be significantly associated with MS in this Black dataset. In addition, correlations in HLA genotypes with MS phenotypes in Black PwMS who were reported carriers for DRB1*15 alleles were twice more likely to have classic MS and have an earlier age of onset, whereas those following an opticospinal MS were less likely to carry DRB1*15.[60] DRG1*15:01 and

DQB1*06:02 were found to independently contribute to MS risk in Black and Hispanic samples from a large multiethnic cohort study.[61] This study also found a decrease in Native American ancestry across Black and particularly Hispanic MS cases, suggesting a protective mechanism.[61] Another study suggested that the serine threonine kinase 11 (STK11) gene SNP may be a risk factor for Blacks with secondary progressive MS, with an association of older age at symptom onset and diagnosis.[62] Efforts in determining other susceptible genes that may be unique to Blacks and Hispanics and better understanding phenotypic variability within and from Whites continue, attempting to bridge this large knowledge gap.

### *Social Determinants of Health and Disparities*

SDOH are the conditions in which people are born, grow, work, live, and age that influence health outcomes.[63] In the United States, socioeconomic factors alone were estimated to account 47% of the variability in health outcomes.[64] Health behaviors are estimated to account for another 34% of observed variability and are heavily influenced by SDOH. Globally, a social gradient is observed in which those of lower socioeconomic status have worse health outcomes, including more accelerated disease progression among PwMS.[65–67] Inequitable distribution of SDOH gives rise to health disparities, which adversely affect those who have systematically experienced greater obstacles to health based on their racial or ethnic group; religion; socioeconomic status; gender; age; mental health; cognitive, sensory, or physical disability; sexual orientation or gender identity; geographic location; or other characteristics historically linked to discrimination or exclusion.[68]

Profound[69] differences in socioeconomic advantage and other inequities exist in the United States along racial and ethnic lines, including among PwMS. Studies have demonstrated that Black and Hispanic PwMS are more likely than White PwMS to reside in neighborhoods with greater socioeconomic deprivation,[59] have lower educational attainment,[26,70,71] be unemployed,[25,40,71] and have Medicaid or Medicare rather than private insurance.[2,6,13,14,23] It is likely that these and other SDOH are key drivers of disparate MS risk and outcomes among racial and ethnic groups. Importantly, SDOH represent modifiable risk factors, the amelioration of which may result in transformative benefit for disadvantaged populations.[72]

Illustrative examples of the importance of SDOH in understanding racial and ethnic MS disparities have been published. A study of patients enrolled in the North American Research Committee (NARCOMS) registry found that the odds of having severe versus mild disability after adjustment for clinical factors were greater for Black patients compared with White patients (odds ratio [OR] 1.72, 95% CI 1.43–2.08), but the association was markedly attenuated by additional adjustment for socioeconomic status (OR 1.37, CI 1.11–1.67).[70] A study of cognitive symptoms of MS among KPSC patients demonstrated that lower cognitive assessment scores among Black and Hispanic PwMS were attributable to baseline population-level differences, suggesting that MS disease did not differ between the 2 groups in such a way as to produce quantifiably different levels of cognitive impairment.[37] In addition, a national web-based survey investigating the mental health of PwMS found that psychiatric symptom burden was associated with socioeconomic status but not with race and ethnicity.[73] In both examples outcomes are better predicted by inequitable SDOH than by race and ethnicity themselves, suggesting that SDOH have an important and likely causative role in observed disparities.

The mechanisms by which socioeconomic status and other SDOH influence disparate risk and disability accumulation among Black, Hispanic, and White PwMS are likely complex, and at present they are incompletely understood.[72] Available evidence suggests that health care access, health literacy, illness perception, immigration, and acculturation may be part of a web of interrelated phenomena (**Fig. 1**).

*Health care access* is likely a major mediator of the effects of systemic inequities on racial and ethnic MS disparities. An analysis of data from Medical Expenditure Panel Survey reflecting patients with MS and other chronic disabling neurologic disease found that Black and Hispanic patients were 30% (OR 0.72, CI 0.64–0.81) and 40% (OR 0.61, CI 0.54–0.69), respectively, less likely to see an outpatient neurologist, even in regression models controlling for age, sex, activity limitation, self-reported health status, health insurance coverage, family income, education, and region.[27] A survey of low-income Black and Hispanic PwMS enrolled in the Independence Care System (ICS), a Medicaid long-term managed care plan in New York, found that 32% of patients had never seen an MS specialist, and a similar number were not receiving disease-modifying therapy (DMT).[74]

Unequal access to other specialists and services important for successful management of MS has also been documented. Hispanic patients enrolled in the NARCOMS registry were less likely to receive mental health care or see a rehabilitation specialist.[40] A study of patients with MS who received Medicaid home and community-based services found that African American patients were less likely to receive case management, equipment, technology and modification services, and nursing services compared with White patients.[75] A nationwide survey of patients with MS noted that those who were not seen by a neurologist were also less likely to be seen by a rehabilitation specialist or urologist.[76] Deficiencies in preventive care such as osteoporosis screening among low-income Black and Hispanic PwMS have also been documented.[74]

*Health literacy* has also been implicated as a mediator of the effects of socioeconomic inequity on health disparities.[77] In the aforementioned survey of Black and Hispanic ICS patients, the most common reasons for discontinuing medication suggested that patients had not received adequate education regarding the role of DMT and realistic expectations for anticipated benefits and side effects.[74] The fact that many patients had never seen an MS specialist suggests that a lack of specialized care may contribute to gaps in health literacy. This idea is supported by an analysis of NARCOMS enrollment data that observed PwMS receiving MS care from a neurologist to have a greater understanding of MS disease and its effects on their lives than those with principal care physicians specializing in other fields.[78] It is likely that additional factors contribute to differences in health literacy, including, but not limited to, the previously described differences in educational attainment.[26,70,71,79]

*Illness perceptions* differ among racial and ethnic groups of PwMS, and although they are related to health literacy, they are influenced by other factors as well. Studies of illness perception among Black PwMS have found that religious and spiritual beliefs may influence ideas of illness causation[80] and inform patients' coping strategies.[81] Black women with MS interviewed about their experiences felt that physicians' assumptions about MS among Black persons may have delayed diagnosis.[81] They also emphasized that maintaining their identity as strong Black women was central to the way they coped with their condition. Racial identity, religious and spiritual beliefs, and other ideas with differing patterns among racial and ethnic groups seem to have a profound effect on patients' experiences in all phases of the MS disease experience.

*Immigration and acculturation* among Hispanic PwMS are likely important influences on illness perception, health care access, and other determinants of health care access and risk. The circumstances leading to immigration and the immigration process itself have been shown to influence both health status and psychological distress among Hispanic persons in the United States.[82] Acculturation also has complex effects on the

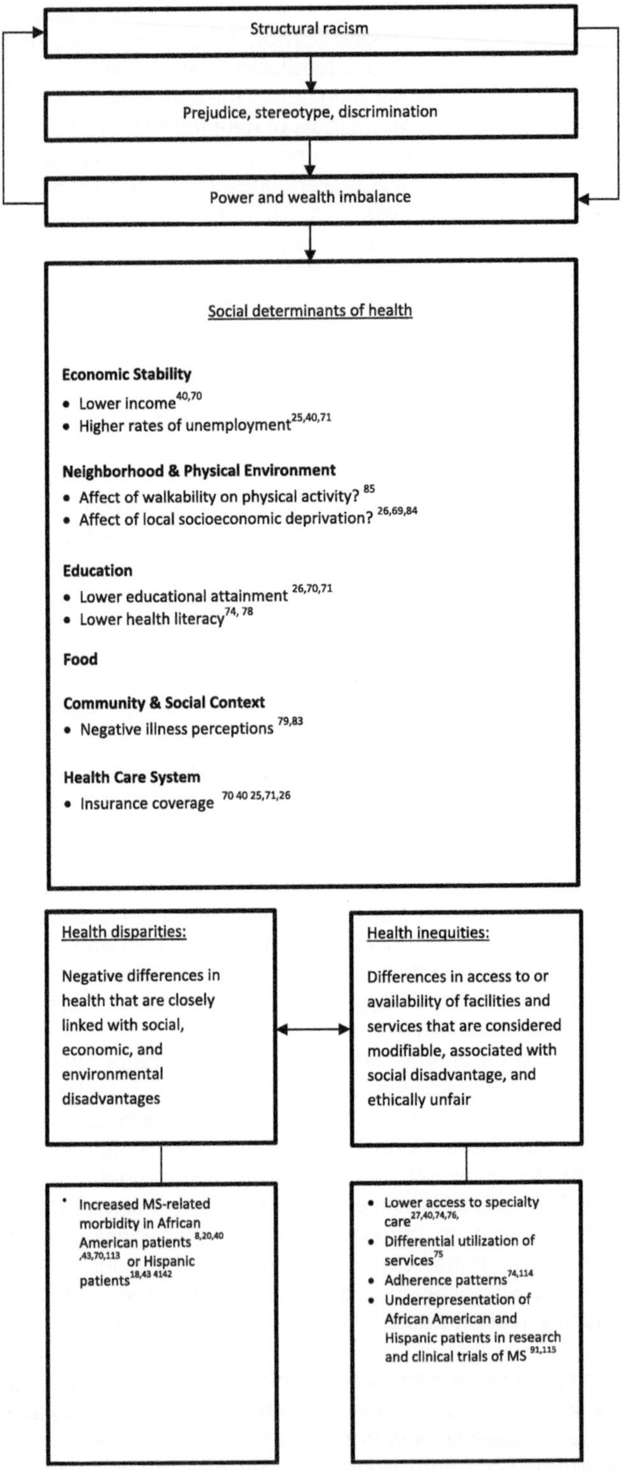


**Fig. 1.** Social determinants of health and health disparities and inequities in multiple sclerosis.

health of Hispanic persons, and evidence of both positive and negative effects is found in the research literature.[79] In one study of Hispanic PwMS in the United States, being a later immigrant was independently associated with greater disability (OR 2.3, CI 1.07–4.82; $P = .03$) compared with being born in the United States.[15] In another study, nonimmigrant Hispanic patients with MS or other chronic disabling neurologic condition were more likely to have been seen by a neurologist compared with immigrants (OR 2.85, CI 2.72–2.98).[27] A study of illness perception among Hispanic American PwMS reported that immigrants were 4 times more likely than nonimmigrants to view sociocultural factors such as strong emotions as having a causative role in MS.[83] The mechanisms by which immigration, acculturation, citizenship status, early childhood exposures, and cultural background affect illness perception, health care access, and disease physiology among Hispanic PwMS are likely important to the observed disparities in MS-related disability and warrant additional investigation.

*Neighborhood conditions and the built environment* may also play a role, although present data are lacking.[72] Black and Hispanic PwMS tend to live in more socioeconomically disadvantaged neighborhoods than White PwMS, and neighborhood-level socioeconomic disadvantage is broadly associated with poorer clinical outcomes among patients with MS.[26,59,84] Although this again highlights the importance of SDOH, these studies have not been able to elucidate whether this is due to the strong correlation between individual- and neighborhood-level socioeconomic status or due to conditions of the neighborhood itself that affect health. A study of physical activity among patients with MS found relationships with activity level and social support and neighborhood characteristics affecting walkability.[85] Given the degree of residential segregation that exists in the United States,[69] it would not be surprising to find differences in these characteristics between neighborhoods of Black, Hispanic, and White PwMS, but an investigation of such has not been published to date.

*Clinicians' racial bias* occurs both implicitly (without conscious choice or awareness) and explicitly and has been linked to the perpetuation of racial health disparities.[86] Many ideas that individuals of a certain race or ethnicity are more or less susceptible to certain diseases persist in medicine, despite evidence to the contrary.[87] These ideas may give rise to differences among racial and ethnic groups in the frequency with which people are diagnosed with certain diseases that are incongruent with the true prevalence of the diseases. Black women with MS who participated in a study of their experiences with their disease felt that their diagnosis had been delayed because physicians failed to consider MS and focused on other conditions perceived as more common among Black people.[81] Further research might investigate physicians' understanding of racial and ethnic differences in the epidemiology of MS and how implicit bias might lead to delays in diagnosis or treatment of MS beyond those attributable to insurance coverage and other inequities in health care access.

Addressing the fundamental inequities that drive racial and ethnic health disparities will require societal change, but smaller scale interventions that can be successfully deployed in communities and clinical settings have been investigated. Clinical care navigators can facilitate access to multidisciplinary specialized care and have been effective in reducing racial and ethnic disparities among patients with other diseases.[88,89] A short narrative film used to deliver information about MS culturally tailored to Hispanic/Latinx audiences has been shown to improve understanding of the disease and perceptions of its treatment.[90] Research recruitment efforts that account for concerns expressed by underrepresented groups may help to remedy the present lack of clinical trial data among these populations, improve access to care, and develop mechanisms through which SDOH can be studied and addressed.[91,92]

### *Creating Awareness Among Underrepresented Racial/Ethnic Groups and Increasing Participation in Clinical Research*

Ethnic minorities are known to have lower enrollment in health research.[93] Some of the common barriers to participation include the delivery of culturally sensitive and competent care to underserved, lower income, and the less acculturated.[94] In addition, deficiency in the patient-physician relationship and mistrust of the medical community have been reported as barriers.[95] A study conducted by Pimentel Maldonado and colleagues surveyed more than 2000 PwMS about attitudes toward research involvement and found that although there were concerns about mistrust, an overwhelming majority of patients surveyed had positive attitudes toward research involvement.[92] Important concerns that were raised by Hispanic participants, regardless of socioeconomic status, were risk of research participation on their job or legal status, as well as risk of losing health insurance coverage. The risk of personal information being released without permission, and the risk of receiving poor-quality health care, were more common among the Black participants independent of socioeconomic status. Other identified barriers included that participants were not asked to participate and they did not know where to find information about research being conducted in their areas.[92]

Increasing diversity in clinical research will involve the input of multiple stakeholders. Potential strategies will include assessing where studies are conducted to ensure that diverse populations are being reached, addressing overly restrictive inclusion/exclusion criteria that may exclude minoritized groups, and creating lasting community partnerships to raise awareness about the importance and benefits of research participation.[96] By developing patient navigation and educational opportunities that merge the patients and caregivers, the community, policy makers, health care professionals, and researchers, we might be able to increase participation of minorities in MS projects.[94,97]

Patient registries provide a robust educational hub and research opportunity for population-based studies. The Alliance for Research in Hispanic MS (arhms.org) was created as a multiinstitutional collaboration consortium dedicated to epidemiologic and genetic studies to better understand MS in people of Hispanic background living in the United States and Puerto Rico.[98] Pivotal studies specific to Hispanic people with MS supporting clinical and genetic diversity have been published. The National African Americans with MS Registry[99] was created to be an educational resource for MS in the Black community for both patients and providers, with objectives to increase opportunities for clinical trial participation. This registry seeks to answer vital questions such as estimates and geographic distribution of Black PwMS in the United States. Regarding recruitment of diverse participants for genetic studies, it is important to consider thoughtful approaches. It is possible that indirect efforts from ARHMS, Hispanic PwMS are more motivated to participate in genetic studies by their personal experience with MS.[100]

Methods for improving diversity in clinical trials include addressing resource constraints and providing culturally sensitive educational trial materials.[101] The CHIMES trial is a phase IV study evaluating ocrelizumab treatment response in Black and Hispanic patients, which intentionally addressed these barriers with accessible study sites, enhanced scheduling flexibility, and translated patient materials in Spanish. This study also used a unique collaborative approach with patient and advocacy organization input during the conception and protocol creation phases. [102] Although previous trials have relatively low inclusion of Black and Hispanic participants, they do suggest efficacy of the available DMTs (**Table 4**). Continued efforts addressing

**Table 4**
**Analyses of multiple sclerosis phase III disease-modifying therapy trials**

| DMT/Trial | Population | Sample Size | Main Findings |
|---|---|---|---|
| Alemtuzumab (CARE-MS I and II, and extension)[103] | African descent | n = 43 | Alemtuzumab vs IFN beta-1a: year 2: ARR (0.09 vs 0.42), improved EDSS (18% vs 11%), NEDA (55% vs 13%), brain volume loss (0.55% vs 1.32%) |
| Dimethyl Fumarate (DEFINE, CONFIRM)[104] | Black, Hispanic, Asian | n = 219 | DMF vs placebo: ARR (AA 0.01 vs 0.27, Hispanic 0.15 vs 0.49, Asian 0.14 vs 0.21) |
| Dimethyl Fumarate (ESTEEM interim analysis)[105] | African descent | n = 187 | 12 mo before DMF vs 36 mo post DMF: ARR (0.68 vs 0.07) |
| Fingolimod (FREEDOMS, FREEDOMS II, TRANSFORMS)[106] | Hispanic | n = 181 | Fingolimod vs interferon beta-1a/placebo: ARR (0.22 vs 0.34/0.46) |
| Fingolimod (PREFERMS)[107] | African descent | n = 141 | Fingolimod vs injectables (IFN beta-1a/b, glatiramer acetate): ARR (0.13 vs 0.23), patient satisfaction (80.6% vs 49.3%) |
| Interferon beta-1a (EVIDENCE)[108] | African descent | n = 36 | Black vs white: at 24 wk—ARR (0.47 vs 0.33), new lesions (1.37 v s 0.97), at 48 wk—ARR (0.73 vs 0.57), new lesions (2.00 vs 1.10) |
| Natalizumab (AFFIRM and SENTINEL)[109] | African descent | n = 49 | Natalizumab vs placebo: ARR (0.21 vs 0.53), gad lesions over 2 y (0.19 vs 0.91), new or enlarged T2 lesions (0.88 vs 8.52) |
| Ocrelizumab (OPERA I, OPERA II)[110–114] | African descent | n = 72 | Ocrelizumab vs interferon beta-1a: ARR (0.13 vs 0.26), gad lesions (0.03 vs 0.72), new or enlarging T2 lesions (0.37 vs 2.65), NEDA (67.7% vs 26.1%) |

*Abbreviations:* ARR, annualized relapse risk; Black, African American or African ancestry persons; DMF, dimethyl fumarate; DMT, disease-modifying therapy; IFN, interferon; NEDA, no evidence of disease activity.

the barriers to participation are needed to best address low enrollment that could represent a bioethical concern in the care and treatment of MS.

## SUMMARY

Black and Hispanic people could be at risk of greater MS disease burden early in the disease course. The higher percentage presenting at a younger age, the higher degree of lesion burden, and faster disability progression, all have the capacity to contribute to disparate outcomes. Although the most sensitive of the determinants in MS are considered to be biology and genetics, due to low clinical trial enrollment, there is poor understanding of how the interplay of these factors may affect disease course in minoritized groups. Also, other social determinants of health including implicit bias, socioeconomic status, and health literacy contribute to the disparities in overall health among different racial and ethnic groups in the United States. With an increasing understanding of the relationship between these genetic factors and health outcomes, we see greater opportunities to intervene. As we move toward personalized health care, health disparities will continue to be of importance in the management of MS.

## CLINICS CARE POINTS

- The fact that many patients had never seen a MS specialist suggests that a lack of specialized care may contribute to gaps in health literacy among minoritized groups.
- Addressing the fundamental inequities that drive racial and ethnic health disparities will require societal change, but smaller scale interventions that can be successfully deployed in communities and clinical settings have been investigated.
- By developing patient navigation and educational opportunities that merge the patients and caregivers, the community, policy makers, health care professionals, and researchers, we might be able to increase participation of minorities in MS studies.

## DISCLOSURE

Dr M.J. Williams received honoraria for Advisory Boards and Consulting from Alexion, Biogen, Bristol-Myers Squibb, EMD Serono, Horizon, Genentech, Novartis, Octave Bioscience, Sanofi Genzyme; TG Therapeutics. Dr M.J. Williams participated in Speaker's Bureau's for Biogen, EMD Serono, Genentech, TG Therapeutics. L. Amezcua has research support from the National MS Society, United States, NIH NINDS, Bristol-Myers Squibb Foundation, United States, Race to Erase MS Foundation and Biogen Idec. She is a local PI for commercial trials funded by Genentech and Sanofi, Genzyme, United States, and consulting fees from Biogen Idec, Novartis, Genentech, and EMD Serono.

## REFERENCES

1. Wallin MT, Culpepper WJ, Coffman P, et al. The Gulf War era multiple sclerosis cohort: age and incidence rates by race, sex and service. Brain 2012;135(6):1778–85.
2. Langer-Gould AM, Brara SM, Beaber BE, et al. Incidence of multiple sclerosis in multiple racial and ethnic groups. Neurology 2013;80(19):1734–9.
3. Walton C, King R, Rechtman L, et al. Rising prevalence of multiple sclerosis worldwide: Insights from the Atlas of MS, 3rd edition. Multiple Sclerosis Journal 2020;26(14):1816–21.

4. Wallin MT, Culpepper WJ, Campbell JD, et al. The prevalence of MS in the United States: A population-based estimate using health claims data. Neurology 2019;92(10). https://doi.org/10.1212/WNL.0000000000007035.
5. Wallin MT, Kurtzke JF, Culpepper WJ, et al. Multiple Sclerosis in Gulf War Era Veterans. 2. Military Deployment and Risk of Multiple Sclerosis in the First Gulf War. Neuroepidemiology 2014;42(4):226–34.
6. Negrotto L, Correale J. Evolution of multiple sclerosis prevalence and phenotype in Latin America. Mult Scler Relat Disord 2018;22:97–102.
7. Langer-Gould AM, Brara SM, Beaber BE, et al. The incidence of clinically isolated syndrome in a multi-ethnic cohort. J Neurol 2014;261(7):1349–55.
8. Romanelli RJ, Huang Q, Lacy J, et al. Multiple sclerosis in a multi-ethnic population from Northern California: a retrospective analysis, 2010–2016. BMC Neurol 2020;20(1):163.
9. Langer-Gould AM, Gonzales EG, Smith JB, et al. Racial and Ethnic Disparities in Multiple Sclerosis Prevalence. Neurology 2022;98(18):e1818–27.
10. Redelings MD, McCoy L, Sorvillo F. Multiple Sclerosis Mortality and Patterns of Comorbidity in the United States from 1990 to 2001. Neuroepidemiology 2006; 26(2):102–7.
11. Amezcua L, Rivas E, Joseph S, et al. Multiple Sclerosis Mortality by Race/Ethnicity, Age, Sex, and Time Period in the United States, 1999–2015. Neuroepidemiology 2018;50(1–2):35–40.
12. Marrie RA, Cohen J, Stuve O, et al. A systematic review of the incidence and prevalence of comorbidity in multiple sclerosis: overview. Mult Scler 2015; 21(3):263–81.
13. Conway DS, Thompson NR, Cohen JA. Influence of hypertension, diabetes, hyperlipidemia, and obstructive lung disease on multiple sclerosis disease course. Mult Scler 2017;23(2):277–85.
14. Conway DS, Briggs FB, Mowry EM, et al. Racial disparities in hypertension management among multiple sclerosis patients. Mult Scler Relat Disord 2022;64: 103972.
15. Amezcua L, Conti DV, Liu L, et al. Place of birth, age of immigration, and disability in Hispanics with multiple sclerosis. Mult Scler Relat Disord 2015; 4(1):25–30.
16. Robers MV, Chan C, Vajdi B, et al. Hypertension and hypertension severity in Hispanics/Latinx with MS. Multiple Sclerosis Journal 2021;27(12):1894–901.
17. Sahai-Srivastava S, Wang SL, Ugurlu C, et al. Headaches in multiple sclerosis: Cross-sectional study of a multiethnic population. Clin Neurol Neurosurg 2016 Apr;143:71–5.
18. Ventura RE, Antezana AO, Bacon T, et al. Hispanic Americans and African Americans with multiple sclerosis have more severe disease course than Caucasian Americans. Mult Scler 2016;23(11):1554–7.
19. Kister I, Chamot E, Bacon JH, et al. Rapid disease course in African Americans with multiple sclerosis. Neurology 2010;75(3):217–23.
20. Cree BAC, Khan O, Bourdette D, et al. Clinical characteristics of African Americans vs Caucasian Americans with multiple sclerosis. Neurology 2004;63(11): 2039–45.
21. Naismith RT TK, Cross AH. Phenotype and prognosis in African-Americans with multiple sclerosis: a retrospective chart review: Mult Scler.
22. Naismith RT, Trinkaus K, Cross AH. Phenotype and prognosis in African-Americans with multiple sclerosis: a retrospective chart review. Mult Scler 2006; 12(6):775–81.

23. Cipriani VP, Klein S. Clinical Characteristics of Multiple Sclerosis in African-Americans. Curr Neurol Neurosci Rep 2019;19(11):87.
24. Howard J, Battaglini M, Babb JS, et al. MRI correlates of disability in African-Americans with multiple sclerosis. PLoS One 2012;7(8):e43061.
25. Weinstock-Guttman B, Jacobs LD, Brownscheidle CM, et al. Multiple sclerosis characteristics in African American patients in the New York State Multiple Sclerosis Consortium. Mult Scler 2003;9(3):293–8.
26. Gray-Roncal K, Fitzgerald KC, Ryerson LZ, et al. Association of Disease Severity and Socioeconomic Status in Black and White Americans With Multiple Sclerosis. Neurology 2021;97(9):e881–9.
27. Saadi A, Himmelstein DU, Woolhandler S, et al. Racial disparities in neurologic health care access and utilization in the United States. Neurology 2017;88(24): 2268–75.
28. Reder AT, Centonze D, Naylor ML, et al. COVID-19 in Patients with Multiple Sclerosis: Associations with Disease-Modifying Therapies. CNS Drugs 2021;35(3): 317–30.
29. Rinker JR 2nd TK, Naismith RT, Cross AH. Higher IgG index found in African Americans versus Caucasians with multiple sclerosis: Neurology.
30. Weinstock-Guttman B, Ramanathan M, Hashmi K, et al. Increased tissue damage and lesion volumes in African Americans with multiple sclerosis. Neurology 2010; 74(7):538–44.
31. Fisniku LK, Brex PA, Altmann DR, et al. Disability and T2 MRI lesions: a 20-year follow-up of patients with relapse onset of multiple sclerosis. Brain 2008;131(Pt 3):808–17.
32. Caldito NG, Saidha S, Sotirchos ES, et al. Brain and retinal atrophy in African-Americans versus Caucasian-Americans with multiple sclerosis: a longitudinal study. Brain 2018;141(11):3115–29.
33. Darin T Okuda TS, Morgan McCreary , Alexander Smith, Andrew Wilson, Marco C Pinho, Fang F Yu, Thibo Billiet , Wim Van Hecke, Annemie Ribbens, Burcu Zeydan OK, Xiaohu Guo and Tatum M Moog. Selective vulnerability of brainstem and cervical spinal cord regions in people with non-progressive multiple sclerosis of Black or African American and European ancestry.
34. Moog TM, McCreary M, Stanley T, et al. African Americans experience disproportionate neurodegenerative changes in the medulla and upper cervical spinal cord in early multiple sclerosis. Mult Scler Relat Disord 2020;45:102429.
35. Kimbrough DJ, Sotirchos ES, Wilson JA, et al. Retinal damage and vision loss in African American multiple sclerosis patients. Ann Neurol 2015;77(2):228–36.
36. Seraji-Bozorgzad N, Reed S, Bao F, et al. Characterizing retinal structure injury in African-Americans with multiple sclerosis. Mult Scler Relat Disord 2016;7: 16–20.
37. Amezcua L, Smith JB, Gonzales EG, et al. Race, ethnicity, and cognition in persons newly diagnosed with multiple sclerosis. Neurology 2020;94(14):e1548–56.
38. Petracca M, Palladino R, Droby A, et al. Disability outcomes in early-stage African American and White people with multiple sclerosis. Mult Scler Relat Disord 2023;69:104413.
39. Bureau USC. 2017 national population projections. United States Census Bureau; 2018.
40. Buchanan RJ, Zuniga MA, Carrillo-Zuniga G, et al. Comparisons of Latinos, African Americans, and Caucasians with multiple sclerosis. Ethnic Dis 2010;20(4): 451–7.

41. Hadjixenofontos A, Beecham AH, Manrique CP, et al. Clinical Expression of Multiple Sclerosis in Hispanic Whites of Primarily Caribbean Ancestry. Neuroepidemiology 2015;44(4):262–8.
42. Amezcua L, Lund BT, Weiner LP, et al. Multiple sclerosis in Hispanics: a study of clinical disease expression. Mult Scler 2011;17(8):1010–6.
43. Kister I, Bacon T, Cutter GR. How Multiple Sclerosis Symptoms Vary by Age, Sex, and Race/Ethnicity. Neurology: Clin Pract 2021;11(4):335–41.
44. Langille MM, Islam T, Burnett M, et al. Clinical Characteristics of Pediatric-Onset and Adult-Onset Multiple Sclerosis in Hispanic Americans. J Child Neurol 2016; 31(8):1068–73.
45. Amezcua L, Beecham AH, Delgado SR, et al. Native ancestry is associated with optic neuritis and age of onset in hispanics with multiple sclerosis. Ann Clin Transl Neurol 2018;5(11):1362–71.
46. Amezcua L, Lerner A, Ledezma K, et al. Spinal cord lesions and disability in Hispanics with multiple sclerosis. J Neurol 2013;260(11):2770–6.
47. Tan CT, Mao Z, Wingerchuk DM, et al. International consensus diagnostic criteria for neuromyelitis optica spectrum disorders. Neurology 2016;86(5):491–2.
48. Banwell B, Bennett JL, Marignier R, et al. Diagnosis of myelin oligodendrocyte glycoprotein antibody-associated disease: International MOGAD Panel proposed criteria. Lancet Neurol 2023;22(3):268–82.
49. Bryc K, Durand EY, Macpherson JM, et al. The genetic ancestry of African Americans, Latinos, and European Americans across the United States. Am J Hum Genet 2015;96(1):37–53.
50. Millstein JCD, Gilliland FD, Gauderman WJ. A Testing Framework for Identifying Susceptibility Genes in the Presence of Epistasis. Am J Hum Genet 2006.
51. Tishkoff SA, Reed FA, Friedlaender FR, et al. The genetic structure and history of Africans and African Americans. Science 2009;324(5930):1035–44.
52. Ordoñez G, Romero S, Orozco L, et al. Genomewide admixture study in Mexican Mestizos with multiple sclerosis. Clin Neurol Neurosurg 2015;130: 55–60.
53. Oksenberg JR, Barcellos LF, Cree BA, et al. Mapping multiple sclerosis susceptibility to the HLA-DR locus in African Americans. Am J Hum Genet 2004;74(1): 160–7.
54. Isobe N, Madireddy L, Khankhanian P, et al. An ImmunoChip study of multiple sclerosis risk in African Americans. Brain 2015;138(Pt 6):1518–30.
55. Isobe N, Gourraud PA, Harbo HF, et al. Genetic risk variants in African Americans with multiple sclerosis. Neurology 2013;81(3):219–27.
56. Beecham AH, Amezcua L, Chinea A, et al. The genetic diversity of multiple sclerosis risk among Hispanic and African American populations living in the United States. Mult Scler 2020;26(11):1329–39.
57. Nakatsuka N, Patterson N, Patsopoulos NA, et al. Two genetic variants explain the association of European ancestry with multiple sclerosis risk in African-Americans. Sci Rep 2020;10(1):16902.
58. Hafler DA, Compston A, Sawcer S, et al. Risk alleles for multiple sclerosis identified by a genomewide study. N Engl J Med 2007;357(9):851–62.
59. Abbatemarco JR, Carlson A, Ontaneda D, et al. Association of socioeconomic disadvantage and neighborhood disparities with clinical outcomes in multiple sclerosis patients. Mult Scler Relat Disord 2022;61:103734.
60. Johnson BA, Wang J, Taylor EM, et al. Multiple sclerosis susceptibility alleles in African Americans. Genes Immun 2010;11(4):343–50.

61. Beecham AH, Amezcua L, Chinea A, et al. Ancestral risk modification for multiple sclerosis susceptibility detected across the Major Histocompatibility Complex in a multi-ethnic population. PLoS One 2022;17(12):e0279132.
62. Boullerne AI, Wallin MT, Culpepper WJ, et al. Liver kinase B1 rs9282860 polymorphism and risk for multiple sclerosis in White and Black Americans. Mult Scler Relat Disord 2021;55:103185.
63. Social determinants of health. 2023. https://www.who.int/health-topics/social-determinants-of-health#tab=tab_1 (Accessed April 4 2023).
64. Hood CM, Gennuso KP, Swain GR, et al. County Health Rankings: Relationships Between Determinant Factors and Health Outcomes. Am J Prev Med 2016;50(2):129–35.
65. Marmot M, Friel S, Bell R, et al. Closing the gap in a generation: health equity through action on the social determinants of health. Lancet 2008;372(9650):1661–9.
66. Calocer F, Dejardin O, Kwiatkowski A, et al. Socioeconomic deprivation increases the risk of disability in multiple sclerosis patients. Multiple Sclerosis and Related Disorders 2020;40:101930.
67. Harding KE, Wardle M, Carruthers R, et al. Socioeconomic status and disability progression in multiple sclerosis: A multinational study. Neurology 2019;92(13):e1497–506.
68. Promotion OoDP, Health. Health Equity in Healthy People 2030. Healthy People 2030.
69. Bailey ZD, Krieger N, Agénor M, et al. Structural racism and health inequities in the USA: evidence and interventions. Lancet 2017;389(10077):1453–63.
70. Marrie RA, Cutter G, Tyry T, et al. Does multiple sclerosis–associated disability differ between races? Neurology 2006;66(8):1235–40.
71. Wang Y, Tian F, Fitzgerald KC, et al. Socioeconomic status and race are correlated with affective symptoms in multiple sclerosis. Multiple Sclerosis and Related Disorders 2020;41:102010.
72. Amezcua L, Rivera VM, Vazquez TC, et al. Health Disparities, Inequities, and Social Determinants of Health in Multiple Sclerosis and Related Disorders in the US: A Review. JAMA Neurol 2021;78(12):1515–24.
73. Pimentel Maldonado DA, Eusebio JR, Amezcua L, et al. The impact of socioeconomic status on mental health and health-seeking behavior across race and ethnicity in a large multiple sclerosis cohort. Multiple Sclerosis and Related Disorders 2022;58:103451.
74. Shabas D, Heffner M. Multiple sclerosis management for low-income minorities. Multiple Sclerosis Journal 2005;11(6):635–40.
75. Fabius CD, Thomas KS, Zhang T, et al. Racial disparities in Medicaid home and community-based service utilization and expenditures among persons with multiple sclerosis. BMC Health Serv Res 2018;18(1):773.
76. Minden SL, Hoaglin DC, Hadden L, et al. Access to and utilization of neurologists by people with multiple sclerosis. Neurology 2008;70(13, Part 2 of 2):1141–9.
77. Stormacq C, Broucke SVd, Wosinski J. Does health literacy mediate the relationship between socioeconomic status and health disparities? Integrative review. Health Promot Int 2018;34(5):e1–17.
78. Buchanan RJ, Kaufman M, Zhu L, et al. Patient perceptions of multiple sclerosis-related care: comparisons by practice specialty of principal care physician. NeuroRehabilitation 2008;23(3):267–72.

79. Lara M, Gamboa C, Kahramanian MI, et al. Acculturation and Latino health in the United States: a review of the literature and its sociopolitical context. Annu Rev Publ Health 2005;26:367–97.
80. Koffman J, Goddard C, Gao W, et al. Exploring meanings of illness causation among those severely affected by multiple sclerosis: a comparative qualitative study of Black Caribbean and White British people. BMC Palliat Care 2015; 14(1):13.
81. Stuifbergen A, Becker H, Phillips C, et al. The Experience of African-American Women with Multiple Sclerosis. International Journal of MS Care 2020;23(2): 59–65.
82. Torres JM, Wallace SP. Migration circumstances, psychological distress, and self-rated physical health for Latino immigrants in the United States. American Journal of Public Health 2013;103(9):1619–27.
83. Obiwuru O, Joseph S, Liu L, et al. Perceptions of Multiple Sclerosis in Hispanic Americans: Need for Targeted Messaging. International Journal of MS Care 2016;19(3):131–9.
84. Boorgu DSSK, Venkatesh S, Lakhani CM, et al. The impact of socioeconomic status on subsequent neurological outcomes in multiple sclerosis. Multiple Sclerosis and Related Disorders 2022;65:103994.
85. Silveira SL, Motl RW. Environmental correlates of health-promoting leisure physical activity in persons with multiple sclerosis using a social cognitive perspective embedded within social ecological model. Prev Medicine Reports 2019;15: 100921.
86. Dovidio JF, Penner LA, Albrecht TL, et al. Disparities and distrust: The implications of psychological processes for understanding racial disparities in health and health care. Soc Sci Med 2008;67(3):478–86.
87. Hamilton R, Ciccarelli O. Multiple Sclerosis Incidence in Black Patients:†It Is Time to Do Away With a Racial Medical Myth. Neurology 2022;98(18):739–40.
88. Lawthers AG, Pransky GS, Peterson LE, et al. Rethinking quality in the context of persons with disability. Int J Qual Health Care 2003;15(4):287–99.
89. Natale-Pereira A, Enard KR, Nevarez L, et al. The role of patient navigators in eliminating health disparities. Cancer 2011;117(S15):3541–50.
90. Chiong-Rivero H, Robers M, Martinez A, et al. Effectiveness of film as a health communication tool to improve perceptions and attitudes in multiple sclerosis. Multiple Scler J Exp Transl Clin 2021;7(1). 2055217321995947.
91. Avasarala J. FDA-approved drugs for multiple sclerosis have no efficacy or disability data in non-Caucasian patients. CNS Spectr 2019;24(3):279–80.
92. Pimentel Maldonado DA, Moreno A, Williams MJ, et al. Perceptions and Preferences Regarding Multiple Sclerosis Research Among Racial and Ethnic Groups. International Journal of MS Care 2021;23(4):170–7.
93. Heller C, Balls-Berry JE, Nery JD, et al. Strategies addressing barriers to clinical trial enrollment of underrepresented populations: a systematic review. Contemp Clin Trials 2014;39(2):169–82.
94. Salman A, Nguyen C, Lee YH, et al. A Review of Barriers to Minorities' Participation in Cancer Clinical Trials: Implications for Future Cancer Research. J Immigr Minor Health 2016;18(2):447–53.
95. Schmotzer GL. Barriers and facilitators to participation of minorities in clinical trials. Ethn Dis 2012;22(2):226–30.
96. Garrick O, Mesa R, Ferris A, et al. Advancing Inclusive Research: Establishing Collaborative Strategies to Improve Diversity in Clinical Trials. Ethn Dis 2022; 32(1):61–8.

97. Jandorf L, Fatone A, Borker PV, et al. Creating alliances to improve cancer prevention and detection among urban medically underserved minority groups. The East Harlem Partnership for Cancer Awareness. Cancer 2006;107(8 Suppl):2043–51.
98. Amezcua L, Oksenberg JR, McCauley JL. MS in self-identified Hispanic/Latino individuals living in the US. Mult Scler J Exp Transl Clin 2017;3(3). 2055217317725103.
99. The National African Americans with MS Registry (NAAMSR) https://naamsr.org/(Accessed April 12, 2023 2023).
100. Cuccaro ML, Manrique CP, Quintero MA, et al. Understanding Participation in Genetic Research Among Patients With Multiple Sclerosis: The Influences of Ethnicity, Gender, Education, and Age. Front Genet 2020;11:120.
101. Clark LT, Watkins L, Pina IL, et al. Increasing Diversity in Clinical Trials: Overcoming Critical Barriers. Curr Probl Cardiol 2019;44(5):148–72.
102. Amezcua L, Okai AF, Cross AH, et al. Demographics and Baseline Disease Characteristics of Black and Hispanic Patients With Multiple Sclerosis in the CHIMES Trial (P4-4.005). Neurology 2022;98(18 Supplement):3257.
103. Okai AF, Amezcua L, Berkovich RR, et al. Efficacy and Safety of Alemtuzumab in Patients of African Descent with Relapsing-Remitting Multiple Sclerosis: 8-Year Follow-up of CARE-MS I and II (TOPAZ Study). Neurol Ther 2019;8(2):367–81.
104. Fox RJ, Gold R, Phillips JT, et al. Efficacy and Tolerability of Delayed-release Dimethyl Fumarate in Black, Hispanic, and Asian Patients with Relapsing-Remitting Multiple Sclerosis: Post Hoc Integrated Analysis of DEFINE and CONFIRM. Neurol Ther 2017;6(2):175–87.
105. Williams MJ, Amezcua L, Okai A, et al. Real-World Safety and Effectiveness of Dimethyl Fumarate in Black or African American Patients with Multiple Sclerosis: 3-Year Results from ESTEEM. Neurol Ther 2020;9(2):483–93.
106. Chinea Martinez AR, Correale J, Coyle PK, et al. Efficacy and safety of fingolimod in Hispanic patients with multiple sclerosis: pooled clinical trial analyses. Adv Ther 2014;31(10):1072–81.
107. Cascione M, Tenenbaum N, Wendt J, et al. Treatment retention on fingolimod compared with injectable multiple sclerosis therapies in African-American patients: A subgroup analysis of a randomized phase 4 study. Mult Scler Relat Disord 2018;25:50–6.
108. Cree BAC, Al-Sabbagh A, Bennett R, et al. Response to Interferon Beta-1a Treatment in African American Multiple Sclerosis Patients. Arch Neurol 2005;62(11):1681–3.
109. Cree BAC, Stuart WH, Tornatore CS, et al. Efficacy of Natalizumab Therapy in Patients of African Descent With Relapsing Multiple Sclerosis: Analysis of AFFIRM and SENTINEL Data. Arch Neurol 2011;68(4):464–8.
110. Cree BAC, Pradhan A, Pei J, et al. Efficacy and safety of ocrelizumab vs interferon beta-1a in participants of African descent with relapsing multiple sclerosis in the Phase III OPERA I and OPERA II studies. Mult Scler Relat Disord 2021;52:103010.
111. Hofrichter R, Bhatia R, County NAo, et al. Tackling health inequities through public health practice: theory to action. 2nd edition. Oxford ; New York: Oxford University Press; 2010.
112. Wallin MT, Culpepper WJ, Maloni H, et al. The Gulf War era multiple sclerosis cohort: 3. Early clinical features. Acta Neurol Scand 2018;137(1):76–84.

113. Perez CA, Lincoln JA. Racial and ethnic disparities in treatment response and tolerability in multiple sclerosis: A comparative study. Mult Scler Relat Disord 2021;56:103248.
114. Avasarala J. Inadequacy of Clinical Trial Designs and Data to Control for the Confounding Impact of Race/Ethnicity in Response to Treatment in Multiple Sclerosis. JAMA Neurol 2014;71(8):943–4.

# Era of COVID-19 in Multiple Sclerosis Care

Jonathan D. Krett, MD[a], Amber Salter, PhD[b],
Scott D. Newsome, DO[a,*]

**KEYWORDS**

• COVID-19 • Multiple sclerosis • Telemedicine • Registries
• Disease-modifying therapy • Vaccination

**KEY POINTS**

- People with multiple sclerosis (PwMS) experienced disruptions in their care and everyday lives during the coronavirus disease 2019 (COVID-19) pandemic.
- Innovations such as telemedicine helped preserve access to clinicians, whereas its optimal application to future MS care remains a topic of debate.
- Data from large MS registries proved to be informative regarding risks associated with COVID-19 and interactions with MS disease-modifying therapies.
- Many of the risk factors for poor outcomes in COVID-19 for PwMS are similar to those in the general population (eg, older age, black race); among PwMS, greater disability and B cell depleting therapies are associated with increased risk.
- Vaccines against COVID-19 are safe and effective for PwMS, although humoral responses to vaccination are blunted by certain disease-modifying therapies.

## INTRODUCTION

As of April 2023, there have been more than 760 million confirmed cases and 6.8 million deaths worldwide due to coronavirus disease 2019 (COVID-19).[1] In the United States, there have been more than 100 million cases and 1 million deaths.[2] The pandemic resulted in profound disruptions to society and healthcare systems globally.

For people with multiple sclerosis (PwMS) and their clinicians, the COVID-19 pandemic presented significant challenges. It not only affected the psychosocial well-being of PwMS but also caused major interruptions in routine MS care.[3] For

[a] Division of Neuroimmunology and Neurological Infections, Department of Neurology, Johns Hopkins University School of Medicine, 600 North Wolfe Street, Pathology 627, Baltimore, MD 21287, USA; [b] Section on Statistical Planning & Analysis, Department of Neurology, University of Texas Southwestern Medical Center, 5323 Harry Hines Boulevard, Dallas, TX 75390, USA
* Corresponding author. Division of Neuroimmunology and Neurological Infections, Johns Hopkins Hospital, 600 North Wolfe Street, Pathology 627, Baltimore, MD 21287.
*E-mail address:* snewsom2@jhmi.edu

Neurol Clin 42 (2024) 319–340
https://doi.org/10.1016/j.ncl.2023.06.006

example, missed clinical, laboratory, and imaging appointments related to the pandemic made it more difficult for clinicians to monitor disease activity and quality-of-life issues in PwMS.[4] Uncertainty surrounding the safety of MS disease-modifying therapies (DMTs) due to their varied effects on the immune system was also a major concern.

In this review, we will discuss the broad impact of the COVID-19 pandemic on MS care. We will highlight lessons learned by the MS community regarding delivery of care, COVID-19 risks, DMT selection, and strategies to optimize the efficacy of vaccinations against severe acute respiratory syndrome coronavirus 2 (SARS-CoV-2). We will conclude by examining implications for future care as we transition from the COVID-19 global health emergency to a phase of endemic and seasonal infection.[5]

## DISRUPTIONS ALONG THE CONTINUUM OF MULTIPLE SCLEROSIS CARE DUE TO COVID-19

The COVID-19 pandemic caused significant disruption for PwMS and the public. Lockdowns and physical distancing measures, which were implemented for public safety, made it difficult to access routine care for chronic conditions such as MS. Naturally, there was uncertainty about which activities outside the home could be done safely and, in some jurisdictions, PwMS may not have been permitted to leave home, with rare exceptions.

Interruptions along the continuum of MS care were common during the pandemic. A cross-sectional survey of more than 1000 PwMS conducted in April 2020 found that 22% cancelled a visit with their neurologist, 11% cancelled an MRI, 21% cancelled a laboratory test, and 10% altered the administration schedule of their DMT.[6] Another study of more than 4000 individuals with autoimmune disorders, of whom more than 800 were PwMS showed that nearly half experienced an interruption in health-care services.[7] Delays in infusions and lost rehabilitation visits were frequent sources of disruption.[8] Surveys of MS care providers confirmed that postponements in usual care were common and that providers were concerned about the risk COVID-19 posed to PwMS and themselves.[9,10] Along with consternation about being able to safely monitor PwMS, many providers expressed misgivings about the risk–benefit ratio of using higher efficacy DMTs in the context of the pandemic.[9,10] Whether disruptions in MS care resulted in any long-lasting consequences at an individual level is currently unknown.

Several studies also showed that changes to daily activities including work and socialization because of the pandemic were common among PwMS (ie, remaining at home, using virtual methods), similar to the general population.[8,11] Despite the heterogeneity of PwMS regarding health-related quality of life and disability, it was suggested that substantial psychosocial and occupational change might have a greater impact for PwMS, particularly those with preexisting activity limitations.[11,12] In one such study, women with MS were more likely than men with MS to experience job termination or furlough during the pandemic and expressed greater concern about the risk posed by COVID-19 to their health.[6] Moreover, psychological distress among PwMS pertaining to COVID-19 risk adversely affected their well-being, particularly when few effective treatments and no vaccines were available during the early pandemic.[13]

Altogether, public health measures put in place to protect us from COVID-19 no doubt had unintended impacts on MS care and required compensatory strategies to counterbalance them (**Fig. 1**). The next section will explore innovative care delivery

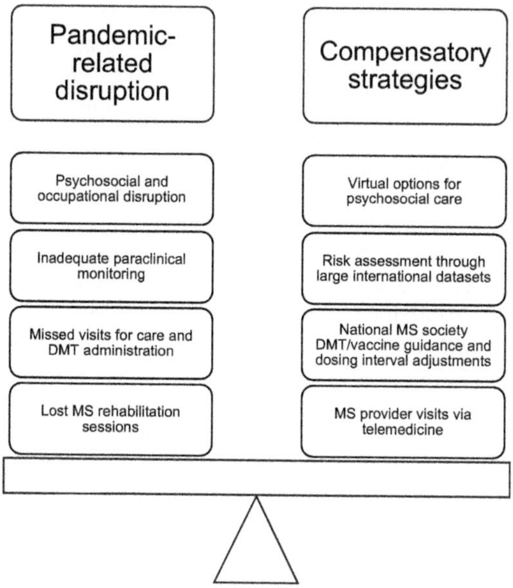


**Fig. 1. Disruptions and compensatory strategies in the COVID-19 era of MS care.** Examples provided depict how compensatory strategies and innovations by the MS community helped counterbalance pandemic-related disruptions to care.

methods that were accelerated during the pandemic to keep PwMS connected with their providers.

## BRINGING CARE TO PEOPLE WITH MULTIPLE SCLEROSIS USING TELEMEDICINE

Telemedicine, or telehealth, leverages the ability for individuals and their providers to connect despite not being physically present in the same location. Telemedicine was already being used for chronic and acute medical care before the COVID-19 pandemic and can take a variety of forms. These include synchronous contact over an audiovisual platform using the Internet, or asynchronous methods such as prerecorded or other electronic communication.[14] Studies before the COVID-19 pandemic demonstrated that assessment of PwMS, including disability measures, is feasible in a virtual format.[15,16] In response to pandemic-related disruptions, many MS centers started conducting most visits using telemedicine.[17,18]

Several studies highlighted benefits of telemedicine for PwMS, including improved access for those who live far from an MS center and those with mobility issues.[17,19] Some PwMS have greater comfort being in their home environment and having additional carers present virtually who may not otherwise be present at in-person visits.[20] Additionally, those with higher disability may benefit from more frequent clinical touchpoints by supplementing in-person visits with telemedicine appointments. Surveys suggest that most neurologists and PwMS who used telemedicine during the COVID-19 pandemic were satisfied with its use but we do not yet know whether this translates to better MS disease outcomes.[17,21] Of great concern is that subtle changes on neurological examination could be missed when using a virtual platform, resulting in inappropriately maintaining therapies that have suboptimal effectiveness.

There are other concerns that telemedicine could make accessing care harder for certain PwMS. For example, persons of lower socioeconomic status (SES), health literacy, and skill with technology may have more difficulty using telemedicine.[3] In at least one study, this concern did not bear out given that providers were able to conduct follow-up visits using mainly smartphones (and these are globally available at relatively low cost).[15,20] It is notable that most surveys examining satisfaction with telemedicine sampled individuals who were of higher SES and may not be generalizable to marginalized populations.[3,12]

Arguably, qualitative evaluation of telemedicine during the exceptional circumstance of the COVID-19 pandemic may have been more focused on its feasibility rather than what might be optimal in the long-term care of PwMS. We can be reassured that most studies viewed the use of telemedicine positively and suggested that no major short-term complications arose because of its widespread use.[17,20,22,23] It is worth carefully considering how best to integrate this knowledge into future clinical practice. For example, it is unclear whether exclusive use of telemedicine for both new and follow-up visits is ideal as opposed to the use of telemedicine only for follow-ups. One study from Norway suggested that some clinicians were dissatisfied completing new patient visits using telemedicine and looked on telemedicine more favorably for follow-up visits.[19] Furthermore, ensuring universal access remains a concern in jurisdictions with multiple healthcare payers such as the United States.[14] Lingering concerns also exist pertaining to cybersecurity and privacy due to use of Internet-based platforms.[14]

Overall, the rapid uptake of telemedicine during the COVID-19 pandemic may result in lasting changes in MS practice. The use of telemedicine is fluid and ever changing based on regulations around its use and uncertainty on how best to apply it. Future research is needed to elucidate the full range of implications associated with short-term and long-term use of telemedicine.

## THE POWER OF LARGE REGISTRIES FOR ASSESSING COVID-19 RISK IN PEOPLE WITH MULTIPLE SCLEROSIS

During the early part of the COVID-19 pandemic, MS researchers recognized the need for large studies to answer key questions. The Global Data Sharing Initiative developed a data sharing process to study the effects of COVID-19 in PwMS across small and large efforts globally.[24] This provided harmonized data across multiple countries and helped determine potential risk factors using large registries. Registry data was ideal for this purpose because large populations could be studied while adjusting for confounders and examining for rare outcomes. **Table 1** summarizes key contributions from several databases.

A crucial question was whether PwMS possessed any unique risk factors for poor outcomes with COVID-19. Several registry-based MS studies found that many of the risk factors were similar to individuals in the general population, including older age and the presence of specific medical comorbidities (eg, diabetes).[25–27] Data from the North American COVID-19 Infections in MS and related diseases (COViMS) registry showed a 30% increase in the risk of hospitalization and intensive care unit (ICU) admission and/or need for artificial ventilation for every 10-year increase in age, with a 76.5% increased risk of death for every 10-year age epoch.[25] Hypertension, diabetes, and morbid obesity also increased the risk of poor outcomes. Greater levels of ambulatory disability (eg, Expanded Disability Status Scale [EDSS] > 6 or requiring any assistance to walk) more than double the odds of more severe COVID-19 outcomes.[25,27,28] Being nonambulatory was associated with a 25-fold increased odds of death compared with fully ambulatory PwMS and black race was

**Table 1**
**Selected registries and key contributions to COVID-19 risk assessment in multiple sclerosis**

| Registry | Country of Origin | Largest MS Cohort | Key Contributions |
|---|---|---|---|
| Multiple Sclerosis International Federation Global Data Sharing Initiative | Global (HQ in UK) | 5648 | Harmonized data collection through multiple pooled registries[24,26] |
| North American Research Committee on Multiple Sclerosis (NARCOMS) | United States | 4955 | Survey showed high rates (84.1%) of SARS-CoV-2 vaccination and determined reasons for vaccine hesitancy in PwMS[96] |
| COVID-19 Infections in Multiple Sclerosis and Related Diseases (COViMS) | United States | 1626 | Risk factors for poor outcome with COVID-19 include increased disability, older age, hypertension, diabetes, obesity, black race, anti-CD20 DMT, and recent corticosteroid treatment[25]; pregnancy outcomes are no worse in PwMS[35] |
| Multiple Sclerosis and COVID-19 (MuSC-19) | Italy | 1362 | Increased risk of poor COVID-19 outcome in PwMS with EDSS >3 or at least 1 comorbidity[28] and use of anti-CD20 DMT[32] |
| Covisep | France | 347 | Age, EDSS 6 or higher, and obesity were found to be independent risk factors for hospitalization with COVID-19[27] |
| German MS Register | Germany | Hundreds | Contributed to the Global Data Sharing Initiative, and provided evidence that SARS-CoV-2 vaccination does not increase risk of relapse[83] |
| UK MS Register | UK | 404 | Multiple studies, including those that described common symptoms of self-diagnosed COVID-19 in PwMS[38] and determined that PwMS commonly experienced amplification of MS symptoms during COVID-19 infection; an effect that was attenuated by DMT[46] |
| Swedish MS Registry | Sweden | 17692 | Corroborated increased risk of hospitalization with COVID-19 in PwMS on anti-CD20 DMT but suggested that this risk may be more modest than the risk associated with older age, increased disability, and medical comorbidities[34] |
| MSBase COVID-19 Substudy | Australia | Thousands | Most notable publications relating to COVID-19 were under the auspices of the Global Data Sharing Initiative above |

*Abbreviations:* DMT, disease-modifying therapy; HQ, headquartered; PwMS, people with MS.

associated with more than 40% increased odds of being hospitalized (but not with an increased risk of death).[25]

Determining the risk of poor COVID-19 outcomes related to MS DMTs was also an intense focus of investigation. Smaller registries, such as those with hundreds rather than thousands of patients, initially found no effect of DMT exposure.[27,29,30] Revisiting this using larger datasets revealed that anti-CD20 monoclonal antibody therapies were associated with increased risk.[25,26,31,32] Rituximab was associated with 4.5-fold increased odds of hospitalization with COVID-19.[25] Pooled international data confirmed that ocrelizumab and rituximab (compared with other DMTs) increased the odds of hospitalization and ICU admission but not death.[31] This is consistent with data from other patients with immune-mediated disorders included in the Global Rheumatology Alliance registry, which found that rituximab was associated with 4-fold increased odds of death compared with methotrexate-treated individuals.[33]

DMT-treated status in isolation is not sufficient to risk stratify PwMS. Investigators in Italy found that COVID-19 risk was confined to PwMS in a "higher risk" group, defined as those with EDSS greater than 3 or with at least 1 comorbidity.[28] Conversely, PwMS with EDSS 3 or less and no comorbidities had a risk of severe COVID-19 outcome similar to age-matched and sex-matched controls.[28] Of note, untreated PwMS seem to have a higher risk of poor outcome[31] that is variably present in different studies following adjustment for factors such as age and MS phenotype.[27,32] This may reflect that this group consists of both individuals who are untreated due to having milder MS and those with more severe disability or progressive course who do not benefit from DMT (and may be at higher baseline risk of severe COVID-19 due to ambulatory status). A study of more than 17,000 PwMS from Sweden further supported the notion that premorbid disability and progressive MS course were likely more predictive of poor COVID-19 outcome compared with DMT type; an increased risk in rituximab-treated PwMS was again seen (although to a lesser degree than in smaller studies).[34] Pregnant and postpartum PwMS and children with MS do not seem to be at higher risk of poor COVID-19 outcomes; however, conclusions are limited by small sample size and underrepresentation of pregnant/young PwMS with high levels of ambulatory disability/comorbidities.[35,36] In general, pregnant women who develop COVID-19 may have a higher risk of preterm birth,[37] so individualized counseling remains important.

Data from the United Kingdom (UK) MS Register suggested that the likelihood of developing COVID-19 is not influenced by DMT-treated status or premorbid disability; however, these conclusions are limited by patient self-reporting.[38]

COVID-19 risk also relates to treatments used for MS relapses. Glucocorticoid use in the 2 months preceding infection was associated with a doubling of the odds of hospitalization and quadrupling the risk of death among PwMS with COVID-19.[25] Intravenous (IV) methylprednisolone use in the month preceding COVID-19 increases the risk but it is unknown whether lower doses typically used as premedication interacts with the increased risk observed with anti-CD-20 monoclonal antibodies.[32] The reasons for this observation are not well understood, given that dexamethasone is beneficial in severe acute COVID-19 respiratory infection.[39] The timing, dose, and duration of corticosteroid administration relative to pathogen exposure may determine the net immunomodulatory and therefore clinical effects.

In summary, pooled data from large registries has proven instrumental for informing the MS community about risk factors for poor outcomes secondary to COVID-19. Harmonized data using variables that were readily collected at the point of care enabled conclusions about clinically relevant risk factors for PwMS that seem consistent across studies. Possible limitations relate to voluntary reporting of data, use of variables only included a priori in the register, and lack of potentially relevant details such as DMT dose/frequency and MS disease activity.

## SYMPTOMATIC MANIFESTATIONS OF COVID-19 IN PEOPLE WITH MULTIPLE SCLEROSIS

Studies based on patient self-report found that COVID-19 symptoms experienced by PwMS (eg, ageusia, hyposmia, and upper respiratory tract symptoms) are no different than those experienced by individuals in the general population.[40–42] In a study assessing postacute symptoms in PwMS, nearly 30% of 8000 respondents reported COVID-19 symptoms lasting more than 1 month.[43] The risk was higher in those with severe preexisting neurological disability and mental health comorbidities.[43] Many persistent manifestations such as lower respiratory tract symptoms (eg, cough) and nondescript muscle aches were not consistent with MS; however, new or worsened fatigue had a prevalence of nearly 70% among those with postacute COVID-19 sequelae.[43] Because symptoms such as fatigue and cognitive impairment are common to both MS and postacute COVID-19, any pathogenetic interaction between the 2 disorders remains speculative currently.[44]

Evidence is sparse regarding whether COVID-19 produces durable changes in inflammatory disease activity in MS. It is common for PwMS to experience neurological symptoms during acute COVID-19; however, in these studies, self-reported data limit the ability to conclusively distinguish pseudoexacerbations from new focal CNS inflammation due to MS.[45–47]

## IMPACT OF COVID-19 ON DISEASE-MODIFYING THERAPY SELECTION

The expanding landscape of DMTs for PwMS has provided hope in terms of controlling the macroscopic neuroinflammatory component of MS (relapses and new lesions on MRI). Because many DMTs modulate, suppress, or reconstitute components of the immune system, concerns about safety came up early in the COVID-19 pandemic. Practical recommendations were needed to balance infectious safety concerns with preserving efficacy for people with active MS. We will focus on key lessons about DMT selection in the context of COVID-19. For an in-depth review of SARS-CoV-2 pathogenesis and its relationship to DMT mechanisms, we direct the reader to other published literature.[48–52]

So far, no MS DMT has proven to be protective against COVID-19. There was initially optimism that beta interferons could counteract SARS-CoV-2 through antiviral effects and possibly by dampening proinflammatory host responses.[53] Following one study which showed a nonstatistically significant trend toward lower rates of hospitalization for PwMS on beta interferon[25], further studies found no significant beneficial effect.[31,53,54] Hypotheses that other DMTs could attenuate COVID-19 severity through immunomodulatory mechanisms,[55] particularly in the case of fingolimod and natalizumab, have not borne out in large datasets.[26,31,48,56,57]

During the pandemic, recommendations for DMT prescribing and risk assessments were largely based on expert consensus or experience with other infectious diseases.[51,58] Changes in DMT use by PwMS were considered for some patients based on survey data and presumably related to concern about COVID-19.[6,8–10] Many MS providers remained comfortable with new DMT starts during the pandemic if appropriate based on MS severity, and only a small minority (8%) recommended postponing all DMT administrations.[59] This comfort level may have been enhanced by the larger

COVID-19 MS registries highlighting that the majority of DMTs did not seem to increase the risk of contracting SARS-CoV-2 or experiencing more severe COVID-19 outcomes.[26,31,32] Some PwMS may have had new MS disease activity and/or progression due to a change or discontinuation in therapy; however, evidence is lacking in this regard.

Prescribing patterns for DMTs were altered during the COVID-19 pandemic. A study from the UK showed a steady trend to increasing monoclonal antibody DMT prescriptions from 2016 to 2019 that was reversed in 2020 at the start of the pandemic (except for natalizumab) with a 16.7% reduction in new starts.[60] A similar trend was observed in Spain with decreases in prescriptions for anti-CD20 therapies and an increase in new natalizumab prescriptions, ostensibly due to lesser peripheral immunosuppression with natalizumab.[61] A study of 670 PwMS prescribed DMT in the United States showed a 10% reduction in IV infusion DMT prescriptions with an increase in oral DMT prescriptions (+7%), which persisted from the prevaccine to the postvaccine period of the pandemic.[62] Delays in infused DMT (mostly B cell therapies) were more common than switches in DMT class or type. Prescribing patterns of self-injected therapies remained stable, although the study overlapped with a time where ofatumumab (a self-injected anti-CD20 DMT) was becoming more widely prescribed.[62]

Although the global health emergency has been declared over, endemic COVID-19 risk will continue to factor into therapeutic shared decision-making along with the perceived benefits of treatment. This will require similar "risk calculus" as was used by experienced MS clinicians in the past. Before the COVID-19 pandemic, a qualitative study reinforced the idea that providers should engage PwMS in personalized discussions about risk tolerance when prescribing a DMT.[63] In this study, many PwMS would accept a risk of non–life-threatening infection in order to better control their MS and preserve function.[63]

We direct the reader to other excellent resources for a more detailed discussion about starting or sequencing DMTs in the era of COVID-19.[52,58,64–66] Some general recommendations from the National MS Society apply including the following: (1) PwMS currently on a DMT should not stop the treatment unless instructed to do so; (2) PwMS with COVID-19 symptoms or with a positive COVID-19 test should speak with their provider(s) (primary care and neurology clinicians); and (3) individualized decisions should be made regarding initiating or switching DMTs.[64] Practical recommendations for use of approved DMTs, including when to consider interrupting treatment can be found in **Table 2**.

Most of the COVID-19-specific concern surrounds cell-depleting DMTs such as anti-CD20 monoclonal antibodies. Theoretical concern surrounds the induction phase of alemtuzumab and cladribine treatment due to their respective mechanisms but they were not shown to be associated with increased risk in studies that included patients in the postinduction phase.[27,31,32,67] Interferons, glatiramer acetate, fumarates, teriflunomide, sphingosine-1-phosphate (S1P) receptor modulators and natalizumab were not shown to be associated with an increased risk of COVID-19 severity.[27,31,32,67] Lymphopenia with absolute lymphocyte counts (ALC) less than 800 cells/mm$^3$ can occur rarely with fumarates and with cladribine or alemtuzumab treatment and should be monitored because severe lymphopenia may increase risk.[48,50,51,68] Lymphocytes are peripherally sequestered by S1P modulators (eg, fingolimod), so low-lymphocyte counts likely represent a functional lymphopenia and may not increase risk unless the measured ALC is severely reduced (<200 cells/mm$^3$).[69,70]

Even though the anti-CD20 infusions are dosed intermittently, this results in maintenance of a B cell-depleted state and may result in hypogammaglobulinemia.[50]

**Table 2**
**Summary of recommendations for commercially available multiple sclerosis disease-modifying therapies in the COVID-19 era**

| DMT Class | Brief Mechanism of Action | Mode of Administration | Effect on COVID-19 Outcome | Recommendation in SARS-CoV-2 Infected PwMS |
| --- | --- | --- | --- | --- |
| Beta interferon | Inhibits proinflammatory cytokines | SQ or IM | No increased risk. Protective effect has not been proven[53] | Continue treatment |
| Glatiramer acetate | Modulates T cell cytokine profile to increased Th2; promotes Treg cells | SQ | No increased risk[26] | Continue treatment |
| Teriflunomide | Inhibits reactive lymphocyte proliferation | Oral | No increased risk[26] | Continue treatment |
| Fumarates | Enhances Nrf2 pathway, improves oxidative stress response, and limits survival/activation of T cell subsets | Oral | No increased risk, except rarely if lymphopenic (ALC <800 cells/$mm^3$)[104] | Continue; consider suspending if severe infection or ALC <800 cells/$mm^3$ |
| S1P receptor modulators | Inhibits lymphocyte trafficking out of peripheral lymph nodes | Oral | No evidence of direct increased risk[26] but may impair response to vaccines[92] | Continue; consider suspending if ALC <200 cells/$mm^3$ |
| Natalizumab | Prevents leukocyte trafficking across the blood-CNS barrier by targeting alpha-4 integrins | IV | No evidence of increased risk.[26] Extended interval dosing may reduce risk of infusion center exposure[71] | Continue; may consider delaying infusion if critically ill |
| Anti-CD20 monoclonal antibodies | Lyses and depletes B lymphocytes by targeting CD20 on their surface | IV (eg, ocrelizumab) or SQ (ofatumumab) | Increased risk of hospitalization estimated in the range of 2 to 5-fold.[25,26,67] May impair response to vaccines[86,94] | Suspend/delay dosing |

(*continued on next page*)

Table 2
(*continued*)

| DMT Class | Brief Mechanism of Action | Mode of Administration | Effect on COVID-19 Outcome | Recommendation in SARS-CoV-2 Infected PwMS |
|---|---|---|---|---|
| Cladribine | Inhibits DNA synthesis and depletes B > T lymphocytes | Oral—2 cycles separated by 1 year | Likely only at increased risk when severely lymphopenic[26,51] | Suspend/delay dosing |
| Alemtuzumab | Lyses and depletes mature T and B lymphocytes and several innate immune cells by targeting CD52 on their surface | IV—2 cycles separated by 1 year | Likely only at increased risk when severely lymphopenic/leukopenic[26,51] | Suspend/delay dosing |

*Abbreviations:* ALC, absolute lymphocyte count; DMT, disease-modifying therapy; IM, intramuscular; IV, intravenous; Nrf2, nuclear factor erythroid 2-related factor 2; PwMS, people with MS; S1P, sphingosine-1 phosphate; SQ, subcutaneous; Th2, T helper-2 cytokine profile; Treg, T regulatory cells.

Immune reconstitution therapies (alemtuzumab and cladribine) possibly carry a greater peak risk during induction but may be appealing options for some PwMS who prefer their risk to be frontloaded.[31,48] Although large observational studies did not show statistically significant increases in COVID-19 risk with immune reconstitution therapies, this does not necessarily indicate superior safety, especially since the number of patients on these therapies was small in comparison to the other DMTs.[26]

Autologous hematopoietic stem cell transplant remains an option for treatment of refractory MS.[64] COVID-19 risk is likely elevated for several months following the immunoablative phase of treatment but this has not been well studied.[64] Despite the increased risk of COVID-19 severity with some of the MS DMTs, available data along with expert opinion suggests that some PwMS should continue to use these therapies in the proper clinical context.[64] PwMS should also adhere to routine precautions to reduce risk of infection and exposure to COVID-19.[64] These therapies remain an effective option for reducing disease activity and undertreating MS may present a greater risk than COVID-19.

During the pandemic, some MS providers preferentially used natalizumab in John Cunningham virus seronegative patients who had active disease given lower COVID-19 risks and less impact on vaccination response.[30,69] The exposure risk of frequent visits to the infusion center can likely be mitigated by extended interval dosing.[50,71] Extended interval dosing for ocrelizumab and rituximab (ie, delaying maintenance redosing by 4 or more weeks or personalized redosing based on CD19 cell count) was found not to be associated with increased MS disease activity in the short-term.[72–75] However, a single cohort study of extended interval ocrelizumab dosing raised concern about increased MRI activity without an increase in confirmed disability progression,[76] emphasizing that the long-term safety and efficacy of this off-label approach need to be confirmed with prospective studies.

When PwMS are diagnosed with COVID-19, several Food and Drug Administration (FDA)-approved antiviral treatments may be available to them depending on their baseline risk factors and severity of illness.[77] Of note, Evusheld and REGEN-COV are not authorized by the FDA anymore because they no longer cover dominant circulating SARS-CoV-2 variants.[77]

## VACCINATION AGAINST SARS-CoV-2 FOR PEOPLE WITH MULTIPLE SCLEROSIS

Since their advent in August 2021, large population-based data show that SARS-CoV-2 mRNA vaccines are safe and effective in PwMS, as in the general population.[78–82] Adverse effects are typically mild and self-limited (injection site reaction, malaise, headache, fever) and are not associated with increased short-term risk of MS relapse.[80,81,83]

Early on, it was not known whether PwMS treated with certain DMT classes (eg, cell-depleting therapies) would mount adequate immune responses, including memory B cell responses to SARS-CoV-2 vaccination. Multiple studies confirmed that those on cell-depleting therapies (anti-CD20, alemtuzumab) and those on S1P receptor modulators have diminished humoral responses to SARS-CoV-2 vaccination.[84–88] However, T cell-mediated adaptive responses are preserved in many patients on anti-CD20 therapy and may be more robust, suggesting that other immune mechanisms may compensate for a blunted humoral response.[86,89–91] These effects persist in the long term and affect memory B cells.[84] It has become evident that timing of vaccine and DMT administration (**Table 3**) influences the magnitude of serologic immune response observed.[92–94] However, it is unknown whether these suspected

**Table 3**
**Summary of recommendations for SARS-CoV-2 vaccination in people with multiple sclerosis by treatment status**

| MS Treatment | Negative Effect on SARS-CoV-2 Vaccine Response? | Timing of Vaccine Before Starting Treatment | Timing of Vaccine After Treatment Started[a] |
|---|---|---|---|
| No DMT | None: having MS in isolation does not affect ability to mount a humoral response to available SARS-CoV-2 vaccines[78] | SARS-CoV-2 vaccines are safe and effective for PwMS and recommended for all patients[81] | N/A |
| Beta interferon | None[78,93] | Do not delay starting for vaccine | No adjustments required; vaccinate when able |
| Glatiramer acetate | None[78,93] | Do not delay starting for vaccine | No adjustments required; vaccinate when able |
| Teriflunomide | No data to suggest impaired response[78,93] | Do not delay starting for vaccine | No adjustments required; vaccinate when able |
| Fumarates | No reduction in humoral or T cell-dependent responses for dimethyl fumarate; unknown for other fumarate DMTs[93,105] | Do not delay starting for vaccine | No adjustments required; vaccinate when able |
| S1P receptor modulators | Impairment in humoral response in PwMS on fingolimod[92] | Vaccinate at least 2 wk before starting | Continue taking the medication as prescribed and vaccinate when able |
| Natalizumab | No data to suggest impaired responses for SARS-CoV-2 vaccines[93,105] | Do not delay starting for vaccine | No adjustments required; vaccinate when able |
| Anti-CD20 monoclonal antibodies | Impairment in humoral response was observed in several studies, however certain T cell responses were found to be more robust[78,86,87,90,106] | Vaccinate at least 2 wk before starting | Ideal timing to vaccinate is 4 wk before next infusion or 4 wk after last dose of ofatumumab |
| Cladribine | Empiric data suggest no impairment in humoral antibody responses; theoretical concern during lymphodepletive treatment phase[84] | Vaccinate at least 2 wk before starting | No adjustments required; vaccinate when able |

| | | | |
|---|---|---|---|
| Alemtuzumab | Empiric data suggest no impairment in humoral antibody responses; theoretical concern during lymphodepletive treatment phase[93] | Vaccinate at least 4 wk before starting | Consider vaccination 24 wk or more after the last infusion |
| High-dose corticosteroids | Not demonstrated with empirical data but theoretical concern exists given mechanism of action | Vaccinate 3–5 d after last dose | Vaccinate 3–5 d after the last dose |

*Abbreviations:* DMT, disease-modifying therapy; PwMS, people with MS; S1P, sphingosine-1 phosphate.
[a] Note that ideal timing of therapy with vaccination may not be possible.

compensatory immune mechanisms or DMT timing result in preventing SARS-CoV-2 infections and/or severe COVID-19 outcomes.

It is recommended that all PwMS receive vaccination against SARS-CoV-2 unless there is a contraindication (eg, allergic reaction) and keep their vaccinations up to date when they are able to receive boosters.[82,95] **Table 3** summarizes recommendations regarding the optimal timing of SARS-CoV-2 vaccinations with various DMTs.

Addressing concerns PwMS may have about vaccination is paramount. Surveys suggest that most PwMS are willing to receive SARS-CoV-2 vaccines (>75%–90% depending on the study).[96,97] The most prevalent concerns relate to long-term safety and efficacy.[96,98,99] In one large patient survey (n = ~5000), factors that increased the likelihood of receiving the SARS-CoV-2 vaccine included obtaining influenza vaccine, older age (≥65 years), higher SES, physical activity, and use of DMT.[96] People with MS were less likely to be vaccine hesitant when explicitly counseled by their MS provider about risks and benefits.[100] Overall, providers should continue to individualize counseling to promote vaccination wherever possible to reduce long-term COVID-19 risk as the pandemic shifts to a more endemic/seasonal pattern globally.

## DISCUSSION

With the end of the COVID-19 global health emergency, it remains unknown whether changes to MS care will persist. A shift to endemic patterns of infection likely means that a degree of normalcy will return. However, the field has demonstrated that MS care can be adapted to meet PwMS in their home environments with telemedicine. Prospective investigation will be required to clarify the extent telemedicine should be used in routine practice based on patient care outcomes.

As efficacious DMTs continue to be developed, the MS community can incorporate lessons learned during the COVID-19 pandemic to develop contingency plans in the event of future viral pandemics. DMT and vaccination guidelines will need to discuss suggested actions in the event of future viral outbreaks. PwMS will require information about risk while on DMTs and how vaccine responses may be impacted.

Finally, the long-term effects of widespread COVID-19 on PwMS are not yet fully understood. The degree to which long-COVID might interact with MS fatigue and other symptomatology has been explored[101,102] but relationships have not been conclusively demonstrated. It will also take time to study sustained effects of pandemic-related occupational and psychosocial disruption, which may have disproportionately affected certain PwMS,[11,13,68,103] particularly those who were already vulnerable socioeconomically. Observational studies should continue to monitor the long-term impact of the COVID-19 pandemic on MS incidence and disease activity, although preliminary data suggest that its short-term impacts are no different than those of other respiratory viruses.[40,102] As we enter the post-pandemic COVID-19 era, the future of person-centered MS care looks as promising as ever.

## SUMMARY

Despite multiple COVID-19 pandemic-related disruptions along the continuum of MS care, providers and PwMS collaborated to develop innovative solutions. There were unprecedented efforts across the MS community to work together to collect as much information as possible to make informed decisions in the care of PwMS. We reviewed considerations for DMT prescription and vaccination for PwMS in the era of COVID-19 and speculate on questions for future research in this area.

## CLINICS CARE POINTS

- Until more data are available, use of telemedicine for MS care should be based on the preferences of people with MS and providers along with local regulations.
- Considering currently available safety data, DMTs can be started and sequenced similarly postpandemic compared with the prepandemic era, assuming risks and benefits are discussed in detail with each person with MS.
- Anti-CD20 monoclonal antibody therapies remain first-line options for some, and people on these therapies should be counseled about increased infection risk along with the possibility of impaired vaccine responses. Extended interval dosing requires further investigation, should be considered in select cases, and has relevance beyond the scope of COVID-19.
- SARS-CoV-2 vaccines are recommended for people with MS and do not seem to be associated with an increased risk of relapse.

## DISCLOSURES

J.D. Krett: receives fellowship funding (paid directly to institution) provided by the National Multiple Sclerosis Society and a University of Calgary Medical Group Helios Advanced Training Award. A. Salter: receives research funding (paid directly to institution) from Multiple Sclerosis Canada, National Multiple Sclerosis Society, Consortium of Multiple Sclerosis Centers and the Department of Defense Congressionally Directed Medical Research Program and is a member of the editorial board for Neurology. She serves as a consultant for Gryphon Bio, LLC. She is a member of the Data and Safety Monitoring Board for Premature Infants Receiving Milking or Delayed Cord Clamping (PREMOD2), Central Vein Sign: A Diagnostic Biomarker in Multiple Sclerosis (CAVS-MS), and Methotrexate treatment of Arthritis caused by Chikungunya virus (MARCH). She is supported (in part) by a Biostatistics/Informatics Junior Faculty Award (BI-2105-37656) from the National Multiple Sclerosis Society, United States. She holds the Kenney Marie Dixon-Pickens Distinguished Professorship in Multiple Sclerosis Research. S.D. Newsome received consultant fees for scientific advisory boards from Biogen, Genentech, Bristol Myers Squibb, EMD Serono, Greenwich Biosciences, Horizon Therapeutics, Novartis, TG Therapeutics; study lead PI for a Roche clinical trial program; advisor to Autobahn; received research funding (paid directly to institution) from Biogen, United States, Lundbeck, Denmark, Roche, Switzerland, Genentech, United States, National MS Society, United States, The Stiff Person Syndrome Research Foundation, Department of Defense, and Patient Centered Outcomes Research Institute.

## REFERENCES

1. World Health Organization Coronavirus Dashboard (Internet). Internet. Updated 2023 Feb 8.Available at: https://covid19.who.int/. Accessed 2023 Feb 8.
2. Centers for Disease Control and Prevention, COVID Data Tracker (Internet). Internet. Accessed 2023 Feb 8. Available at: https://covid.cdc.gov/covid-data-tracker/#datatracker-home. Accessed 2023 Feb 8.
3. Chen MH, Goverover Y, Botticello A, et al. Healthcare disruptions and use of telehealth services among people with multiple sclerosis during the COVID-19 pandemic. Arch Phys Med Rehabil 2022;103(7):1379–86.

4. Zhang Y, Staker E, Cutter G, et al. Perceptions of risk and adherence to care in MS patients during the COVID-19 pandemic: a cross-sectional study. Mult Scler Relat Disord 2021;50:102856.
5. Harris E. WHO declares end of COVID-19 global health emergency. JAMA 2023. https://doi.org/10.1001/jama.2023.8656.
6. Vogel AC, Schmidt H, Loud S, et al. Impact of the COVID-19 pandemic on the health care of >1,000 People living with multiple sclerosis: A cross-sectional study. Mult Scler Relat Disord 2020;46:102512.
7. Fitzgerald KC, Mecoli CA, Douglas M, et al. Risk factors for infection and health impacts of the coronavirus disease 2019 (COVID-19) pandemic in people with autoimmune diseases. Clin Infect Dis 2022;74(3):427–36.
8. Moss BP, Mahajan KR, Bermel RA, et al. Multiple sclerosis management during the COVID-19 pandemic. Mult Scler 2020;26(10):1163–71.
9. Mateen FJ, Rezaei S, Alakel N, et al. Impact of COVID-19 on U.S. and Canadian neurologists' therapeutic approach to multiple sclerosis: a survey of knowledge, attitudes, and practices. J Neurol 2020;267(12):3467–75.
10. Morrison EH, Michtich K, Hersh CM. How the COVID-19 Pandemic has changed multiple sclerosis clinical practice: Results of a nationwide provider survey. Mult Scler Relat Disord 2021;51:102913.
11. Goverover Y, Chen MH, Botticello A, et al. Relationships between changes in daily occupations and health-related quality of life in persons with multiple sclerosis during the COVID-19 pandemic. Mult Scler Relat Disord 2022;57:103339.
12. Parkinson A, Drew J, Hall Dykgraaf S, et al. 'They're getting a taste of our world': a qualitative study of people with multiple sclerosis' experiences of accessing health care during the COVID-19 pandemic in the Australian Capital Territory. Health Expect 2021;24(5):1607–17.
13. Alschuler KN, Roberts MK, Herring TE, et al. Distress and risk perception in people living with multiple sclerosis during the early phase of the COVID-19 pandemic. Mult Scler Relat Disord 2021;47:102618.
14. Hatcher-Martin JM, Busis NA, Cohen BH, et al. American academy of neurology telehealth position statement. Neurology 2021;97(7):334–9.
15. Bove R, Bevan C, Crabtree E, et al. Toward a low-cost, in-home, telemedicine-enabled assessment of disability in multiple sclerosis. Mult Scler 2019;25(11): 1526–34.
16. Bove R, Garcha P, Bevan CJ, et al. Clinic to in-home telemedicine reduces barriers to care for patients with MS or other neuroimmunologic conditions. Neurol Neuroimmunol Neuroinflamm 2018;5(6):e505.
17. Abbatemarco JR, Hartman J, McGinley M, et al. Providing person-centered care via telemedicine in the era of COVID-19 in multiple sclerosis. J Patient Exp 2021; 8. https://doi.org/10.1177/2374373520981474. 2374373520981474.
18. McGinley MP, Ontaneda D, Wang Z, et al. Teleneurology as a solution for outpatient care during the COVID-19 pandemic. Telemed J e Health 2020;26(12): 1537–9.
19. Kristoffersen ES, Sandset EC, Winsvold BS, et al. Experiences of telemedicine in neurological out-patient clinics during the COVID-19 pandemic. Ann Clin Transl Neurol 2021;8(2):440–7.
20. Corea F, Ciotti S, Cometa A, et al. Telemedicine during the coronavirus disease (COVID-19) pandemic: a multiple sclerosis (MS) outpatients service perspective. Neurol Int 2021;13(1):25–31.

21. McGinley MP, Gales S, Rowles W, et al. Expanded access to multiple sclerosis teleneurology care following the COVID-19 pandemic. Mult Scler J Exp Transl Clin 2021;7(1). https://doi.org/10.1177/2055217321997467. 2055217321997467.
22. Keszler P, Maloni H, Miles Z, et al. Telemedicine and multiple sclerosis: a survey of health care providers before and during the COVID-19 pandemic. Int J MS Care 2022;24(6):266–70.
23. Li V, Roos I, Monif M, et al. Impact of telehealth on health care in a multiple sclerosis outpatient clinic during the COVID-19 pandemic. Mult Scler Relat Disord 2022;63:103913.
24. Peeters LM, Parciak T, Walton C, et al. COVID-19 in people with multiple sclerosis: a global data sharing initiative. Mult Scler 2020;26(10):1157–62.
25. Salter A, Fox RJ, Newsome SD, et al. Outcomes and risk factors associated with SARS-CoV-2 infection in a north american registry of patients with multiple sclerosis. JAMA Neurol 2021;78(6):699–708.
26. Simpson-Yap S, Pirmani A, Kalincik T, et al. Updated results of the COVID-19 in MS global data sharing initiative: anti-CD20 and other risk factors associated with COVID-19 severity. Neurol Neuroimmunol Neuroinflamm 2022;9(6). https://doi.org/10.1212/NXI.0000000000200021.
27. Louapre C, Collongues N, Stankoff B, et al. Clinical characteristics and outcomes in patients with coronavirus disease 2019 and multiple sclerosis. JAMA Neurol 2020;77(9):1079–88.
28. Sormani MP, Schiavetti I, Carmisciano L, et al. COVID-19 severity in multiple sclerosis: putting data into context. Neurol Neuroimmunol Neuroinflamm 2022; 9(1). https://doi.org/10.1212/NXI.0000000000001105.
29. Bsteh G, Assar H, Hegen H, et al. COVID-19 severity and mortality in multiple sclerosis are not associated with immunotherapy: Insights from a nation-wide Austrian registry. PLoS One 2021;16(7):e0255316.
30. Arrambide G, Llaneza-Gonzalez MA, Costa-Frossard Franca L, et al. SARS-CoV-2 Infection in Multiple Sclerosis: Results of the Spanish Neurology Society Registry. Neurol Neuroimmunol Neuroinflamm 2021;8(5). https://doi.org/10.1212/NXI.0000000000001024.
31. Simpson-Yap S, De Brouwer E, Kalincik T, et al. Associations of disease-modifying therapies with COVID-19 severity in multiple sclerosis. Neurology 2021;97(19):e1870–85.
32. Sormani MP, Salvetti M, Labauge P, et al. DMTs and Covid-19 severity in MS: a pooled analysis from Italy and France. Ann Clin Transl Neurol 2021;8(8): 1738–44.
33. Strangfeld A, Schafer M, Gianfrancesco MA, et al. Factors associated with COVID-19-related death in people with rheumatic diseases: results from the COVID-19 global rheumatology alliance physician-reported registry. Ann Rheum Dis 2021;80(7):930–42.
34. Longinetti E, Bower H, McKay KA, et al. COVID-19 clinical outcomes and DMT of MS patients and population-based controls. Ann Clin Transl Neurol 2022;9(9): 1449–58.
35. Salter A, Cross AH, Cutter GR, et al. COVID-19 in the pregnant or postpartum MS patient: symptoms and outcomes. Mult Scler Relat Disord 2022;65:104028.
36. Oncel I, Alici N, Solmaz I, et al. The outcome of COVID-19 in pediatric-onset multiple sclerosis patients. Pediatr Neurol 2022;134:7–10.
37. Yam C, Jokubaitis V, Hellwig K, et al. MS, pregnancy and COVID-19. Mult Scler 2020;26(10):1137–46.

38. Evangelou N, Garjani A, dasNair R, et al. Self-diagnosed COVID-19 in people with multiple sclerosis: a community-based cohort of the UK MS Register. J Neurol Neurosurg Psychiatry 2020;92(1):107–9.
39. Group RC, Horby P, Lim WS, et al. Dexamethasone in hospitalized patients with covid-19. N Engl J Med 2021;384(8):693–704.
40. Sepulveda M, Llufriu S, Martinez-Hernandez E, et al. Incidence and impact of COVID-19 in MS: a survey from a barcelona MS unit. Neurol Neuroimmunol Neuroinflamm 2021;8(2). https://doi.org/10.1212/NXI.0000000000000954.
41. Schiavetti I, Carmisciano L, Ponzano M, et al. Signs and symptoms of COVID-19 in patients with multiple sclerosis. Eur J Neurol 2022;29(12):3728–36.
42. Parrotta E, Kister I, Charvet L, et al. COVID-19 outcomes in MS: observational study of early experience from NYU multiple sclerosis comprehensive care center. Neurol Neuroimmunol Neuroinflamm 2020;7(5). https://doi.org/10.1212/NXI.0000000000000835.
43. Garjani A, Middleton RM, Nicholas R, et al. Recovery from COVID-19 in multiple sclerosis: a prospective and longitudinal cohort study of the United Kingdom multiple sclerosis register. Neurol Neuroimmunol Neuroinflamm 2022;9(1). https://doi.org/10.1212/NXI.0000000000001118.
44. Bellucci G, Rinaldi V, Buscarinu MC, et al. Multiple sclerosis and SARS-CoV-2: has the interplay started? Front Immunol 2021;12:755333.
45. Etemadifar M, Sedaghat N, Aghababaee A, et al. COVID-19 and the risk of relapse in multiple sclerosis patients: a fight with no bystander effect? Mult Scler Relat Disord 2021;51:102915.
46. Garjani A, Middleton RM, Hunter R, et al. COVID-19 is associated with new symptoms of multiple sclerosis that are prevented by disease modifying therapies. Mult Scler Relat Disord 2021;52:102939.
47. Kataria S, Tandon M, Melnic V, et al. A case series and literature review of multiple sclerosis and COVID-19: Clinical characteristics, outcomes and a brief review of immunotherapies. eNeurologicalSci 2020;21:100287. https://doi.org/10.1016/j.ensci.2020.100287.
48. Cabreira V, Abreu P, Soares-Dos-Reis R, et al. Multiple Sclerosis, Disease-Modifying Therapies and COVID-19: A Systematic Review on Immune Response and Vaccination Recommendations. Vaccines (Basel) 2021;9(7). https://doi.org/10.3390/vaccines9070773.
49. Chaudhry F, Jageka C, Levy PD, et al. Review of the COVID-19 Risk in Multiple Sclerosis. J Cell Immunol 2021;3(2):68–77. https://doi.org/10.33696/immunology.3.080.
50. Zheng C, Kar I, Chen CK, et al. Multiple Sclerosis Disease-Modifying Therapy and the COVID-19 Pandemic: Implications on the Risk of Infection and Future Vaccination. CNS Drugs 2020;34(9):879–96. https://doi.org/10.1007/s40263-020-00756-y.
51. Giovannoni G, Hawkes C, Lechner-Scott J, et al. The COVID-19 pandemic and the use of MS disease-modifying therapies. Mult Scler Relat Disord 2020;39:102073. https://doi.org/10.1016/j.msard.2020.102073.
52. Hollen C, Bernard J. Multiple Sclerosis Management During the COVID-19 Pandemic. Curr Neurol Neurosci Rep 2022;22(8):537–43. https://doi.org/10.1007/s11910-022-01211-9.
53. Simpson-Yap S, Pirmani A, De Brouwer E, et al. Severity of COVID19 infection among patients with multiple sclerosis treated with interferon-beta. Mult Scler Relat Disord 2022;66:104072. https://doi.org/10.1016/j.msard.2022.104072.

54. Freedman MS, Jack D, Murgasova Z, et al. Outcomes of COVID-19 among patients treated with subcutaneous interferon beta-1a for multiple sclerosis. Mult Scler Relat Disord 2021;56:103283. https://doi.org/10.1016/j.msard.2021.103283.
55. Mohn N, Konen FF, Pul R, et al. Experience in Multiple Sclerosis Patients with COVID-19 and Disease-Modifying Therapies: A Review of 873 Published Cases. J Clin Med 2020;9(12). https://doi.org/10.3390/jcm9124067.
56. Tasat DR, Yakisich JS. Rationale for the use of sphingosine analogues in COVID-19 patients. Clin Med (Lond) 2021;21(1):e84–7. https://doi.org/10.7861/clinmed.2020-0309.
57. Teymouri S, Pourbayram Kaleybar S, Hejazian SS, et al. The effect of Fingolimod on patients with moderate to severe COVID-19. Pharmacol Res Perspect 2023; 11(1):e01039. https://doi.org/10.1002/prp2.1039.
58. Ciotti JR, Grebenciucova E, Moss BP, et al. Multiple Sclerosis Disease-Modifying Therapies in the COVID-19 Era. Ann Neurol 2020;88(6):1062–4. https://doi.org/10.1002/ana.25907.
59. Portaccio E, Fonderico M, Hemmer B, et al. Impact of COVID-19 on multiple sclerosis care and management: Results from the European Committee for Treatment and Research in Multiple Sclerosis survey. Mult Scler 2022;28(1): 132–8. https://doi.org/10.1177/13524585211005339.
60. Williams T, Mishra R, Bharkhada B, et al. Impact of the COVID-19 pandemic on the prescription of disease-modifying therapy for multiple sclerosis in England: a nationwide study. J Neurol Neurosurg Psychiatry 2022;93(11):1229–30. https://doi.org/10.1136/jnnp-2021-328340.
61. Cobo-Calvo A, Zabalza A, Rio J, et al. Impact of COVID-19 pandemic on frequency of clinical visits, performance of MRI studies, and therapeutic choices in a multiple sclerosis referral centre. J Neurol 2022;269(4):1764–72. https://doi.org/10.1007/s00415-021-10958-z.
62. Zaheer R, Amin R, Riddick L, et al. Impact of COVID-19 on prescribing patterns and treatment selection of disease modifying therapies in multiple sclerosis. Mult Scler Relat Disord 2023;71:104575. https://doi.org/10.1016/j.msard.2023.104575.
63. Fox RJ, Cosenza C, Cripps L, et al. A survey of risk tolerance to multiple sclerosis therapies. Neurology 2019;92(14):e1634–42. https://doi.org/10.1212/WNL.0000000000007245.
64. National MS Society, Disease Modifying Therapy Guidance During COVID-19 (Internet). Updated 2023. Available at: https://www.nationalmssociety.org/coronavirus-covid-19-information/ms-treatment-guidelines-during-coronavirus. Accessed June 1, 2023.
65. MS International Federation, MS, COVID-19 and Vaccines - Updated Global Advice (Internet). Updated 2022 May 24. Available at: https://www.msif.org/news/2020/02/10/the-coronavirus-and-ms-what-you-need-to-know/. Accessed June 1, 2023.
66. Pugliatti M, Berger T, Hartung HP, et al. Multiple sclerosis in the era of COVID-19: disease course, DMTs and SARS-CoV2 vaccinations. Curr Opin Neurol 2022;35(3):319–27.
67. Sormani MP, De Rossi N, Schiavetti I, et al. Disease-modifying therapies and coronavirus disease 2019 severity in multiple sclerosis. Ann Neurol 2021;89(4): 780–9.

68. Abbadessa G, Lavorgna L, Trojsi F, et al. Understanding and managing the impact of the Covid-19 pandemic and lockdown on patients with multiple sclerosis. Expert Rev Neurother 2021;21(7):731–43.
69. Luna G, Alping P, Burman J, et al. Infection risks among patients with multiple sclerosis treated with fingolimod, natalizumab, rituximab, and injectable therapies. JAMA Neurol 2020;77(2):184–91.
70. Sullivan R, Kilaru A, Hemmer B, et al. COVID-19 infection in fingolimod- or siponimod-treated patients: case series. Neurol Neuroimmunol Neuroinflamm 2021;9(1).
71. Foley JF, Defer G, Ryerson LZ, et al. Comparison of switching to 6-week dosing of natalizumab versus continuing with 4-week dosing in patients with relapsing-remitting multiple sclerosis (NOVA): a randomised, controlled, open-label, phase 3b trial. Lancet Neurol 2022;21(7):608–19. https://doi.org/10.1016/S1474-4422(22)00143-0.
72. Maarouf A, Rico A, Boutiere C, et al. Extending rituximab dosing intervals in patients with MS during the COVID-19 pandemic and beyond? Neurol Neuroimmunol Neuroinflamm 2020;7(5). https://doi.org/10.1212/NXI.0000000000000825.
73. Rolfes L, Pawlitzki M, Pfeuffer S, et al. Ocrelizumab extended interval dosing in multiple sclerosis in times of COVID-19. Neurol Neuroimmunol Neuroinflamm 2021;8(5). https://doi.org/10.1212/NXI.0000000000001035.
74. Sahi NK, Abidi SMA, Salim O, et al. Clinical impact of Ocrelizumab extended interval dosing during the COVID-19 pandemic and associations with CD19(+)B-cell repopulation. Mult Scler Relat Disord 2021;56:103287.
75. van Lierop ZY, Toorop AA, van Ballegoij WJ, et al. Personalized B-cell tailored dosing of ocrelizumab in patients with multiple sclerosis during the COVID-19 pandemic. Mult Scler 2022;28(7):1121–5.
76. Zanghi A, Avolio C, Signoriello E, et al. Is It Time for Ocrelizumab Extended Interval Dosing in Relapsing Remitting MS? Evidence from An Italian Multicenter Experience During the COVID-19 Pandemic. Neurotherapeutics 2022;19(5):1535–45.
77. National MS Society, Medicines to Prevent and Treat COVID-19 (Internet). Updated 2023 January 27. Available at: https://www.nationalmssociety.org/coronavirus-covid-19-information/suspected-covid-19-and-ms. Accessed June 1, 2023.
78. Achiron A, Dolev M, Menascu S, et al. COVID-19 vaccination in patients with multiple sclerosis: What we have learnt by February 2021. Mult Scler 2021;27(6):864–70.
79. Garjani A, Patel S, Bharkhada D, et al. Impact of mass vaccination on SARS-CoV-2 infections among multiple sclerosis patients taking immunomodulatory disease-modifying therapies in England. Mult Scler Relat Disord 2022;57:103458.
80. Lotan I, Wilf-Yarkoni A, Friedman Y, et al. Safety of the BNT162b2 COVID-19 vaccine in multiple sclerosis (MS): early experience from a tertiary MS center in Israel. Eur J Neurol 2021;28(11):3742–8.
81. Stefanou MI, Palaiodimou L, Theodorou A, et al. Safety of COVID-19 vaccines in multiple sclerosis: a systematic review and meta-analysis. Mult Scler 2023;29(4–5):585–94.
82. Coyle PK, Gocke A, Vignos M, et al. Vaccine considerations for multiple sclerosis in the COVID-19 era. Adv Ther 2021;38(7):3550–88.
83. Frahm N, Fneish F, Ellenberger D, et al. Frequency and predictors of relapses following SARS-CoV-2 vaccination in patients with multiple sclerosis: interim

results from a longitudinal observational study. J Clin Med 2023;12(11). https://doi.org/10.3390/jcm12113640.
84. Disanto G, Galante A, Cantu M, et al. Longitudinal postvaccine SARS-CoV-2 immunoglobulin G titers, memory B-cell responses, and risk of COVID-19 in multiple sclerosis over 1 year. Neurol Neuroimmunol Neuroinflamm 2023;10(1). https://doi.org/10.1212/NXI.0000000000200043.
85. Wu X, Wang L, Shen L, et al. Response of COVID-19 vaccination in multiple sclerosis patients following disease-modifying therapies: A meta-analysis. EBioMedicine 2022;81:104102.
86. Brill L, Rechtman A, Zveik O, et al. Humoral and T-cell response to SARS-CoV-2 vaccination in patients with multiple sclerosis treated with ocrelizumab. JAMA Neurol 2021;78(12):1510–4.
87. Kornek B, Leutmezer F, Rommer PS, et al. B cell depletion and SARS-CoV-2 vaccine responses in neuroimmunologic patients. Ann Neurol 2022;91(3): 342–52.
88. Cohen JA, Bermel RA, Grossman CI, et al. Immunoglobulin G immune response to SARS-CoV-2 vaccination in people living with multiple sclerosis within multiple sclerosis partners advancing technology and health solutions. Mult Scler 2022; 28(7):1131–7.
89. Ali A, Dwyer D, Wu Q, et al. Characterization of humoral response to COVID mRNA vaccines in multiple sclerosis patients on disease modifying therapies. Vaccine 2021;39(41):6111–6.
90. Apostolidis SA, Kakara M, Painter MM, et al. Cellular and humoral immune responses following SARS-CoV-2 mRNA vaccination in patients with multiple sclerosis on anti-CD20 therapy. Nat Med 2021;27(11):1990–2001.
91. Gadani SP, Reyes-Mantilla M, Jank L, et al. Discordant humoral and T cell immune responses to SARS-CoV-2 vaccination in people with multiple sclerosis on anti-CD20 therapy. EBioMedicine 2021;73:103636.
92. Achiron A, Mandel M, Gurevich M, et al. Immune response to the third COVID-19 vaccine dose is related to lymphocyte count in multiple sclerosis patients treated with fingolimod. J Neurol 2022;269(5):2286–92.
93. Tallantyre EC, Vickaryous N, Anderson V, et al. COVID-19 vaccine response in people with multiple sclerosis. Ann Neurol 2022;91(1):89–100.
94. Disanto G, Sacco R, Bernasconi E, et al. Association of disease-modifying treatment and anti-CD20 Infusion timing with humoral response to 2 SARS-CoV-2 vaccines in patients with multiple sclerosis. JAMA Neurol 2021;78(12):1529–31.
95. National MS Society, COVID-19 Vaccine Guidance for People Living with MS (Internet). Updated February 23, 2023. Available at: https://www.nationalmssociety.org/coronavirus-covid-19-information/covid-19-vaccine-guidance.
96. Marrie RA, Dolovich C, Cutter GR, et al. Attitudes toward coronavirus disease 2019 vaccination in people with multiple sclerosis. Mult Scler J Exp Transl Clin 2022;8(2). https://doi.org/10.1177/20552173221102067. 20552173221102067.
97. Ciotti JR, Perantie DC, Moss BP, et al. Perspectives and experiences with COVID-19 vaccines in people with MS. Mult Scler J Exp Transl Clin 2022;8(1). https://doi.org/10.1177/20552173221085242. 20552173221085242.
98. Ehde DM, Roberts MK, Humbert AT, et al. COVID-19 vaccine hesitancy in adults with multiple sclerosis in the United States: a follow up survey during the initial vaccine rollout in 2021. Mult Scler Relat Disord 2021;54:103163.
99. Uhr L, Mateen FJ. COVID-19 vaccine hesitancy in multiple sclerosis: a cross-sectional survey. Mult Scler 2022;28(7):1072–80.

100. Yap SM, Al Hinai M, Gaughan M, et al. Vaccine hesitancy among people with multiple sclerosis. Mult Scler Relat Disord 2021;56:103236.
101. Barzegar M, Mirmosayyeb O, Gajarzadeh M, et al. COVID-19 among patients with multiple sclerosis: a systematic review. Neurol Neuroimmunol Neuroinflamm 2021;8(4). https://doi.org/10.1212/NXI.0000000000001001.
102. Bsteh G, Assar H, Gradl C, et al. Long-term outcome after COVID-19 infection in multiple sclerosis: a nation-wide multicenter matched-control study. Eur J Neurol 2022. https://doi.org/10.1111/ene.15477.
103. Chiaravalloti ND, Amato MP, Brichetto G, et al. The emotional impact of the COVID-19 pandemic on individuals with progressive multiple sclerosis. J Neurol 2021;268(5):1598–607.
104. Mehta D, Miller C, Arnold DL, et al. Effect of dimethyl fumarate on lymphocytes in RRMS: Implications for clinical practice. Neurology 2019;92(15):e1724–38.
105. Levit E, Longbrake EE, Stoll SS. Seroconversion after COVID-19 vaccination for multiple sclerosis patients on high efficacy disease modifying medications. Mult Scler Relat Disord 2022;60:103719.
106. Bar-Or A, Calkwood JC, Chognot C, et al. Effect of ocrelizumab on vaccine responses in patients with multiple sclerosis: The VELOCE study. Neurology 2020;95(14):e1999–2008.

Printed and bound by CPI Group (UK) Ltd, Croydon, CR0 4YY
03/10/2024
01040466-0006